Metabolic and Bariatric Surgery Exam and Board Review

NOTICE

Metabolic and Bariatric Surgery Exam and Board Review

Robert B. Lim, MD

Professor of Surgery, Vice Chair of Education
George Kaiser Family Foundation Chair in Surgery
Residency Program Director
University of Oklahoma School of Medicine at Tulsa
Tulsa, Oklahoma

Daniel B. Jones, MD, MS

Professor and Chair of Surgery
Department of Surgery
Rutgers New Jersey Medical School
Newark, New Jersey

Mc Graw Hill

New York Chicago San Francisco Athens London Madrid Mexico City
Milan New Delhi Singapore Sydney Toronto

Metabolic and Bariatric Surgery Exam and Board Review

1 2 3 4 5 6 7 8 9 DSS 27 26 25 24 23 22

ISBN 978-1-260-46806-9
MHID 1-260-46806-2

The editors were Jason Malley and Christina M. Thomas.
The production supervisor was Catherine Saggese.
Project management was provided by Poonam Bisht, MPS Limited.

Library of Congress Control Number: 2021947609

I would like to dedicate this textbook to my wonderful wife Lisa and to my amazing children, Luke, Alec, Viktoria, and Grace, I'm so very proud of you all. You bring me so much joy and happiness.

—Robert B. Lim

I am indebted to Dr. George Blackburn, MD, PHD, and Ed Hatchigian who cofounded the multidisciplinary bariatric surgery program at Beth Israel Deaconess Medical Center at Harvard Medical School.

—Daniel B. Jones, MD

Contents

Section 4: Surgical

Section 5: Outcomes Short-Term

Section 6: Preoperative Preparation

Section 9: Other Issues

Contributors

Mohammad Abu Hilal, MD, PhD
Professor of Hepatobiliary and Pancreas Surgery
Poliambulanza Foundation Hospital
Brescia, Italy

Souheil Adra, MD, FACS, FASMBS, ABOM
Director, Metabolic and Bariatric Surgery Program
Beth Israel Deaconess Milton Hospital, Harvard Medical School
Boston, Massachusetts

Eric Ahnfeldt, DO
Associate Professor of Surgery
Landstuhl Regional Medical Center
Landstuhl, Germany

Adnan Alseidi, MD, EdM
Professor of Hepatobiliary and Pancreas Surgery
University of California San Francisco
San Francisco, California

Katherine Aucoin, MD, MSc
Advanced GI MIS Surgery Fellow
Dalhousie University
Halifax, Nova Scotia, Canada

Jesse Bandle, MD
Chair of Surgery
Naval Medical Center
San Diego, California

Limaris Barrios, MD
Clinical Assistant Professor in Surgery
Nova Southeastern University Dr. Kiran C. Patel College of Allopathic Medicine
Mercy Hospital
Miami, Florida

Christopher Barton, MD
Fellow, Critical Care
Oregon Health & Science University
Portland, Oregon

Jordan D. Bohnen, MD, MBA
Assistant Professor of Surgery
Beth Israel Deaconess Medical Center, Harvard Medical School
Boston, Massachusetts

Kliment Bozhilov, MD
General Surgery Resident
University of Hawaii
Honolulu, Hawaii

Morgan Bresnick, MD
Instructor in Surgery
Beth Israel Deaconess Medical Center, Harvard Medical School
Boston, Massachusetts

Joel Brockmeyer, MD
Associate Program Director, General Surgery
Dwight D. Eisenhower Army Medical Center
Fort Gordon, Georgia

Andrew M. Brown, MD
Assistant Professor of Surgery
St. Luke's University Health Network
Temple University
Bethlehem, Pennsylvania

Racquel Bueno, MD
Associate Clinical Professor of Surgery
University of Hawaii
Honolulu, Hawaii

Jonathan Carter, MD, FACS, FASMBS
Associate Professor of Surgery
University of California San Francisco
San Francisco, California

Julietta Chang, MD, FACS
Bariatric Surgeon
Washington Permanente Medical Group
Bellevue, Washington

Kyle Checchi, MD
Assistant Professor of Surgery
Uniformed Services University
Navy Medicine Readiness & Training Command
San Diego, California

Judy YR Chen, MD
Assistant Professor of Surgery
University of Washington, Department of Surgery
Seattle, Washington

Yong Choi, MD
Associate Professor of Surgery
Baylor College of Medicine
Houston, Texas

Geoffrey S. Chow, MD
Assistant Professor of Surgery
University of Oklahoma School of Medicine at Tulsa
Tulsa, Oklahoma

Alex Clem, MD
General Surgeon
Evans Army Community Hospital
Colorado Springs, Colorado

Jesse R. Conner, MD
General Surgery Resident
University of Oklahoma
Oklahoma City, Oklahoma

Kim Danbee, MD
Clinical Fellow of MIS and Bariatric Surgery
Beth Israel Deaconess Medical Center, Harvard Medical School
Boston, Massachusetts

Paul Davidson, PhD
Director of Behavioral Services
Center for Weight Management and Wellness
Brigham and Women's Hospital, Harvard Medical School
Boston, Massachusetts

James Dickerson, MD
Minimally Invasive and Bariatric Surgeon
Baylor St. Luke's Medical Group
Houston, Texas

Derek T. Dirks, MD
Bariatric Surgeon
Northwest Bariatrics
Post Falls, Idaho

Colston Edgerton, MD
Assistant Professor of Surgery
Medical University of South Carolina
Charleston, South Carolina

Anne P. Ehlers, MD, MPH
Assistant Professor of Surgery
University of Michigan Medical School
Ann Arbor, Michigan

Dan Eisenberg, MD, MS
Associate Professor of Surgery
Stanford Medical Center and VA Palo Alto Health Care System
Palo Alto, California

James Ellsmere, MD, MS, FRCSC, FACS
Associate Professor of Surgery
Dalhousie University
Halifax, Nova Scotia, Canada

COL Byron Faler, MD
Program Director, General Surgery Residency
Dwight D. Eisenhower Army Medical Center
Fort Gordon, Georgia

Laura E. Fischer, MD, MS
Assistant Professor of Surgery
University of Oklahoma
Oklahoma City, Oklahoma

Ondria C. Gleason, MD
Professor of Psychiatry
University of Oklahoma School of Medicine at Tulsa
Tulsa, Oklahoma

Rahul Gupta, MBBS
Instructor in Surgery
Beth Israel Deaconess Medical Center, Harvard Medical School
Boston, Massachusetts

Samar Hafida, MD
Assistant Medical Director, Adult Diabetes Section
Joslin Diabetes Center, Harvard Medical School
Boston, Massachusetts

Caitlin Halbert, DO, MS
Medical Director Bariatric Surgery Program
Christiana Care Health System
Wilmington, Delaware

Xiao-Yue Han, MD
General Surgery Resident
Oregon Health & Science University
Portland, Oregon

Daniel M. Herron, MD
Professor of Surgery
Icahn School of Medicine at Mount Sinai
New York, New York

Farah A. Husain, MD
Associate Professor of Surgery
Oregon Health & Science University
Portland, Oregon

James Jarvis, MD
General Surgery Resident
Christiana Care Health System
Newark, Delaware

Darya D. Kazei, MD
Research Fellow
BIDMC Plastic and Reconstructive Surgery
Boston, Massachusetts

Timothy Kelly, MD
Bariatric Surgeon
Baylor Scott and White Center for Bariatric Surgery
Waxahachie, Texas

Brittany Kern, MD
Assistant Professor of Surgery
Indiana University Health Ball Memorial
Muncie, Indiana

Zhamak Khorgami, MD
Assistant Professor of Surgery
University of Oklahoma School of Medicine at Tulsa
Tulsa, Oklahoma

Danbee Kim, MD
Clinical Fellow of MIS and Bariatric Surgery
Beth Israel Deaconess Medical Center
Boston, Massachusetts

Marina Kurian, MD
Clinical Professor of Surgery
NYU Grossman School of Medicine
New York, New York

Teresa LaMasters, MD
Medical Director Bariatric Surgery
UnityPoint Clinic Bariatric Surgery
West Des Moines, Iowa

Henry Lin, MD
Bariatric & Minimally Invasive Surgeon
Erie County Medical Center
Buffalo, New York

Samuel J. Lin, MD, MBA
Program Director, BIDMC/HMS Plastic Surgery Residency Training
Program, Associate Professor of Surgery (Plastic Surgery, Otolaryngology)
Boston, Massachusetts

Victoria Lyo, MD, MTM
Assistant Professor of Surgery
University of California, Davis
Sacramento, California

Tessa L. Manning, MD
Assistant Professor of Psychiatry
University of Oklahoma School of Medicine at Tulsa
Tulsa, Oklahoma

Samuel M. Manstein, MD
Research Fellow
BIDMC Plastic and Reconstructive Surgery
Boston, Massachusetts

Matthew N. Marturano, MD
Resident, General Surgery
Atrium Health Carolinas Medical Center
Charlotte, North Carolina

Pamela Masella, MD
General and Bariatric Surgeon
Brooke Army Medical Center
San Antonio, Texas

Brent D. Matthews, MD
Professor and Chair
Department of Surgery
Surgeon-in-Chief
Atrium Health Carolinas Medical Center
Charlotte, North Carolina

Laura M. Mazer, MD
Assistant Professor of Surgery
University of Michigan Medical School
Ann Arbor, Michigan

Sarah McClanahan, DO
Associate Professor of Psychiatry
University of Oklahoma School of Medicine at Tulsa
Tulsa, Oklahoma

Ozanan R. Meireles, MD
Assistant Professor of Surgery
Massachusetts General Hospital, Harvard Medical School
Boston, Massachusetts

W. James Melvin, MD
Chief Resident in General Surgery
University of Michigan Medical School
Ann Arbor, Michigan

Andrea Moon, MD
General Surgery Resident
Tripler Army Medical Center
Honolulu, Hawaii

Rachel L. Moore, MD
Bariatric Surgeon
Moore Metabolics
New Orleans, Louisiana

Michael Mulcahy, MD
Assistant Professor of Surgery
Tripler Army Medical Center
Honolulu, Hawaii

Christopher Mulla, MD, MS
Division Chief of Endocrinology, Assistant Professor of Medicine
Landstuhl Regional Medical Center
Landstuhl, Germany

Alex Myers, MD
General Surgery Resident
William Beaumont Army Medical Center
El Paso, Texas

Keitaro Nakamoto, MD
Acute Care Surgeon
MedStar Health Baltimore
Baltimore, Maryland

Philip Omotosho, MD
Associate Professor of Surgery
Rush University
Chicago, Illinois

Chan W. Park, MD
Associate Professor of Surgery
Tripler Army Medical Center
Honolulu, Hawaii

Carl M. Pesta, DO
Associate Professor of Surgery
Michigan State University
Mount Clemens, Michigan

Eduardo Pirolla, MD, PhD
Assistant Professor of Surgery
Heart Institute, University of São Paulo
São Paulo, Brazil

Kinga A. Powers, MD, PhD
Associate Professor of Surgery
Stony Brook Medicine
Stony Brook, New York

Janey S.A. Pratt, MD, FACS, FASMBS
Clinical Professor of Surgery
Stanford University School of Medicine
Lucille Packard Children's Hospital
Palo Alto, California

Aurora D. Pryor, MD
Professor of Surgery
Stony Brook University
Stony Brook, New York

Nikdokht Rashidian, MD, PhD
Hepatobiliary and Pancreas Surgeon
Ghent University
Ghent, Belgium

Michael Logan Rawlins, MD
Bariatric Surgery Fellowship Program Director
Allegheny Health Network
Pittsburgh, Pennsylvania

Kevin M. Reavis, MD
Associate Professor of Surgery
The Oregon Clinic
Portland, Oregon

Angel Reyes, MD
General and Bariatric Surgeon
St. Michael Medical Center
Silverdale, Washington

Jesse Richards, DO, ABOM
Assistant Professor of Medicine
University of Oklahoma School of Medicine at Tulsa
Tulsa, Oklahoma

Angel J. Rivera Aponta, MD
General Surgery resident
Valley Health System
Las Vegas, Nevada

John R. Romanelli, MD
Professor of Surgery
University of Massachusetts Chan Medical School – Baystate Medical Center
Springfield, Massachusetts

Amy Rosenbluth, MD
Clinical Assistant Professor of Surgery
Stony Brook School of Medicine
Stony Brook, New York

Oleg Ryabinin, MD
General Surgery Resident
Navy Medicine Readiness & Training Command
San Diego, California

Ben Schwab, MD
Attending Surgeon
John Muir Health System
Walnut Creek, California

Daniel J. Scott, MD
Frank J. Kidd, Jr. MD Distinguished Professorship in Surgery
University of Texas Southwestern Medical Center
Dallas, Texas

Kevin K. Seeras, DO
South Shore Surgical Specialists
Minimally Invasive General and Bariatric Surgeon
Sun City, Florida

Nargiz Seyidova MD, MHQS
Research Fellow
BIDMC Plastic and Reconstructive Surgery
Boston, Massachusetts

Juliana Simonetti, MD
Director, Medical Bariatric Program
University of Utah
Salt Lake City, Utah

Kevin Smith, DO
Assistant Professor of Internal Medicine
University of Oklahoma School of Medicine at Tulsa
Tulsa, Oklahoma

Andrea Stroud, MD, MS
Assistant Professor of Surgery
Oregon Health & Science University
Portland, Oregon

Ali Tavakkoli, MD
Associate Professor of Surgery
Brigham and Women's Hospital, Harvard Medical School
Boston, Massachusetts

Dana Telem, MD, MPH
Associate Professor of Surgery
University of Michigan Medical School
Ann Arbor, Michigan

Samantha Terranella, MD
General Surgery Resident
Rush University
Chicago, Illinois

Stephanie Therrien, BSc
Senior Administrative Manager
Massachusetts General Hospital
Boston, Massachusetts

Hung Truong, MD
Bariatric and General Surgeon
Scripps Clinic Medical Group
San Diego, California

Shawn Tsuda, MD, MBA, FACS
Surgeon
Valley Health System
Las Vegas, Nevada

Laure-Anne Van Loon, MD
Research Fellow
BIDMC Plastic and Reconstructive Surgery
Boston, Massachusetts

Ashley E. Walker, MD
Associate Professor of Psychiatry
University of Oklahoma School of Medicine at Tulsa
Tulsa, Oklahoma

Gordon G. Wisbach, MD, MBA
Associate Professor of Surgery
Uniformed Services University
Navy Medicine Readiness & Training Command
San Diego, California

Lye-Yeng Wong, MD
General Surgery Resident
Oregon Health & Science University
Portland, Oregon

Christopher Yheulon, MD
Associate Professor of Surgery
Tripler Army Medical Center
Honolulu, Hawaii

Phylicia Yorgure, MD
Bariatric/General Surgeon
Baylor Scott & White
Killeen, Texas

Linda P. Zhang, MD
Associate Professor of Surgery, Director of Global Surgery
Mount Sinai Hospital
New York, New York

Preface

Over the last four decades, bariatric surgery has emerged as a defined surgical specialty within a multidisciplinary team. Today, over 900 bariatric surgery programs in the United States are accredited jointly by the ASMBS and the American College of Surgeons. Every operation is entered into the MBSAQIP database and quarterly reports provide benchmarks to assure patient safety and best outcomes.

Despite obesity being the number one preventable disease, obesity experts are not sure what exactly causes obesity and why it is so hard to lose weight once a patient becomes obese. There are genetic, environmental, and behavioral factors but there are also bacterial, biochemical, and hormonal aspects at play. Bariatric and Metabolic Surgeons, for their part, are not sure why the surgery works against diseases like type 2 diabetes mellitus and why it does not always sustain weight loss for all patients.

The sleeve gastrectomy is the most popular operation this year. The Roux-en-Y gastric bypass is still considered the operation against which all other operations are compared for efficacy, but why does it work for some but not for others. How might the microbiome affect weight? How much and what kind of exercise does one need to maintain weight loss? How does NAFLD and renal disease improve after surgery? What surgical operation is best for which patient?

Bariatric Surgery Examination and Review covers the material that every health provider caring for patients of size should know. It addresses when to refer patients for medical weight loss or evaluation for surgical options; preoperative, intraoperative and postoperative care pathways are explored; the potential risks, benefits, and long-term outcomes of the adjustable gastric band, the sleeve gastrectomy, the gastric bypass, and other common procedures are compared.

We think this review book is also a value to medical students and surgical residents rotating on the Bariatric Surgery Service. Topics include how to evaluate tachycardia in a post op patient, manage a leak after gastric bypass, or management options for a stenosis after sleeve gastrectomy. It also covers questions such as what is the role of ghrelin, PPY, and new medical treatment options. Many of the review questions will appear on National Board Part 3, ABSITE and ABS General Surgery board exams. We believe this answer key of the review book is also helpful to the bariatric fellow and surgeon in-practice preparing to take the new American Board of Surgery Focused Designation Exam in Bariatric Surgery.

Robert B. Lim, MD, FASMBS
Daniel B. Jones, MD, MS

Acknowledgment

The editors would like to acknowledge Cierra Gleason for helping bring this textbook to completion. Thank you so much for your work.

SECTION 1

Obesity

1

The Theory of Obesity and Epidemiology

Stephanie Therrien, BSc, and Juliana Simonetti, MD

1. **Homeostatic control of satiety and food intake is a complex system that involves the hypothalamus in the central nervous system and peripheral signals from fat cells and the gastrointestinal tract. As the regulation center of both appetite and energy expenditure, the hypothalamus consists of several interconnecting nuclei.**

   Which area of the hypothalamus is considered to be the primary region for sensing the peripheral metabolic signals that lead to feeding behavior and appetite regulations?

   A. Arcuate nucleus (ARC)
   B. Hypothalamic nuclei
   C. Paraventricular nucleus
   D. Dorsal vagal complex (DVC)

2. **The gastrointestinal tract, whose primary role is to digest and absorb nutrients, also plays a role in energy homeostasis through mechanoreceptors and chemo sensors.**

   Which of the following are satiety signals secreted by the small intestine?

   A. Ghrelin
   B. Leptin (LEP)
   C. Glucagon-like peptide-1 (GLP-1)
   D. Octreotide

3. **Both monogenic and polygenic forms of obesity result in an impairment in the hypothalamus ability to control energy expenditure, food intake, and other metabolic actions.**

   Which of the following syndromes presents with early onset of obesity, hyperphagia, visual impairment, and polydactyly?

   A. Prader–Willi syndrome (PWS)
   B. Proopiomelanocortin (POMC) gene mutation
   C. Bardet-Biedl syndrome (BBS)
   D. Melanocortin-4-receptor (MC4R) deficiency

4. **Adipose tissue was previously thought of as a site for energy storage. However, we now know it as an endocrine organ that is metabolically dynamic. Adipocytes are capable of synthesizing a number of hormones and cytokines (adipokines) that regulate metabolic homeostasis.**

   Which of the following are adipokines that cross the blood-brain barrier, work on anorexigenic neurons [proopiomelanocortin/cocaine- and amphetamine-regulated transcript (POMC/CART)] to decrease hunger, and have a strong association with obesity, elevated cardiovascular risk, and morbidity?

   A. Leptin (LEP)
   B. Ghrelin
   C. Interleukin-1 (IL-6)
   D. Tumor necrosis factor–alpha (TNF-α)

5. **A decrease in which of the following gut microbiota is thought to be responsible for adverse metabolic outcomes in the offspring of mothers with obesity?**

   A. Proteobacteria
   B. Firmicutes
   C. Bacteroidetes
   D. Actinobacteria

6. It has been found that adipocytes in visceral fat produce adipokines comprised of bioactive peptides, immune molecules, and inflammatory mediators more actively than subcutaneous adipose tissue. Elevated levels of abdominal adiposity in the visceral depot increases an individual's risk for developing metabolic and cardiovascular problems.

Macrophages within the adipose tissue play an important role in the low-grade systemic inflammation that is associated with obesity. Which one of the cytokines listed here has been found to be elevated in those with obesity compared to lean individuals?

A. Interleukin-1 (IL-1)
B. Interferon gamma (IFN-γ)
C. Granulocyte-macrophage colony-stimulating factor (GM-CSF)
D. Interleukin-6 (IL-6)

ANSWERS

1. A. The hypothalamus, in particular the ARC within it, is thought to play an essential role in appetite regulation (see Figure 1-1). The ARC senses peripheral metabolic signals from the gastrointestinal tract and adipocytes. Within the ARC, there are two discrete groups of neurons. The first is the orexigenic group, which increases or stimulates the appetite via the activation of neuropeptide Y (NPY) and agouti-related peptide (AgRP) neurons.[1] These neurons are activated by ghrelin (also known as the hunger hormone), which is released by enteroendocrine cells in the stomach. The second group is comprised of anorexigenic neurons that contain POMC and CART (see Figure 1-2). POMC is a precursor of alpha-melanocyte-stimulating hormone (α-MSH), which acts on melanocortin receptors (mainly MC4R) to reduce food intake and increase energy expenditure.[2,3] POMC is activated by insulin and LEP, an adipokine (a peptide hormone released by adipocytes) that is released in response to excess energy. Lesions of the ARC result in hyperphagia and obesity in mice.[4]

2. C. Ghrelin is a gut-derived hormone that plays an important role in appetite stimulation, while most of the other intestinal hormones, including cholecystokinin (CCK), peptide YY (PYY), and GLP-1, are appetite inhibitors. These important peptides with opposing roles help regulate food intake and energy balance.[5] They affect brain centers involved in the

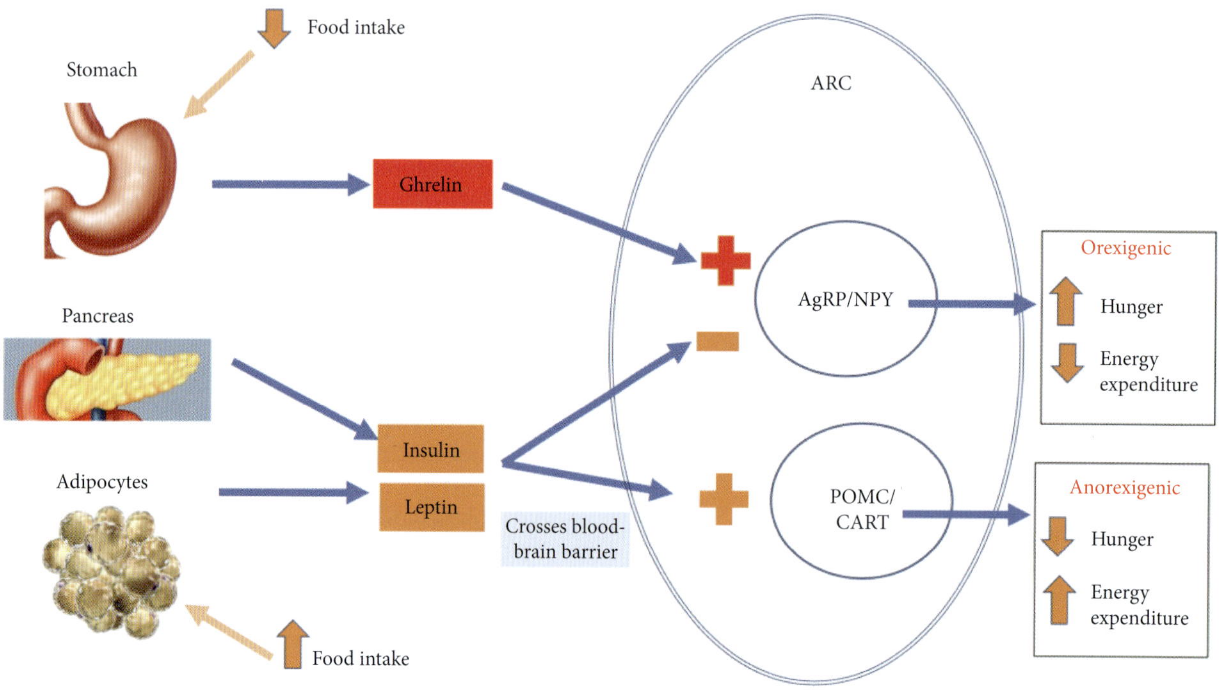

Figure 1-1 Brain appetite control center.

central control of hunger and satiety via the gut-brain axis through crossing of the blood-brain barrier and targeting the ARC of the hypothalamus, or via the vagus nerve to reach the nucleus of the solitary tract (NTS) of the brainstem.

Ghrelin is produced by closed-type enteroendocrine cells in the gastric fundus. It is a short-term hormone secreted by the stomach just before an expected meal, and it strongly promotes food intake.

With ingestion of food, gastric mechano-receptors are activated when the stomach is distended, which are relayed via vagal nerves to the NTS in the brainstem. The amount of gastric distension due to food intake is partly influenced by the rate of gastric emptying, which in turn affects postprandial glycemic excursions.[6,7] Gastric emptying, which controls the rate of appearance of ingested food in the small intestine, intestinal transit, the rate of digestion, and small intestinal nutrient sensing, is the major determinant of the inhibition of ghrelin secretion and the stimulation of CCK, GLP-1, and PYY secretion during and after meals.[5]

Intestinal CCK is secreted in response to luminal nutrients, especially lipids and proteins. GLP-1 is produced primarily by L cells in the distal small intestine and colon, where it colocalizes with oxyntomodulin and PYY. Ingested nutrients, especially fats and carbohydrates, stimulate GLP-1 secretion by indirect, duodenally activated neurohumoral mechanisms, as well as by direct contact within the distal intestine.[8,9] LEP is believed (by experts) to be secreted by adipose cells and not enterocytes. Octreotide does increase satiety, but it is secreted by the pancreas.

3. C. Monogenic forms of obesity are usually characterized by hyperphagia and early-onset obesity associated with endocrine disorders. Mutations are known to occur in several genes implicated in the LEP-melanocortin pathway, which is involved in food intake regulation. Most of these mutations have been found to result in autosomal-recessive forms of obesity, such as LEP, leptin receptor (LEPR), MC4R, and POMC.[10] Variants in the *MC4R* gene represent the most common cause of monogenic obesity.[11,12]

Syndromic obesity can be defined as the presence of obesity, along with additional characteristics, including intellectual disability, dysmorphic features, and congenital abnormalities affecting specific organ systems.[13] Two examples are PWS and BBS.

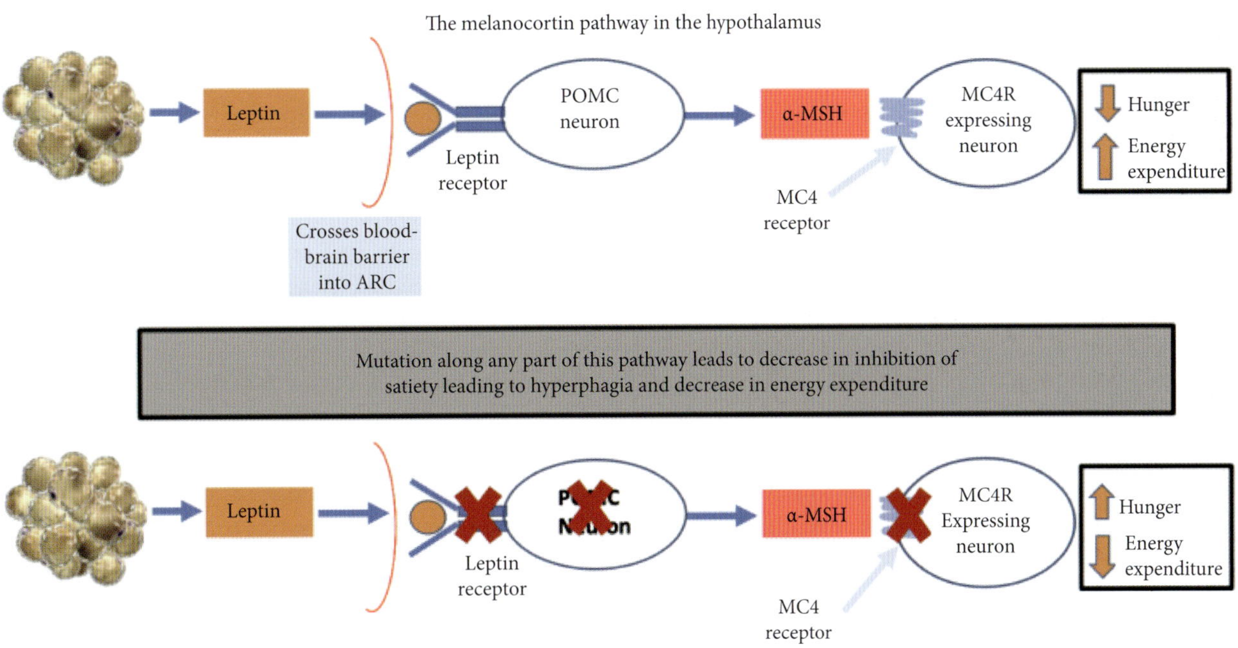

Figure 1-2 Satiety: Melanocortin pathway and the hypothalamus.

PWS is a complex genetic disorder that, in addition to cognitive impairment, is characterized by hyperphagia, obesity, hypogonadism, and growth impairment.[10] This disorder usually results from chromosome 15 deletion or due to having both members of the chromosome 15 pair derived from one parent, a condition known as *uniparental disomy.*[13]

In BBS, mutations in BBS genes (there are 14 such genes) lead to problems with the structure and function of cilia, which disrupts important chemical-signaling pathways, including the LEPR in the ARC.[13] This in turn leads to increased hunger and decreased energy expenditure, leading to hyperphagia and severe obesity. This syndrome is also hallmarked by polydactyly and visual impairment.

4. **A.** LEP is produced by adipose tissue in response to excess energy. It is a peptide hormone and a major regulator of lipid metabolism. There is a strong relationship between body fat mass and the amount of LEP synthesized and secreted. LEP is considered to be an antiobesity hormone due to its ability to promote satiety and increase metabolism.

A major action of LEP is the control of body weight and fat deposition through its effects on hypothalamic receptors in the ARC. LEP has an inhibitory effect on orexigenic neurons to decrease appetite and a stimulating effect on anorexigenic neurons to stimulate satiety via POMC/CART neurons. It also stimulates metabolic rate and thermogenesis. LEP levels decrease during fasting and increase after several days of overfeeding in a mechanism that helps to regulate energy balance in humans. Thus, increased LEP concentrations would be expected to correlate with decreased weight. However, serum LEP levels are increased in those with obesity and strongly correlates with body fat mass. Recent studies suggest the existence of an endogenous LEP-resistance mechanism in obesity that may explain this unexpected correlation. LEP has also been found to have a strong association with elevated cardiovascular risk and morbidity (see Figure 1-3).[14]

Ghrelin is not secreted by adipocytes. IL-6 and TNF are secreted by adipocytes, and they contribute to the pro-inflammatory state of obesity, leading to vascular disease and osteoarthritis, and have less to do with satiety and hunger control.

5. **B.** Gut microbiota and their role as a potential factor in the pathophysiology of obesity have been the center of a growing body of research over the last 10 years.[15,16] We recognize gut microbiota for their role in protecting gastrointestinal mucosa and regulation of fermentation and absorption of polysaccharides. Although the composition of intestinal microbiota is highly diverse in healthy individuals, those exhibiting overall adiposity, insulin resistance, and dyslipidemia are characterized by low bacterial richness.[17]

Although conclusions from recent studies may conflict, it has repeatedly been found that in lean individuals, there is an abundance of Firmicutes and Bacteroidetes bacterial divisions. In obese individuals, lower levels of these bacterial divisions are found, which has led experts to believe that they may play a significant role in how gut microbes influence body mass index (BMI).[15,18]

6. **D.** Obesity is characterized by low-grade, systemic inflammation. Inflammatory markers such as C-reactive protein (CRP) and IL-6 are increased in individuals with obesity compared with lean subjects, although not to the same extent observed in classic inflammatory conditions. The presence of systemic inflammation has been linked to the increased risk of development of cardiovascular disease (CVD) and type 2 diabetes in obese individuals, particularly in the case of visceral adiposity.[19,22]

Expansion of adipose tissue with obesity leads to increased macrophage infiltration and inflammation, with enhanced production of pro-inflammatory cytokines such as TNF and IL-6.[21] This is accompanied by an increased release of free fatty acids and dysregulated secretion of LEP, adiponectin, resistin, and retinol binding protein-4 (RBP4) (see Figure 1-3).[21] Together, these adipocyte- and macrophage-derived substances can act in a paracrine or autocrine fashion to further exacerbate adipose tissue inflammation. On the systemic level, altered adipokine secretion can lead to increased food intake and reduced energy expenditure through actions in the hypothalamus, as well as to decreased muscle and liver insulin sensitivity through enhanced ectopic lipid deposition and inflammation.[19]

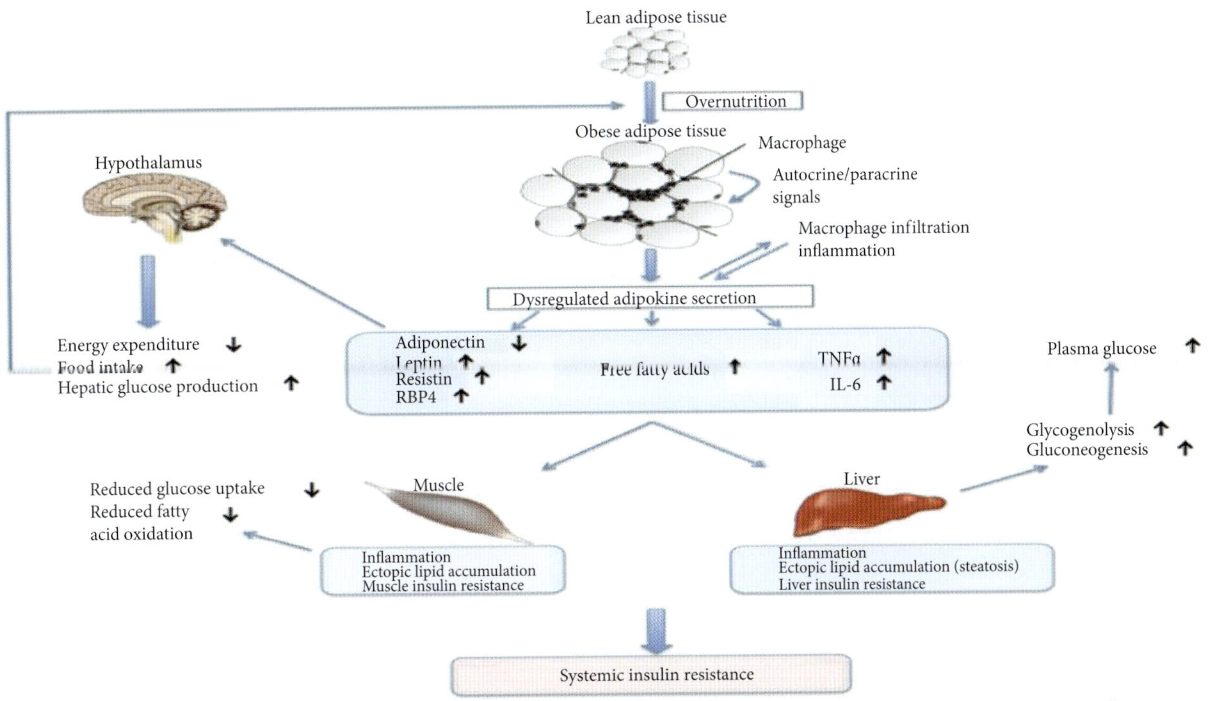

Figure 1-3 Adipokine pathway and metabolic abnormalities: adipose tissue hypertrophy leads to dysfunctions in adipokine pathways, which often result in impaired organ communications and metabolic abnormalities in multiple tissues. Reproduced with permission from Galic S, Oakhill JS, Steinberg GR. Adipose tissue as an endocrine organ. *Mol Cell Endocrinol.* 2010;316(2):129-139.

REFERENCES

1. Schwartz MW, Woods SC, Porte D Jr, Seeley RJ, Baskin DG. Central nervous system control of food intake. *Nature.* 2000;404:661-671.
2. De Silva A, Bloom SR. Gut hormones and appetite control: a focus on PYY and GLP-1 as therapeutic targets in obesity. *Gut and Liver.* 2012;6(1):10-20. https://doi.org/10.5009/gnl.2012.6.1.10.
3. Dodd GT, Decherf S, Loh K, et al. Leptin and insulin act on POMC neurons to promote the browning of white fat. *Cell.* 2015;160(1-2):88-104. https://doi.org/10.1016/j.cell.2014.12.022.
4. Leibowitz SF, Hammer NJ, Chang K. Hypothalamic paraventricular nucleus lesions produce overeating and obesity in the rat. *Physiol Behav.* 1981;27(6):1031-1040. doi:10.1016/0031-9384(81)90366-8.
5. Joly-Amado A, Cansell C, Denis RG, et al. The hypothalamic arcuate nucleus and the control of peripheral substrates. *Best Pract Res Clin Endocrinol Metab.* 2014;28(5):725-737. doi:10.1016/j.beem.2014.03.00.
6. Steinert RE, Feinle-Bisset C, Asarian L, et al. Ghrelin, CCK, GLP-1, and PYY (3-36): Secretory controls and physiological roles in eating and glycemia in health, obesity, and after RYGB. *Phys Rev.* 2017;97(1):411-463. https://doi.org/10.1152/physrev.00031.2014.
7. Cummings DE, Overduin J. Gastrointestinal regulation of food intake. *J Clin Invest.* 2007;117(1):13-23. https://doi.org/10.1172/JCI30227.
8. Blanco AM, Bertucci JI, Valenciano AI, et al. Ghrelin suppresses cholecystokinin (CCK), peptide YY (PYY) and glucagon-like peptide-1 (GLP-1) in the intestine, and attenuates the anorectic effects of CCK, PYY and GLP-1 in goldfish (Carassius auratus). *Horm Behav.* 2017;93:62-71.
9. Dailey MJ, Moran TH. Glucagon-like peptide 1 and appetite. *Trends Endoc Metab.* 2013;24(2):85-91.
10. Prinz P, Stengel A. Control of food intake by gastrointestinal peptides: Mechanisms of action and possible modulation in the treatment of obesity. *J Neurogastroent Motil.* 2017;23(2):180-196.
11. Ramos-Molina B, Molina-Vega M, Fernández-García JC, et al. Hyperphagia and obesity in Prader-Willi Syndrome: PCSK1 deficiency and beyond? *Genes.* 2018;9:288. doi:10.3390/genes9060288.
12. Vollbach H, Brandt S, Lahr G, et al. Prevalence and phenotypic characterization of MC4R variants in a large pediatric cohort. *Int J Obes.* 2017;41:13-22.
13. Kaur Y, de Souza RJ, Gibson WT, Meyre D. A systematic review of genetic syndromes with obesity. *Obes Rev.* 2017;18:603-634.
14. Cassidy SB, Schwartz S. Prader-Willi and Angelman syndromes: disorders of genomic imprinting. *Medicine (Baltimore).* 1998;77(2):140-151. doi:10.1097/00005792-199803000-0000.
15. Ekmen N, Helvaci A, Gunaldi M, Sasani H, Yildirmak ST. Leptin as an important link between obesity and cardiovascular risk factors in men with acute myocardial

infarction. *Ind H J* 2016;68(2):132-137. https://doi.org/10.1016/j.ihj.2015.07.03.

16. Gohir W, Ratcliffe E., Sloboda D. Of the bugs that shape us: maternal obesity, the gut microbiome, and long-term disease risk. *Pediatr Res.* 2015;77:196-204. https://doi.org/10.1038/pr.2014.169.
17. Muscogiuri G, Cantone E, Cassarano S, et al. Gut microbiota: a new path to treat obesity. *Int J Obes Supp.* 2019;9: 10–19. https://doi.org/10.1038/s41367-019-0011-7.
18. Le Chatelier E, Nielsen T, Qin J, et al. Richness of human gut microbiome correlates with metabolic markers. *Nature.* 2013;500:541-546. doi:10.1038/nature12506.
19. Fantuzzi G. Adipose tissue, adipokines, and inflammation. *J Allergy Clin Immun.* 2005;115(5):911-919.
20. Galic, S, Oakhill JS, Steinberg GR. Adipose tissue as an endocrine organ. *Molecular and Cellular Endocrinology.* 2010;316:129-139.
21. Lago F, Dieguez C, Gómez-Reino J, et al. Adipokines as emerging mediators of immune response and inflammation. *Nat Rev Rheumatol.* 2007;3:716-724. https://doi.org/10.1038/ncprheum0674.
22. Wang Z, Nakayama T. Inflammation, a link between obesity and cardiovascular disease. *Mediators Inflamm.* 2010. https://doi.org/10.1155/2010/535918.

2

Set Point Theory

Stephanie Therrien, BSc, and Juliana Simonetti, MD

1. **Which of the following best describes the set point theory?**
   A. A patient who has weighed 58 kg for her entire adult life has gained 11 kg over the last 2 years due to eating more from stress and having a more sedentary lifestyle. She has now significantly decreased her caloric intake and has tried various diets, including juicing, intermittent fasting, and a ketogenic diet. She is extremely frustrated, as she seems to only be able to lose 5 to 7 kg and often will gain the weight back.
   B. A patient who worked out rigorously throughout his college career is experiencing rapid weight gain after starting a job that is mostly sedentary. He has increased his energy expenditure but has not been able to lose the weight.
   C. A patient who started to experience weight gain a year ago has worked on decreasing his caloric intake and increasing his energy expenditure. He was initially able to lose 5 kg, and with the aid of phentermine has been able to lose an additional 11 kg.
   D. A patient has a new diagnosis of type II diabetes and complains of gaining 7 kg after starting glimepiride. She has been trying to decrease her carbohydrate intake and has not been able to lose any weight.
   E. A patient had a sleeve gastrectomy (SG) 2 years ago and was able to lose 70% of her excess weight within the first year after the operation. She comes in for her second-year evaluation, and you noticed a 5-kg weight regain.

2. **A 36-year-old male with a body mass index (BMI) of 36 kg/m^2 presents to your clinic with complaints of excessive weight gain. He has a long-standing history of obesity since his teenage years, but no other obesity-related comorbidities. He informs you that he engages in daily exercise and has been sticking to an 1,800-calorie-a-day diet for close to a month. After further discussion, you learn that he has a long history of dieting that includes intermittent fasting, ketogenic diets, and the Atkins diet, and he has even tried going vegan.**

   What is the next best step to help this person with his weight loss efforts?
   A. Limiting his daily caloric intake to 1,800 calories for at least 6 months prior to discussing other medical treatment options
   B. Referral to an obesity medicine specialist for anti-obesity medication options
   C. Doing high-intensity interval (HIT) exercises for at least 2 days per week to improve his metabolism
   D. Performing indirect calorimetry, so he can know how many calories he should eat every day
   E. Following an intermittent fasting diet

ANSWERS

1. **A.** Several studies have shown that body weight is maintained at a stable range known as the set point, despite variability in energy intake and expenditure.[1–4] The set point theory posits that individuals have a genetically predetermined range of weight

that their metabolism will fight to maintain. The body is efficient at protecting against weight loss during caloric deprivation, suggesting an adaptive role of protection during periods of low food intake. The normal body set point keeps adjusting upward. As someone tries to lose weight by decreasing energy intake and increasing energy expenditure, the body fights to maintain its higher set-point weight by slowing metabolism. Hormonal adaptations, including decreases in leptin (LEP), cholecystokinin (CCK), and insulin and increases in ghrelin, glucagon-like peptide 1 (GLP-1), gastric inhibitory polypeptide, and pancreatic polypeptide, encourage weight gain after diet-induced weight loss and continue for at least 1 year after initial weight reduction. Weight loss also results in adaptive thermogenesis (decreased resting metabolic rate), which is also maintained over the long term. Neural factors such as dopamine also signal the need to respond to an increased desire for fatty foods after weight loss.[3] This is one of the explanations of why it is so difficult to lose weight and maintain weight loss without surgery.

2. **B.** The American Heart Association (AHA), the Obesity Society (TOS), and the American College of Cardiology guidelines for the management of overweight and obesity in adults state that nondrug interventions for the treatment of overweight and obesity should be attempted for at least 6 months before considering pharmacotherapy.[1,6] In the case of this patient, he has spent years trying different diet and exercise programs and would benefit from anti-obesity medication treatment and a referral to an obesity medicine specialist who can offer a comprehensive approach to care, including further guidance on diet, exercise, and medical treatment options.

   Medication options should be offered in combination with diet and exercise as follows:[5]

   - Patients with BMI >27 with concomitant risk factors or diseases including hypertension, dyslipidemia, coronary heart disease (CHD), type 2 diabetes, and sleep apnea,[1] or BMI >30.
   - Medications plus lifestyle changes can result in weight loss of about 3.5 to 10 kg more than lifestyle interventions alone.

Dietary recommendations guidelines for weight loss:

The best diet for weight loss is the one that a patient is able to adhere to. There is strong evidence to recommend any of the following methods to reduce food and calorie intake:[5]

1. Prescribe ingestion of 1,200 to 1,500 kcal/day for women and 1,500 to 1,800 kcal/day for men (kilocalorie levels are usually adjusted for the individual's body weight).
2. Prescribe a 500-kcal/day or 750-kcal/day energy deficit.
3. Prescribe one of the evidence-based diets that restricts certain food types (such as high-carbohydrate foods, low-fiber foods, or high-fat foods) to create an energy deficit by reducing food intake.

REFERENCES

1. Farias MM, Cuevas AM, Rodriguez F. Set-point theory and obesity. *Metab Syndr Relat Disord.* 2011;9(2):85-89. doi:10.1089/met.2010.0090.
2. Müller MJ, Bosy-Westphal A, Heymsfield SB. Is there evidence for a set point that regulates human body weight? *F1000 Med Rep.* 2010;2:59. https://doi.org/10.3410/M2-59.
3. Evert AB, Franz MJ. Why weight loss maintenance is difficult. *Diabetes Spectr.* 2017;30(3):153-156. doi:10.2337/ds017-0025.
4. OAC Article Library. Body weight "set point"—what we know and what we don't know. Retrieved June 15, 2020. https://www.obesityaction.org/community/article-library/body-weight-set-point-what-we-know-and-what-we-dont-know/. Accessed on December 4, 2021.
5. Clinical guidelines on the identification, evaluation, and treatment of overweight and obesity in adults. *WMJ.* 1998;97(9):20-37.
6. Jensen MD, Ryan DH, Apovian CM, et al. AHA/ACC/TOS guideline for the management of overweight and obesity in adults. *Circulation.* 2013;129(25):S102-S138.

3

Obesity Metabolism and Pathophysiology

Samar Hafida, MD

METABOLISM

A 33-year-old male was referred by to you for weight management. He has class III obesity with a body mass index (BMI) of 42 kg/m^2. He has had little success losing weight with lifestyle modifications guided by a team consisting of a registered dietitian, exercise physiologist, and behavioral health specialist. His occupation as a software engineer is mostly sedentary, and he has little opportunity for physical activity. He is married with two children who are in good health. Measurement of his energy expenditure was conducted as part of the workup for obesity to assist with the weight management plan.

1. **Which of the following is true regarding energy expenditure in people with obesity compared to lean individuals of similar age and gender?**
   A. Energy expenditure is lower after adjusting for free fat mass.
   B. Energy expenditure is higher after adjusting for free fat mass.
   C. Energy expenditure is similar to lean individuals after adjusting for free fat mass.
   D. The resting metabolic rate (RMR) is higher in obese people than in lean individuals, but the activity-related energy expenditure (AEE) is lower.

You learn that he has a lifelong history of obesity, and he reports symptoms of hyperphagia and insatiable hunger since early childhood. He is frustrated with his preoccupation with food and reveals a sense of shame that he hides food and is constantly eating, even at night when others are asleep. The physical examination is notable for a middle-aged man with central obesity and acanthosis. Otherwise, it is unremarkable.

2. **The history of early childhood obesity in this patient may be indicative of which of the following?**
   A. Prader-Willi syndrome (PWS)
   B. Mutations in the melanocortin-4-receptor (MC4R) pathway
   C. Cushing's syndrome
   D. Environmental determinants of health

3. **He is interested in pursuing bariatric surgery. Which of the following changes in gut hormones are associated with greater weight loss after bariatric surgery?**
   A. Decreased ghrelin
   B. Decreased cholecystokinin (CCK)
   C. Increased peptide YY (PYY)
   D. Increased fasting insulin

4. **After successfully losing weight with bariatric surgery, the patient returns for follow-up reporting ongoing cravings to calorie-dense, mainly sugar-sweetened foods despite a marked reduction in hunger.**

   Which of the following is true regarding the impact of neural circuitry involving reward systems on the pathophysiology of obesity?
   A. The hedonic drive to eat may override the metabolic signals that control body weight.
   B. Hedonic obesity is independent of metabolic obesity.

C. Hedonic signals driving weight regain can be controlled by willpower.
D. Bariatric surgery has no influence on the hedonic pathways that mediate food intake.

ANSWERS

1. **C.** Energy production is derived from carbohydrates, lipids, proteins, and alcohol. Total energy expenditure is the amount of energy required daily and is the sum of RMR; AEE, which includes exercise and no-exercise activity thermogenesis; and diet-induced thermogenesis.[1,2] Body weight regulation is a complex balance between energy intake and expenditure. The RMR is the amount of energy that an organism spends to support basic bodily activities such as maintaining body temperature, cell growth, and other vital organ function. Body composition (i.e., fat mass and fat-free mass) is the main determinant of RMR; both fat mass and fat-free mass are elevated with obesity. AEE is also elevated in people with obesity compared to their lean counterparts. Thus, people with obesity have a higher absolute energy expenditure than lean individuals, but this difference disappears when fat-free mass is adjusted. Therefore, differences in metabolic rate between those with and without obesity do not adequately explain the pathophysiology of the disease.[3]

2. **B.** Early-onset obesity before the age of 5 years is highly suggestive of a genetic cause of obesity. The hypothalamus and brainstem play a central role in energy balance. It receives and integrates signals both from the central nervous system and the periphery. The arcuate nucleus (ARC) contains two well-defined groups of neurons that have opposing actions.[4] One group is orexigenic (i.e., promotes hunger) and expresses agouti-related peptide (AgRP) and neuropeptide Y (NPY). The other is anorexigenic (i.e., inhibits hunger) and expresses proopiomelanocortin (POMC), as well as cocaine and amphetamine-regulated transcript (CART). When POMC neurons are activated, they lead to release of alpha-melanocyte stimulating hormone (α-MSH), which then binds to its MC4R. Downstream signaling inhibits feeding.[5]

   Rare genetic disorders of obesity can result from mutations in the MC4R pathway affecting the MC4R itself[6] or any of the upstream signals that involve the POMC neurons. Alterations in this pathway may involve POMC gene mutation, leptin (LEP), or PCSK1, which stimulate POMC neurons to produce α-MSH. As a result, anorexic signals are lost, leading to development of obesity in children, usually before the age of 5 years and as early as 1 year. Symptoms are described as hyperphagia, difficulty reaching a state of satiety that lasts for a short duration, food fixation, and recurrent food seeking behavior.[7]

   Prader-Willi syndrome (PWS) is a rare complex genetic disorder caused by lack of expression of genes on the paternal chromosome 15q11.2-q13.[8,9] Manifestations are apparent in infancy and include several endocrine disorders, as well as short stature, developmental delay, cognitive disability, and behavioral disorders.

   Cushing's syndrome is an endocrine disorder characterized by hypercortisolemia secondary to overproduction of cortisol, which manifests as truncal obesity, supraclavicular and dorsal fat pads, moon facies, purple striae, hirsutism, and a host of other metabolic consequences. Excessive cortisol may either originate from a pituitary or adrenal cortex adenoma, or tumors that may result in ectopic production.[10]

3. **C.** The gut is central to metabolic homeostasis. Specialized cells called *enteroendocrine cells,* distributed both in the foregut and hindgut, secrete a host of peptides in response to nutrients that are responsible for energy balance. L-cells produce glucagon-like peptide-1 and 2 (GLP-1 and GLP-2), oxyntomodulin, and PYY. These hormones are derived from the larger preproglucagon in a tissue-specific manner.[11] GLP-1 receptors are abundant in several systems, including those modulating appetite and energy intake.[12] GLP-1 reduces energy intake through multiple mechanisms by binding to receptors in the hypothalamus and hindbrain. It also potentiates insulin secretion from the pancreatic beta cell, which also promotes satiety.[13] PYY levels are increased in the postprandial state and have appetite suppression effects mediated through central appetite-regulating circuits in the hypothalamus and brainstem. Furthermore, it suppresses corticolimbic areas in the brain involved in the food reward.[14] Metabolic surgery is associated with elevations in both GLP-1 and PYY, both after Roux-en-Y gastric bypass (RYGB) and sleeve gastrectomy (SG). Both procedures are associated with up to a 10-fold increase in the absolute levels of GLP1.[15] Similarly, levels of PYY are increased by up to 3.5 times after RYGB in the postprandial state, and for up to 1 year after SG.[16,17] Changes in both these

peptide hormones have been associated with greater weight loss, although the precise mechanisms are yet to be determined.

Ghrelin, a powerful hunger-mediating hormone, is secreted from gastric and duodenal enteroendocrine cells located in the fundus of the stomach. Levels decrease after SG, but not substantially after RGYB. It is not clear, however, to what degree this reduction in ghrelin influences weight loss after metabolic surgery, as rodent studies have shown similar weight loss after SG in those genetically deficient in ghrelin.[18]

Specialized K and I enteroendocrine cells secrete CCK and glucose-dependent insulinotropic peptide (GIP), both of which rise after bariatric surgery. CCK acts as a satiety signal and has been shown in studies to reduce portion size and duration of a meal through exogenous administration.[19] It also promotes contractility of the gall bladder and slows gastric emptying. Levels of CCK have been shown to increase after both RYGB and SG, but this varies according to the procedure, and its exact role in promoting weight loss postoperatively is not fully understood.

Fasting insulin levels decrease after metabolic surgery, a result of elevated GLP-1, improved hepatic and skeletal muscle sensitivity, and improved beta-cell function.[20]

4. **A.** Hedonic or "reward" drives for food intake supersede metabolic signals of satiety in several individuals with obesity. Impulses spawned by reward systems located in the corticolimbic structures of the brain are powerful influences guiding food-seeking behaviors. These reward systems are often subject to higher cortical influences, such as emotion, arousal, stress, and metabolic status[21] which operate at a subconscious level. In simplified terms, the hedonic system mediates cravings and preferences to food. Cravings are influenced by the mesolimbic dopaminergic neurons, which project to the nucleus accumbens (NAc), and preferences to food are mediated by the endocannabinoid system and mu-opiod receptor pathways.[22] Multiple functional magnetic resonance imaging (MRI) studies have demonstrated an altered response to food stimuli in people with obesity, where reward centers were overactivated and the cortical structures responsible for inhibitory impulses were underactivated.[23,24]

Both hedonic and metabolic obesity have distinct mechanisms. However, in the real world, separating the two is arbitrary because both overlap. Determining the dominant influence can be useful clinically to identify which forces are dominant in the pathophysiology of obesity to develop an effective management plan.

Bariatric surgery is a powerful tool for weight management that leads to profound metabolic changes that favor weight loss. Several studies have identified its effect on the reward systems as well. Food preferences are altered after bariatric surgery, where enhanced perception of sweets and decreased consumption of sweet foods and beverages[25-27] have been reported after RYGB. In addition, functional magnetic resonance imaging (fMRI) assessment of reward signals involving the mes olimbic system shows that they are reduced in response to food cues[28] after bariatric surgery. These studies and others demonstrate its potential feasibility to modify hedonic pathways that contribute to obesity.

PATHOPHYSIOLOGY OF OBESITY

A 37-year-old woman with a 10-year history of type 2 diabetes, polycystic ovary syndrome, hypertension, and dyslipidemia presented to the bariatric surgery clinic. Over the years, she has developed microvascular complications due to chronic hyperglycemia, and she now requires multiple daily injections of insulin for diabetes management. Her family history is notable for ischemic heart disease, and she is concerned about her cardiovascular risk. Several attempts at intensive lifestyle modifications to lose weight and improve her risk factors have not led to sustainable results.

Her physical examination is notable for acanthosis. Her height is 152 cm and her weight is 77 kg, for a BMI 33.2 kg/m^2, and her waist circumference is 90 cm.

5. **Which of the following is the best method used clinically to correlate adiposity with metabolic health?**

   A. Waist circumference
   B. BMI
   C. Body weight
   D. Computed tomography (CT)

6. **An abdominal CT scan was ordered as part of the preoperative evaluation (see Figure 3-1). Which of the following is true regarding the fat distribution seen on imaging?**

   A. This adipose tissue is the primary storage depot in the body.
   B. This adipose tissue expands mainly primarily by hyperplasia.

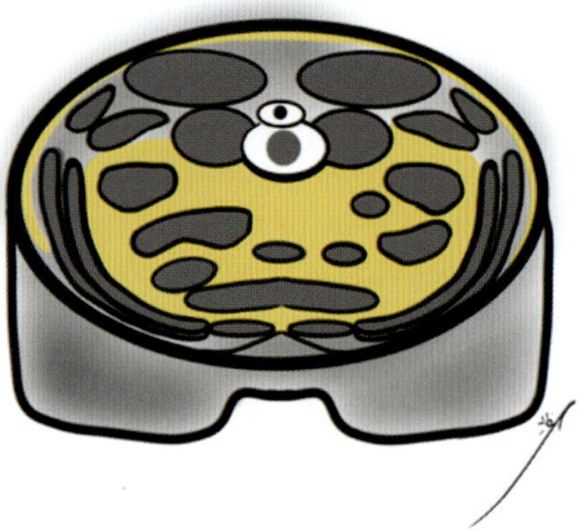

Figure 3-1 Representation of a CT scan of the abdomen showing fat distribution in yellow

C. The fat superficial to the psoas muscles is proinflammatory.
D. The fat of the omentum is associated with metabolic dysfunction.

7. Insulin resistance and cardiovascular disease are linked to accumulation of ectopic adipose tissue, a phenomenon known as *lipotoxicity*. Which of the following is a site of ectopic fat deposition?

A. Epicardial tissue
B. Peribronchial tissue
C. Splenic tissue
D. Pulmonary smooth muscle

8. The patient decides to undergo bariatric surgery. Which of the following is the most likely outcome after metabolic surgery?

A. Loss of more visceral than subcutaneous adipose tissue
B. Loss of both visceral and subcutaneous adipose tissue
C. Gain in visceral adipose tissue
D. Gain in lean muscle mass

ANSWERS

5. A. There are several methods used to estimate total adiposity and how fat mass is distributed. Waist circumference is a clinically useful measurement in individuals with BMI <35 kg/m2. It is easily obtained in the clinical setting, which is associated with central (abdominal) obesity and is considered a useful proxy to metabolic health.[29] It has also been shown to be associated with advanced tools used to assess distribution of adiposity such as abdominal imaging using CT scans and MRIs. Cutoffs used to determine metabolic health differ slightly according to the locations used for measurement. (Table 3-1).[30] So even though this patient's BMI is <35 kg/m^2, because of her waist circumference, she should be considered as someone at risk for the consequences of metabolic syndrome. Moreover, she should be considered as a candidate for metabolic surgery.

The National Institutes of Health (NIH) and National Heart, Lung, and Blood Institute (NHLBI) recommend the use of bony landmarks of the iliac crest as a point of reference due to the lack of change in position with body weight and age.[31,32] The World Health Organization (WHO) bases its cutoffs on the midpoint measurement between the lower rib and iliac crest, which requires two reference points. Although the midpoint is subject to change with body weight and age, its correlation with metabolic risk has been shown to consistent.[33] It is important to note that cutoffs and their association with visceral adiposity are subject to ethnic variations.[34]

BMI is calculated by dividing the weight in kilograms by height in meters squared. It is a simple tool to assess obesity and is widely used in epidemiologic studies, several of which have shown an association between increases in morbidity and mortality where for every 5 kg/m^2 above a BMI of 25, there is a 30% increase in all-cause mortality.[35] Although widely used clinically, BMI does not adequately reflect adiposity and may be misleading in certain

Table 3-1 CUTOFFS FOR WAIST CIRCUMFERENCE CORRELATING WITH CENTRAL ADIPOSITY AND ADVERSE METABOLIC HEALTH

Measurement Locations	Cutoff Men (cm)	Cutoff Women (cm)
Directly above iliac crest	102	93
Midpoint (halfway between lowest rib and iliac crest)	102	90
Point of largest circumference around waist	102	90
Point of minimal circumference around waist	97	87
Umbilicus	100	95

ethnicities or circumstances where lean body mass is low (sarcopenic obesity) or high.[36-38]

Body weight alone is an inaccurate method of estimating adiposity because weight is proportionate to height. CT scan and MRI are two methods that offer an accurate assessment of body composition and fat distribution.[39] However, it is not readily available in all clinical settings and is subject to limitations of cost, availability, and radiation exposure.

6. **D.** Visceral adipose tissue (VAT) is implicated in a number of metabolic disorders, such as insulin resistance as in type 2 diabetes mellitus and polycystic ovarian syndrome, and cardiovascular disease. (Figure 3-2).[40] How VAT adversely impairs metabolic health is multifactorial and related to its proinflammatory and metabolic properties that are unique to each tissue. VAT only comprises 10% to 20% of the total fat in the body, which is predominantly located in the omentum and mesentery.[41] Other significant deposits may occur in the perirenal, retroperitoneal, gonadal, and pericardial regions. When faced with chronic ongoing demand for lipid storage, VAT copes by hypertrophy rather than hyperplasia. This leads to overexpansion of the adipocytes exceeding their blood supply ultimately resulting in hypoxia.[42] Cellular responses to hypoxia then become upregulated, which triggers a host of inflammatory pathways that lead to infiltration of VAT by macrophages and other proinflammatory cells. Recruitment is followed by secretion of interleukin-6 (IL-6), activation of nuclear factor kappa-light-chain-enhancer of activated B cells (NF-κB), TNF alpha (TNF-α), macrophage chemoattractant protein-1 (MCP-1), and alterations in adipokine secretion, all of which contribute to VAT fibrosis, insulin resistance, and cardiovascular disease.[43-45]

Subcutaneous adipose tissue (SAT) is the main storage depot in the body, which plays an important physiologic role as a metabolic sink for excess energy. SAT is able to accommodate storage of fat by both hypertrophy and hyperplasia through recruitment of early-differentiated adipocytes from the stromal vasculature.[46] These small adipocytes have enhanced properties of plasticity and are able to store fat without disrupting their vascular supply. Several factors determine the availability of SAT, including sex dimorphisms, genetic variations, location of fat deposits in the body, and age. It is believed that individuals have their own personal SAT capacity, beyond which a state of overflow into VAT ensues.[47]

Insulin resistance
Impaired fasting Glucose/impaired glucose tolerance
Type 2 diabetes
Atrial fibrillation
Hypertension
Heart failure
Stroke
PVD
Chronic kidney disease
Obstructive sleep apnea
Reactive airway disease
Cancers
Decrease in cognitive function

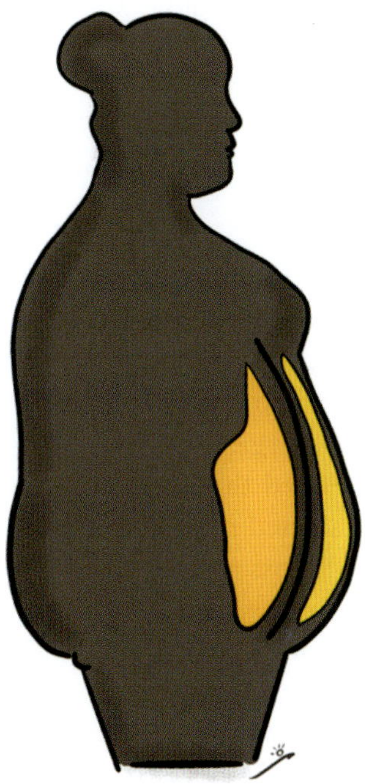

Figure 3-2 Consequences of excessive visceral adipose tissue Polycystic ovary syndrome—PCOS; atherosclerotic cardiovascular disease—ASCVD; coronary artery disease—CAD; peripheral vascular disease—ASCVD; nonalcoholic fatty liver disease—NAFLD; nonalcoholic steatohepatosis—NASH

7. **A.** Ectopic fat is defined as the deposit of triglycerides in nonadipose tissue cells in response to overabundance of energy which exceeds adipose tissue capacity for storage. Organs subject to ectopic fat storage include liver, pancreas, skeletal muscle, renal sinus, and heart and perivascular tissue.[48] Several lipotoxic molecules are generated within

these ectopic sites, causing dysfunction of the host cells by altering mitochondrial function and creating endoplasmic reticulum stress that interferes with protein synthesis and energy balance. Furthermore, disruption of intracellular processes creates a state of inflammation that has negative paracrine and systemic effects. Ramifications of ectopic fat deposits are widespread and include nonalcoholic fatty liver disease and its spectrum (NASH and livery fibrosis), type 2 diabetes, coronary artery disease, atrial fibrillation, and chronic kidney disease.[49-51]

Obesity has both direct and indirect effects on lung function and is associated with several lung diseases. Disorders of respiratory compliance and chest wall mechanics, hyperreactive airway disorders, obstructive sleep apnea, and increased risks of pulmonary infections. However, the lungs and airways are not typical sites for ectopic fat deposits.[52]

8. B. Several studies have examined the effect of weight loss on VAT. A meta-analysis of 89 studies reviewed whether VAT was preferentially targeted by weight loss interventions, including dietary restriction, physical activity (or both), medical weight management, and surgical weight management.[53] The authors concluded that there was no approach that specifically targeted reduction in VAT, and all interventions led to loss of both SAT and VAT. Lifestyle modifications resulting in 5% to 7% weight loss are likely to result in a 15% to 25% reduction in VAT.[54] Because the mass of SAT is greater than VAT, weight loss with any method led to higher percentage of reduction in SAT.[55,56]

REFERENCES

1. Carneiro IP, Elliott SA, Siervo M, et al. Is obesity associated with altered energy expenditure? *Adv Nutr.* 2016;7(3):476–87.
2. Pinheiro Volp AC, Esteves De Oliveira FC, Duarte R, Alves M, Esteves EA, Bressan J. Energy expenditure: components and evaluation methods. *Nutr Hosp.* 2011;26(3): 430-440.
3. Oussaada SM, Van Galen KA, Cooiman MI, et al. The pathogenesis of obesity. *Metabolism.* 2019;92:26-36.
4. Druce M, Bloom SR. The regulation of appetite. *Arch Dis Childhood.* 2006;91:183-187.
5. Wynne K, Stanley S, McGowan B, Bloom SR. Appetite control. *J Endocrinol.* 2005;184:291-318.
6. Ayers KL, Glicksberg BS, Garfield AS, et al. Melanocortin 4 receptor pathway dysfunction in obesity: patient stratification aimed at MC4R agonist treatment. 2018;103(7): 2601–2612.
7. Huvenne H, Dubern B, Clément K, Poitou C. Rare genetic forms of obesity: clinical approach and current treatments in 2016. *Obesity Facts.* 2016;9:158-173.
8. Angulo MA, Butler MG, Cataletto ME. Prader-Willi syndrome: a review of clinical, genetic, and endocrine findings. *J Endocrinol Invest.* 2015;38(12):1249-1263.
9. Heksch R, Kamboj M, Anglin K, Obrynba K. Review of Prader-Willi syndrome: the endocrine approach. *Transl Ped.* 2017;6:274-285.
10. Loriaux DL. Diagnosis and differential diagnosis of Cushing's syndrome [Internet]. *NEJM.* 2017;376:1451-9. http://www.nejm.org/doi/10.1056/NEJMra1505550. Accessed on January 14, 2022.
11. Côté CD, Zadeh-Tahmasebi M, Rasmussen BA, Duca FA, Lam TKT. Hormonal signaling in the gut. *J Biol Chem.* 2014;289:11642-11649.
12. Drucker DJ. Glucagon-like peptide 1—an overview [Internet]. In: Drucker DJ, ed., *Physiology of the Gastrointestinal Tract*, 4th ed. ScienceDirect; 2006. https://www.sciencedirect.com/topics/medicine-and-dentistry/glucagon-like-peptide-1-receptor. Accessed on January 14, 2022.
13. Drucker DJ. Mechanisms of action and therapeutic application of glucagon-like peptide-1. *Cell Metab.* 2018;27(4):740-756.
14. Batterham RL, Ffytche DH, Rosenthal JM, et al. PYY modulation of cortical and hypothalamic brain areas predicts feeding behaviour in humans. *Nature.* 2007;450(7166):106-109.
15. Hutch CR, Sandoval D. The role of GLP-1 in the metabolic success of bariatric surgery. *Endocrinology.* 2017;158(12): 4139-4151.
16. Reinehr T, Roth CL, Schernthaner GH, Kopp HP, Kriwanek S, Schernthaner G. Peptide YY and glucagon-like peptide-1 in morbidly obese patients before and after surgically induced weight loss. *Obes Surg.* 2007;17(12):1571-1577.
17. Korner J, Inabnet W, Febres G, et al. Prospective study of gut hormone and metabolic changes after adjustable gastric banding and Roux-en-Y gastric bypass. *Int J Obes.* 2009;33(7):786-795.
18. Stefater MA, Sandoval DA, Chambers AP, et al. Sleeve gastrectomy in rats improves postprandial lipid clearance by reducing intestinal triglyceride secretion. *Gastroenterology.* 2011;141(3).
19. Lieverse RJ, Jansen JBMJ, Masclee AAM, Lamers CBHW. Satiety effects of a physiological dose of cholecystokinin in humans. *Gut.* 1995;36(2):176-179.
20. Mingrone G, Cummings DE. Changes of insulin sensitivity and secretion after bariatric/metabolic surgery. *Surg Obesity Related Dis.* 2016;12.
21. Yu Y-H, Vasselli JR, Zhang Y, Mechanick JI, Korner J, Peterli R. Metabolic vs. hedonic obesity: a conceptual distinction and its clinical implications. *Obes Rev.* 2015;16(3):234-247.
22. Berridge KC, Robinson TE, Aldridge JW. Dissecting components of reward: "liking," "wanting," and learning. *Curr Op Pharmacol.* 2009;9(1):65-73.
23. Stice E, Spoor S, Bohon C, Veldhuizen MG, Small DM. Relation of reward from food intake and anticipated food

intake to obesity: a functional magnetic resonance imaging study. *J Abnorm Psychol.* 2008;117(4):924-935.
24. Batterink L, Yokum S, Stice E. Body mass correlates inversely with inhibitory control in response to food among adolescent girls: an fMRI study. *Neuroimage.* 2010;52(4):1696-1703.
25. Olbers T, Björkman S, Lindroos A, et al. Body composition, dietary intake, and energy expenditure after laparoscopic Roux-en-Y gastric bypass and laparoscopic vertical banded gastroplasty: a randomized clinical trial. *Ann Surg.* 2006;244(5):715-722.
26. Thirlby RC, Bahiraei F, Randall J, Drewnoski A. Effect of Roux-en-Y gastric bypass on satiety and food likes: the role of genetics. *J Gastrointest Surg.* 2006;10(2):270-277.
27. Schultes B, Ernst B, Wilms B, Thurnheer M, Hallschmid M. Hedonic hunger is increased in severely obese patients and is reduced after gastric bypass surgery. *Am J Clin Nutr.* 2010;92(2):277-283.
28. Ochner CN, Kwok Y, Conceição E, et al. Selective reduction in neural responses to high calorie foods following gastric bypass surgery [Internet]. *Ann Surg.* 2011;253(3):502-507. pmc/articles/PMC3128512/?report=abstract.
29. De Koning L, Merchant AT, Pogue J, Anand SS. Waist circumference and waist-to-hip ratio as predictors of cardiovascular events: meta-regression analysis of prospective studies. *Eur Heart J.* 2007;28(7):850-856.
30. Mason C, Katzmarzyk PT. Waist circumference thresholds for the prediction of cardiometabolic risk: is measurement site important. *Eur J Clin Nutr.* 2010;64(8):862-867.
31. Bosy-Westphal A, Booke C-A, Blöcker T, et al. Measurement site for waist circumference affects its accuracy as an index of visceral and abdominal subcutaneous fat in a Caucasian population. *J Nutr.* 2010;140(5):954-961.
32. NHANES III (1988–1994). Anthropometric procedure videos [Internet]. 2020. https://wwwn.cdc.gov/nchs/nhanes/nhanes3/anthropometricvideos.aspx. Accessed on January 14, 2022.
33. Klein S, Allison DB, Heymsfield SB, et al. Waist circumference and cardiometabolic risk: a consensus statement from Shaping America's Health: Association for Weight Management and Obesity Prevention; NAASO, the Obesity Society; the American Society for Nutrition; and the American Diabetes Association. In: *Diabetes Care* [Internet]. American Diabetes Association; 2007:1647-1652. https://care.diabetesjournals.org/content/30/6/1647. Accessed on January 14, 2022.
34. Gallagher D, Visser M, Sepúlveda D, Pierson RN, Harris T, Heymsfieid SB. How useful is body mass index for comparison of body fatness across age, sex, and ethnic groups? *Am J Epidemiol* [Internet]. 1996;143(3):228-239. https://pubmed.ncbi.nlm.nih.gov/8561156/. Accessed on January 14, 2022.
35. MacMahon S, Baigent C, Duffy S, et al. Body-mass index and cause-specific mortality in 900 000 adults: collaborative analyses of 57 prospective studies. *Lancet* [Internet]. 2009;373(9669):1083-1096. https://pubmed.ncbi.nlm.nih.gov/19299006/. Accessed on January 14, 2022.
36. WHO. Appropriate body-mass index for Asian populations and its implications for policy and intervention strategies: report of a WHO Expert consultation. *Lancet.* 2004;363(9403):157-163.
37. Evans EM, Rowe DA, Racette SB, Ross KM, McAuley E. Is the current BMI obesity classification appropriate for black and white postmenopausal women? *Int J Obes.* 2006;30(5):837-843.
38. Fernández JR, Heo M, Heymsfield SB, et al. Is percentage body fat differentially related to body mass index in Hispanic Americans, African Americans, and European Americans? *Am J Clin Nutr.* 2003;77(1):71-75.
39. Meng K, Lee CH, Saremi F. Metabolic syndrome and ectopic fat deposition: what can CT and MR provide? *Acad Rad.* 2010;17(10):1302-1312.
40. Neeland IJ, Ross R, Després J-P, et al. Visceral and ectopic fat, atherosclerosis, and cardiometabolic disease: a position statement. *Lancet Diabetes-Endocrinol* [Internet]. 2019;7(9):715-725.
41. Palmer BF, Clegg DJ. The sexual dimorphism of obesity [Internet]. *Mole Cell Endocrinol.* 2015;402:113-119. pmc/articles/PMC4326001/?report=abstract.
42. Wang QA, Tao C, Gupta RK, Scherer PE. Tracking adipogenesis during white adipose tissue development, expansion and regeneration. *Nat Med.* 2013;19:1338-1344.
43. Fried SK, Bunkin DA, Greenberg AS. Omental and subcutaneous adipose tissues of obese subjects release interleukin-6: depot difference and regulation by glucocorticoid. *J Clin Endocrinol Metab.* 1998;83(3):847-850.
44. Xu H, Barnes GT, Yang Q, et al. Chronic inflammation in fat plays a crucial role in the development of obesity-related insulin resistance. *J Clin Invest.* 2003;112(12):1821-1830.
45. Fontana L, Eagon JC, Trujillo ME, Scherer PE, Klein S. Visceral fat adipokine secretion is associated with systemic inflammation in obese humans. *Diabetes* [Internet]. 2007;56(4):1010-1013. https://diabetes.diabetesjournals.org/content/56/4/1010. Accessed on January 14, 2022.
46. Cuthbertson DJ, Steele T, Wilding P, et al. What have human experimental overfeeding studies taught us about adipose tissue expansion and susceptibility to obesity and metabolic complications? *Int J Obes.* 2017;41(6):853-865.
47. Taylor R, Holman RR. Normal weight individuals who develop Type 2 diabetes: the personal fat threshold. *Clin Sci.* 2015;128(7):405-410.
48. Ferrara D, Montecucco F, Dallegri F, Carbone F. Impact of different ectopic fat depots on cardiovascular and metabolic diseases. *J Cell Physiol.* 2019;234:21630-21641.
49. Chalasani N, Younossi Z, Lavine JE, et al. The diagnosis and management of nonalcoholic fatty liver disease: practice guidance from the American Association for the Study of Liver Diseases. *Hepatology.* 2018;67(1):328-357.
50. Foster MC, Hwang SJ, Porter SA, Massaro JM, Hoffmann U, Fox CS. Fatty kidney, hypertension, and chronic kidney disease: the Framingham Heart Study. *Hypertension.* 2011;58(5):784-790.
51. Lee JJ, Pedley A, Hoffmann U, Massaro JM, Levy D, Long MT. Visceral and intrahepatic fat are associated with cardiometabolic risk factors above other ectopic fat depots:

the Framingham Heart Study. *Am J Med.* 2018;131(6): 684-692.
52. Dixon AE, Peters U. The effect of obesity on lung function [Internet]. *Exp Rev Resp Med.* 2018;12(9):755-767. pmc/articles/PMC6311385/?report=abstract.
53. Merlotti C, Ceriani V, Morabito A, Pontiroli AE. Subcutaneous fat loss is greater than visceral fat loss with diet and exercise, weight-loss promoting drugs and bariatric surgery: A critical review and meta-analysis [Internet]. *Int J Obes.* 2017;41(5):672-682. https://www-nature-com.ezp-prod1.hul.harvard.edu/articles/ijo201731. Accessed on January 14, 2022.
54. Verheggen RJHM, Maessen MFH, Green DJ, Hermus ARMM, Hopman MTE, Thijssen DHT. A systematic review and meta-analysis on the effects of exercise training versus hypocaloric diet: distinct effects on body weight and visceral adipose tissue. *Obes Rev.* 2016;17(8):664-690.
55. Chaston TB, Dixon JB. Factors associated with percent change in visceral versus subcutaneous abdominal fat during weight loss: findings from a systematic review. *Intl J Obes.* 2008;32(4):619-628.
56. Kay SJ, Fiatarone Singh MA. The influence of physical activity on abdominal fat: a systematic review of the literature. *Obes Rev.* 2006;7(2):183-200.

4

Microbiome Theory of Obesity

Hung Truong, MD

A 50-year-old male with a body mass index (BMI) of 40 kg/m^2, along with type 2 diabetes mellitus, hypertension, and hyperlipidemia, recently completed his preoperative evaluation for surgical management of his obesity and diabetes mellitus. The patient has heard about the restrictive and malabsorptive properties of bariatric surgery, but he also knows that some people do very well with bariatric surgery, while others do not. He also has read that bacteria play a role. He wishes to know more about intestinal microbiome theory and its association with RYGB and SG.

1. Regarding the gut microbiota theory and obesity, which of the following about microbial gene richness is true?

A. Low-grade inflammation/high richness is associated with obesity.
B. Morbid obesity/low richness is seen in normal-weight individuals.
C. Insulin resistance/diabetes mellitus/low richness is seen in inflammatory bowel disease.
D. *Helicobacter pylori* infection tends to cause an increase in microbial diversity.

2. Regarding microbiome diversity in patients after bariatric surgery, which of the following is correct?

A. It increases after bariatric surgery.
B. It decreases after bariatric surgery.
C. It decreases after bariatric surgery in patients with diabetes remission.
D. It changes only after procedures with a malabsorptive component.

3. Which of the following is true regarding changes in intestinal microbiota after bariatric surgery?

A. Changes in diet do not affect the microbiota.
B. The effect that bile acid changes impose are similar between Roux-en-Y gastric bypass (RYGB) and sleeve gastrectomy (SG).
C. Decreased intestinal pH after RYGB causes microbiota changes.
D. A decrease in gut motility can cause bacterial overgrowth, changing the microbiota.

4. Which of the following statements about changes in bile acid metabolism associated with gut microbiota after bariatric surgery is correct?

A. Synthesis of primary and secondary bile acids increases.
B. Synthesis of primary and secondary bile acids decreases.
C. 7α-dehydroxylation activity decreases.
D. Intestinal microbiota only affects secondary bile acids.

ANSWERS

1. Recent studies suggest that a specific composition of gut microbiota is associated with obesity and cardiometabolic diseases such as diabetes.[1,2] These studies consistently have found that obese patients show a low microbial gene richness or less microbial diversity within their gut microbiome. Furthermore, obese patients have less variability in their intestinal microbiota than thin individuals.[3,4] One study found that about 75% of the subjects with severe obesity

exhibit low microbial gene richness, which is far higher than only 40% of overweight or moderately obese subjects.[5] Also, many noncommunicable diseases, such as type 2 diabetes mellitus, asthma, allergies, atopic diseases, inflammatory bowel disease, metabolic syndrome, necrotizing enterocolitis, and atherosclerosis, are closely linked with low intestinal microbiota diversity as well.[4,6]

As a result, it is proposed that low gut microbial gene richness in obesity is strongly associated with metabolic comorbidities such as low-grade inflammation, insulin resistance, dyslipidemia, truncal-adiposity, and cardiometabolic complications such as severity of hypertension, glucose intolerance, and type 2 diabetes.[1,4,5,7,8] *H. pylori* does not increase the diversity of the microbiome.

2. **A.** When discussing gut microbiota versus microbiome, the gut microbiota is defined as the community of microorganisms located in the human intestines. The microbiome is defined as the genetic pool of the microbiota living in a specific place and its relationship with the environment such as the intestine.[9,10] Significant changes in gut microbiota after bariatric surgery have been reported in both human and mouse models.[9] Multiple small studies show increases in gut microbiota after bariatric surgeries of various cohorts who underwent bariatric surgery. One study, based on a direct comparison of patients presurgery and postsurgery, showed that in addition to weight reduction and glucose improvement, the alterations in gut microbiota included increased diversity and altered composition that occurred within 3 months after RYGB.[11] Furthermore, long-term follow-up shows that more than half of the altered species were maintained in relative abundance, which indicates that bariatric surgery results in rapid and sustained changes in the gut microbiome.[11,12] Aron-Wisnewky et al have confirmed lasting increased diversity in gut microbiome changes up to 5 years after bariatric surgery.[13] Moreso et al have found that alterations from bariatric surgery, rather than a low-calorie diet, change the gut microbe profile in obese subjects toward a phenotype similar to normal-weight subjects.[14]

3. **D.** Diet therapy, nutrient malabsorption, bile acid metabolism, and pH are all factors found to be associated with changes in intestinal microbiota. Changes in diet, a decrease in volume of food consumption, and nutrient malabsorption after bariatric surgery can cause rapid changes in the intestinal microbiota.[15,16] Also, variations in fat content, carbohydrates, and glycemic indexes of various diets affect the amounts of specific strains found in the intestinal microbiota.[17] Both complex carbohydrate–rich and simple carbohydrate–rich diets have been associated with Prevotella enterotypes whereas Bacteroides enterotypes are linked with a typical Western diet, which is rich in animal protein and saturated fat.[15,18] Bariatric surgery changes the intestinal microorganism pattern by gastric volume restriction or rearrangement of the intestinal tract.[19] The SG and RYGB alter food digestion, which results in nutrient presentation farther downstream in the gut. These changes in nutritional exposure within the intestinal tract have been found to alter the gut environment and affect the composition of the intestinal bacterial.[19,20]

   Similar differences in gut microbiota have been seen in obese patients with diabetes after RYGB and SG, with studies showing contrasting changes in ratios of Bacteroidetes and Firmicutes. Interestingly, Guo et al found fewer changes in intestinal microbiota after SG than after RYGB, which was consistent with another study carried out in rodents. They proposed that this difference could be attributed to the fact that the SG induces relatively mild physical manipulations of the intestinal tract compared to RYGB.[21] Alteration in intestinal pH is also believed to be associated with intestinal microbiota changes. For example, reduced gastric acid secretion in RYGB can increase pH levels in the distal digestive tract, especially in the colon.[19] Finally, changes in bile acid presentation and metabolism in the intestinal tract can affect gut microbiota after bariatric surgery as well.[15] The absence of food exposure, as well as the decrease in gut motility of the proximal jejunum in RYGB patients, have been found to cause bacterial overgrowth and alterations of bile acid metabolism.[22] Furthermore, changes in bile acid deconjugation also alters the 7α-dehydroxylation capacity of the gut microbiota, which contributes to the synthesis of intermediate bile acids.[15]

4. **A.** Gut microbiota has been shown to play a key role in modulating bile acids after both RYGB and SG.[23,24] Primary and secondary bile acid plasma levels have been found to increase after RYGB and SG in humans compared to weight-matched individuals,

which is believed to contribute to metabolic improvement such as glucose homeostasis and beta-cell function.[25–27]

Previous rat models have shown that 7α-hydroxylase and sterol-27-hydroxylase levels were decreased in livers of conventionally raised mice compared with those in germ-free mice. This implies that gut microbiota play a role in formation of primary bile acids through these mechanisms.[28] Changes in secondary bile acid synthesis in RYGB patients are believed to be related to bacterial overgrowth in the biliopancreatic limb that cause increases in bile salt hydrolases of the gut microbiota and result in an increase of bile acid deconjugation.[29,30] These changes are believed to also affect intestinal microbiota 7α-dehydroxylation activity, which is associated with increase in secondary bile acid synthesis and bile acid diversity. In RYGB patients, increases in 7α-dehydroxylation of bile acids from human gut microbiota and plasma levels of the glycine-conjugated litocholic acid have been observed after surgery.[31]

REFERENCES

1. Cani PD. Severe obesity and gut microbiota: does bariatric surgery really reset the system? *Gut.* 2019;68(1):5-6. doi:10.1136/gutjnl-2018-316815.
2. Lynch SV, Pedersen O. The human intestinal microbiome in health and disease. *NEJM.* 2016;375(24):2369-2379. doi:10.1056/NEJMra1600266.
3. Turnbaugh PJ, Hamady M, Yatsunenko T, et al. A core gut microbiome in obese and lean twins. *Nature.* 2009;457(7228):480-484.
4. Ulker I, Yildiran H. The effects of bariatric surgery on gut microbiota in patients with obesity: a review of the literature. *Biosci Microbiota, Food Heal.* 2019;38(1):3-9. doi:10.12938/bmfh.18-018.
5. Cotillard A, Kennedy SP, Kong LC, et al. Dietary intervention impact on gut microbial gene richness. *Nature.* 2013;500(7464):585-588. doi:10.1038/nature12480.
6. Mangal Patel R, Denning PW. Intestinal microbiota and its relationship with necrotizing enterocolitis. *Pediatr Res.* 2015;78(3):232-238. http://www.nature.com/pr/index.html%5Cnhttp://ovidsp.ovid.com/ovidweb.cgi?T=JS&PAGE=reference&D=emed17&NEWS=N&AN=605680560.
7. Magouliotis DE, Tasiopoulou VS, Sioka E, Chatedaki C, Zacharoulis D. Impact of bariatric surgery on metabolic and gut microbiota profile: a systematic review and meta-analysis. *Obes Surg.* 2017;27(5):1345-1357. doi:10.1007/s11695-017-2595-8.
8. Dao MC, Everard A, Aron-Wisnewsky J, et al. Akkermansia muciniphila and improved metabolic health during a dietary intervention in obesity: relationship with gut microbiome richness and ecology. *Gut.* 2016;65(3):426-436. doi:10.1136/gutjnl-2014-308778.
9. Ulker I, Yildiran H. The effects of bariatric surgery on gut microbiota in patients with obesity: a review of the literature. *Biosci Microbiota, Food Heal.* 2019;38(1):3-9. doi:10.12938/bmfh.18-018.
10. Rautava S. Early microbial contact, the breast milk microbiome and child health. *J Dev Orig Health Dis.* 2016;7(1):5-14. doi:10.1017/S2040174415001233.
11. Liu H, Hu C, Zhang X, Jia W. Role of gut microbiota, bile acids and their cross-talk in the effects of bariatric surgery on obesity and type 2 diabetes. *J Diabetes Investig.* 2018;9(1):13-20. doi:10.1111/jdi.12687.
12. Palleja A, Kashani A, Allin KH, et al. Roux-en-Y gastric bypass surgery of morbidly obese patients induces swift and persistent changes of the individual gut microbiota. *Genome Med.* 2016;8(1). https://doi.org/10.1186/s13073-016-0312-1.
13. Aron-Wisnewsky J, Prifti E, Belda E, et al. Major microbiota dysbiosis in severe obesity: Fate after bariatric surgery. *Gut.* 2019;68(1):70-82. doi:10.1136/gutjnl-2018-316103.
14. Damms-Machado A, Mitra S, Schollenberger AE, et al. Effects of surgical and dietary weight loss therapy for obesity on gut microbiota composition and nutrient absorption. *Biomed Res Int.* 2015. doi:10.1155/2015/806248.
15. Ulker I, Yildiran H. The effects of bariatric surgery on gut microbiota in patients with obesity: a review of the literature. *Biosci Microbiota, Food Heal.* 2019;38(1):3-9. doi:10.12938/bmfh.18-018.
16. Peat CM, Kleiman SC, Bulik CM, Carroll IM. The intestinal microbiome in bariatric surgery patients. *Eur Eat Disord Rev.* 2015;23(6):496-503. doi:10.1002/erv.2400.
17. David LA, Maurice CF, Carmody RN, et al. Diet rapidly and reproducibly alters the human gut microbiome. *Nature.* 2014;505:559-563.
18. Fava F, Gitau R, Griffin BA, et al. The type and quantity of dietary fat and carbohydrate alter faecal microbiome and short-chain fatty acid excretion in a metabolic syndrome "at-risk" population. *Int J Obes.* 2013;37(2):216-223.
19. Liu H, Hu C, Zhang X, Jia W. Role of gut microbiota, bile acids and their cross-talk in the effects of bariatric surgery on obesity and type 2 diabetes. *J Diabetes Investig.* 2018;9(1):13-20. doi:10.1111/jdi.12687.
20. Murphy R, Tsai P, Jüllig M, Liu, A, Plank L, Booth M. Differential changes in gut microbiota after gastric bypass and sleeve gastrectomy bariatric surgery vary according to diabetes remission. *Obes Surg.* 2017;27(4):917-925.
21. Guo Y, Liu CQ, Shan CX, et al. Gut microbiota after Roux-en-Y gastric bypass and sleeve gastrectomy in a diabetic rat model: increased diversity and associations of discriminant genera with metabolic changes. *Diabetes Metab Res Rev.* 2017;33(3). doi:10.1002/dmrr.2857.
22. Aron-Wisnewsky J, Prifti E, Belda E, et al. Major microbiota dysbiosis in severe obesity: Fate after bariatric surgery. *Gut.* 2019;68(1):70-82. doi:10.1136/gutjnl-2018-316103.
23. Liu H, Hu C, Zhang X, Jia W. Role of gut microbiota, bile acids and their cross-talk in the effects of bariatric surgery on obesity and type 2 diabetes. *J Diabetes Investig.* 2018;9(1):13-20. doi:10.1111/jdi.12687.

24. Ulker I, Yildiran H. The effects of bariatric surgery on gut microbiota in patients with obesity: a review of the literature. *Biosci Microbiota, Food Heal.* 2019;38(1):3-9. doi:10.12938/bmfh.18-018.
25. Myronovych A, Kirby M, Ryan KK, et al. Vertical sleeve gastrectomy reduces hepatic steatosis while increasing serum bile acids in a weight-loss-independent manner. *Obesity.* 2014;22 (2):390-400. doi:10.1002/oby.20548.
26. Patti ME, Houten SM, Bianco AC, et al. Serum bile acids are higher in humans with prior gastric bypass: potential contribution to improved glucose and lipid metabolism. *Obesity.* 2009;17 (9):1671-1677. doi:10.1038/oby.2009.102.
27. Jahansouz C, Xu H, Hertzel A V., et al. Bile acids increase independently from hypocaloric restriction after bariatric surgery. *Ann Surg.* 2016;264(6):1022-1028. doi:10.1097/SLA.0000000000001552.
28. Sayin SI, Wahlström A, Felin J, et al. Gut microbiota regulates bile acid metabolism by reducing the levels of tauro-beta-muricholic acid, a naturally occurring FXR antagonist. *Cell Metab.* 2013;17(2):225-235. doi:10.1016/j.cmet.2013.01.003.
29. Aron-Wisnewsky J, Doré J, Clement K. The importance of the gut microbiota after bariatric surgery. *Nat Rev Gastroenterol Hepatol.* 2012;9(10):590-598. doi:10.1038/nrgastro.2012.161.
30. Wahlström A, Sayin SI, Marschall HU, Bäckhed F. Intestinal crosstalk between bile acids and microbiota and its impact on host metabolism. *Cell Metab.* 2016;24(1):41-50. doi:10.1016/j.cmet.2016.05.005.
31. Tremaroli V, Karlsson F, Werling M, et al. Roux-en-Y gastric bypass and vertical banded gastroplasty induce long-term changes on the human gut microbiome contributing to fat mass regulation. *Cell Metab.* 2015;22(2):228-238. doi:10.1016/j.cmet.2015.07.009.

5

Hormones of Obesity Care: PYY, Ghrelin, GLP-1, and GIP

Kevin Smith, DO

A 39-year-old female with a past medical history of type 2 diabetes and obstructive sleep apnea is presenting to a multidisciplinary weight loss center to be evaluated for bariatric surgery. Medications include atorvastatin (40 mg daily), metformin (1,000 mg BID), liraglutide (1.8 mg daily), detemir (25 units nightly), and aspart (10 units TID with meals). She is compliant with her continuous positive airway pressure (CPAP) machine. She follows her current medication regimen and denies any recent complaints.

Despite her compliance with her medications, she states that she feels tired frequently, which she attributes to her lack of physical exercise and decompensation. She works as an accountant and is physically inactive much of the day. She has started intermittent fasting, with allowable food intake from 10 a.m. to 6 p.m., and restricts her caloric intake to 1,500 kcal/day during this time frame.

Social history is negative for alcohol or tobacco use. Family history is positive for coronary artery disease, as manifested by acute myocardial infarction in her father when he was 59 years old. Her mother is healthy but has excess weight.

The patient is 5'10" (178 cm) and weighs 268 lbs (123 kg), with a body mass index (BMI) of 38.8 kg/m^2. Vital signs reveal blood pressure of 133/81 mmHg, heart rate of 77/min, respiratory rate 19/min, and oxygen saturation of 98% on room air. Abdominal circumference is 37 in (94 cm).

Laboratory work reveals an HbA1c of 7.3%, AST 92 U/L, ALT 86 U/L, and vitamin D of 21 ng/mL. Her complete blood count and cholesterol panel are normal. A subsequent right-upper-quadrant ultrasound displays fatty infiltration of the liver without regenerative nodules.

1. The patient states that in order to prevent hunger throughout the night, she eats a snack right before her fasting time begins. The following are meal-terminating hormones or hormones that suppress hunger. Which of the following is most likely elevated, regardless of food intake and slowed gastric motility?

A. Cholecystokinin (CCK)
B. Amylin
C. Glucagon-like peptide-1 (GLP-1)
D. Oxyntomodulin (OXM)
E. Peptide YY (PYY)

2. The patient is interested in a sleeve gastrectomy (SG). If this surgery is performed, which of the following neurohormonal levels will be significantly reduced 1 week postop compared to preop values?

A. Leptin (LEP)
B. Ghrelin
C. Adiponectin
D. GLP-1
E. α-melanocyte-stimulating hormone (α-MSH)

3. Liraglutide should be avoided in those with severe diabetic gastroparesis, as it slows gastric emptying. Which of the following advantages does this medication display in treating obesity?

A. It increases hepatic gluconeogenesis.
B. It stimulates the pancreatic alpha cells.

C. It promotes lipolysis.
D. It suppresses glucagon production.

4. The surgeon discusses with the patient a Roux-en-Y gastric bypass (RYGB) that provides a high rate of diabetes remission/improvement. Improvements of this condition are partly due to a postoperative increase in a specific hormone secreted by the L cells in the small and large bowel. Of the following, which has the most similar mechanism to this hormone in response to glucose ingestion?

A. Glucose-dependent insulinotropic peptide (GIP)
B. CCK
C. OXM
D. PYY
E. Glucagon

ANSWERS

1. E. Meal-terminating gastrointestinal hormones increase in the fed state to suppress appetite through feedback mechanisms in the hypothalamus, in the gastrointestinal tract, and through endocrine and exocrine hormone stimulation. Of these, PYY is the only hormone listed that is secreted regardless of nutritional intake (the other being OXM) and causes slowing of gastric motility (the other being GLP-1). Although PYY is being evaluated as a potential exogenous anti-obesity agent, unacceptable levels of nausea and vomiting have prevented its usefulness at this point.

Of the other options, amylin is cosecreted with insulin from the beta cells of the pancreas in the setting of carbohydrate ingestions, CCK is secreted in response to fat and protein (not carbohydrates), and although GLP-1 causes gastric slowing, it does so in response only to carbohydrates.

Meal-Terminating Intestinal Hormones

Name	Secretion Stimulation	Action
CCK[1]	Fat/protein ingestion and gastric distention	• Stimulates gallbladder contraction • Slows gastric emptying • Reduces appetite
GLP-1[2]	Carbohydrate ingestion	• Incretin effect • Reduction of hepatic gluconeogenesis • Delays gastric emptying
OXM[3]	Any feeding	• Decrease appetite • Increase energy expenditure
Peptide YY (PYY)[3]	Any feeding	• Appetite suppression • Delays gastric and intestinal emptying

2. B. SL has nearly doubled in popularity since 2012, making up the majority of bariatric surgeries (61.4% as of 2018). Although there is some improvement in GLP-1, the most significant neurohormonal change is a significant reduction of ghrelin. This is the only orexogenic (i.e., appetite-simulating) hormone produced in the gastrointestinal tract, and it is found primarily in the gastric fundus and body. During SL, up to 80% of the stomach is removed, including the cells that produce this hormone. This hormone is typically secreted in response to an empty stomach, a fasting state, and weight loss and is suppressed in a stretched stomach and a fed state. In the arcuate nucleus (ARC) of the hypothalamus, ghrelin also stimulates the NPY/AgRP neurons to stimulate appetite and inhibits the pro-opiomelanocortin and cocaine- and amphetamine-regulated transcript (POMC/CART) pathways, which normally inhibits appetite.

Of the other choices, LEP, an adipokin, will decrease in the setting of weight loss, but only once adipose tissue is reduced (which will likely take weeks to months before a significant reduction occurs). Adiponectin will increase in response to weight loss (levels move inversely to adipose tissue quantity), and GLP-1 will increase postoperatively. Here, α-MSH is an anorexogenic pituitary hormone that will increase with the decrease of ghrelin. As ghrelin normally inhibits the anorexogenic pathway, a decrease in ghrelin removes that inhibition, allowing MSH to increase. The POMC/CART pathways secrete α-MSH to suppress appetite.

3. D. Liraglutide, a GLP-1 analog, should be avoided in those with severe diabetic gastroparesis, as it slows gastric emptying and can exacerbate symptoms. Of note, even though GLP-1 is called "glucagon-like," it actually has several mechanisms that decrease blood glucose. GLP-1 has many positive effects, including glucose-dependent insulin stimulation (with insulin being produced in the beta cells of the pancreas), suppressing hepatic gluconeogenesis via suppressing glucagon production (from alpha cells in the pancreas), and stimulating the anorexogenic POMC/CART pathway in the ARC of the hypothalamus to suppress appetite. This hormone level is endogenously increased significantly after RYGB, and to a lesser degree in SL.

4. **F.** The RYGB has high rates of diabetes remission, with a significant factor being the increased level of GLP-1 postoperatively from the L-cells of the distal small bowel and colon. As this question asks which other hormone is similar to GLP-1, the best answer is GIP. This hormone is anorexigenic in conjunction with GLP-1, has an incretin effect, meaning that it decreases blood sugar by enhancing the secretion of insulin, and slows gastric empyting, all of which are similar to GLP-1. It is secreted in the K cells of the duodenum and jejunum, with its release stimulated by glucose and fat intake. As seen with GLP-1, GIP increases in the fed state, decreases in the fasting state, and increases overall after GLP-1.

Of the other options, CCK does cause gastric slowing, but it is secreted by the I cells of the duodenum and jejunum in response to fat and protein intake, not glucose. PYY and OXM are secreted by the distal small bowel in response to any feeding, but they have no incretin effect. Finally, glucagon is secreted by the alpha cells of the pancreas and has an opposite effect of insulin. Further, it is inhibited by GLP-1 and GIP both directly and indirectly via insulin secretion.

REFERENCES

1. Miller GD. Appetite regulation: hormones, peptides, and neurotransmitters and their role in obesity. *Am J Lifestyle Med.* 2017;13(6):586-601. doi:10.1177/1559827617716376.
2. Bays HE, McCarthy W. *Obesity Algorithm.* Centennial, CO: Obesity Medicine Association; 2020.
3. Accrediting Society for Bariatric Surgeons Fellowships (ASMBS). *Estimate of Bariatric Surgery Numbers, 2011–2019.* https://asmbs.org/resources/estimate-of-bariatric-surgery-numbers. Accessed September 3, 2021.

6

Economics of Bariatric Surgery

Amy Rosenbluth, MD

1. **The cost-effectiveness of bariatric surgery is determined by looking at the overall cost of surgery and subsequent care related to the bariatric surgery. To assess cost-effectiveness, reoperations and revisions must be taken into consideration. Which bariatric procedure has the highest rate of reoperation/revision?**
   A. Adjustable gastric band (AGB)
   B. Duodenal switch
   C. Roux-en-Y gastric bypass (RYGB)
   D. Vertical sleeve gastrectomy (SG)

2. **The cost-effectiveness of bariatric surgery is evaluated over time, but it has many variables. In which time period does bariatric surgery offset the surgical cost to payers like insurance companies?**
   A. Immediately after surgery
   B. 6 months after surgery
   C. 1 year after surgery
   D. 2+ years after surgery

3. **Which of the following statements about bariatric surgery is true?**
   A. It is cost-effective for diabetes management in adults.
   B. It is not cost-effective for patients with nonalcoholic steatohepatitis cirrhosis.
   C. It is cost-effective for obesity management in adolescents sooner than in adults.
   D. It is not cost-effective 10 years after surgery in adolescents.

4. **Which of the following is considered an indirect cost of bariatric surgery?**
   A. Diabetic medications
   B. Intravenous (IV) fluid and tubing
   C. Anesthesia charges
   D. Work absence

ANSWERS

1. **A.** Laparoscopic AGBs are generally considered to be the lowest-cost initial surgery. However, they have high long-term associated costs. One study evaluating 10-year outcomes after AGB showed no statistically significant resolution of comorbidities and a high rate of reoperations (60% of patients had their bands removed).[1] Another study evaluating AGB effectiveness over 10 years did show clinically meaningful weight loss and improvement in comorbidities, but it still had a 43% revision rate.[2] Between 2006 and 2013, Medicare payments for AGB-related reoperations totaled $224 million.[3]

   The duodenal switch has a revision/reoperation rate as high as 7%,[4] bypass 4%, and sleeve 1.7%.[5] When considering the cost-effectiveness of bariatric surgery, the goal is to have a good resolution of comorbidities, which reduces healthcare spending. However, that must be balanced by low complication and revision rates. If healthcare spending increases due to surgical revisions, cost effectiveness will be lost.

2. **D.** While there are several factors and definition of cost-effectiveness, most studies are too variable to

estimate cost. One area of more solid research concerns the cost to insurance companies. The return on investment for insurance companies covering bariatric surgery occurs between 2 and 4 years after surgery.[6] Other studies have shown that it can take longer, between 5 and 10 years.[7] When calculating cost-effectiveness, one must take into account the cost of surgery, preoperative visits, medications, hospital stays, and other direct and indirect costs. These costs must be compared with healthcare utilization in nonsurgical patients. Often, this can require complex models looking at quality-adjusted life years and incremental cost-effectiveness ratios.[8]

3. **A.** Bariatric surgery can induce remission of diabetes in up to 90% of patients,[9] and it is a recommended as a cost-effective management for diabetes in the obese population.[10,11] Nonalcoholic steatohepatitis (NASH) can lead to cirrhosis and hepatocellular carcinoma, and weight loss can slow or stop the progression of this disease process. Bariatric surgery is a cost-effective management of obesity and NASH.[12] Like bariatric surgery in general, for adolescents it does not appear cost effective at 1 year; however, at five years it becomes cost effective. The TEEN LABS study shows improvement in quality-adjusted life years and in incremental cost-effectiveness ratios at 5 years postsurgery.[13]

4. **D.** To assess the cost-effectiveness of bariatric surgery, direct and indirect costs of obesity and surgery must be taken into consideration. Direct costs include inpatient and outpatient visits, procedure costs, testing, medication costs, and in general all medical-related costs, which includes equipment and supplies like IV fluids, catheters, and tubing. Indirect costs are related to short- or long-term disability, sickness absences, early mortality, and other forms of productivity loss. Indirect costs are often harder to quantify,[14] but also may add more significantly to the cost effectiveness of bariatric surgery.

REFERENCES

1. Froylich D, Abramovich-Segal T, Pascal G. et al. Long-term (over 10 years) retrospective follow-up of laparoscopic adjustable gastric banding. *OBES SURG*. 2018;28:976-980. https://doi.org/10.1007/s11695-017-2952-7. Accessed on March 1, 2021.
2. Wentworth JM, Cheng C, Laurie C., et al. Diabetes outcomes more than a decade following sustained weight loss after laparoscopic adjustable gastric band surgery. *OBES SURG*. 2018;28:982-989. https://doi.org/10.1007/s11695-017-2944-7. Accessed on March 1, 2021.
3. Ibrahim AM, Thumma JR, Dimick JB. Reoperation and Medicare expenditures after laparoscopic gastric band surgery. *JAMA Surg*. 2017;152(9):835-842. doi:10.1001/jamasurg.2017.1093.
4. Topart PA, Becouarn G. Revision and reversal after biliopancreatic diversion for excessive side effects or ineffective weight loss: a review of the current literature on indications and procedures. *Surg Obes Relat Dis*. 2015;11(4):965-972. doi:10.1016/j.soard.2015.01.015.
5. Li J, Lai D, Lin Z, Jiang T, Zhang A, Dai J. Comparison of the long-term results of Roux-en-Y gastric bypass and sleeve gastrectomy for morbid obesity. *Surg Laparosc, Endosc Percutan Techniques*. 2014;24(1):1-11. doi:10.1097/SLE.0000000000000041.
6. Crémieux PY, Buchwald H, Shikona SA, Ghosh A, Yang HE, Buessing M. A study on the economic impact of bariatric surgery. *Am J Manag Care*. 2008;14(9):589-596.
7. Finkelstein EA, Allaire BT, Globe D, Dixon JB. The business case for bariatric surgery revisited: a non-randomized case-control study. *PLOS ONE*. 2013;8(9):e75498.
8. Hoerger TJ. Economics and policy in bariatric surgery. *Curr DiabRep*.2019;19(29).https://doi.org/10.1007/s11892-019-1148-z. Accessed on March 1, 2021.
9. Affinati AH, Esfandiari NH, Oral EA, Kraftson AT. Bariatric surgery in the treatment of type 2 diabetes. *Curr Diab Rep*. 2019;19(12):156. doi:10.1007/s11892-019-1269-4. PMID: 31802258; PMCID: PMC7522929.
10. American Diabetes Association. Obesity Management for the Treatment of Type 2 Diabetes: *Standards of Medical Care in Diabetes—2020. Diabetes Care*. 2020;43(Suppl. 1):S89-S97. doi:10.2337/dc20-S008
11. Hoerger TJ, Zhang P, Segal JE, Kahn HS, Barker LE, Couper S. Cost-effectiveness of bariatric surgery for severely obese adults with diabetes. *Diabetes Care*. 2010;33(9):1933-1939.
12. Klebanoff MJ, Corey KE, Samur S, et al. Cost-effectiveness analysis of bariatric surgery for patients with nonalcoholic steatohepatitis cirrhosis. *JAMA Netw Open*. 2019;2(2):e190047. doi:10.1001/jamanetworkopen.2019.0047.
13. Klebanoff MJ, Chhatwal J, Nudel JD, Corey KE, Kaplan LM, Hur C. Cost-effectiveness of bariatric surgery in adolescents with obesity. *JAMA Surg*. 2017;152(2):136-141. doi:10.1001/jamasurg.2016.3640. PMID: 27784062.
14. Dee A, Kearns K, O'Neill C, et al. The direct and indirect costs of both overweight and obesity: a systematic review. *BMC Res Notes*. 2014;7(1):1-9.

7

Risks of Obesity

Limaris Barrios, MD

A 33-year-old African American male with a body mass index (BMI) of 45 kg/m^2 is being evaluated for weight loss surgery. His comorbidities include hypertension, obstructive sleep apnea, and diabetes mellitus. He admits to a sedentary lifestyle. He is married, with one child. He finished high school and is now taking night classes to earn a bachelor's degree. He is an atheist, although he was raised in a Presbyterian household. He grew up in a poor family, but he is sound financially and is projected to start earning $75,000 annually in a few years. He is scheduled at your weight loss surgery center for an initial evaluation.

1. **Which of the following puts him at the highest risk for obesity?**
   A. His race
   B. His socioeconomic status
   C. Level of education
   D. Marital status

2. **Which of these is the strongest contributing factor to this patient's increased risk of obesity?**
   A. Increased intake of all types of dietary fat
   B. Increased whole grain intake
   C. Getting 6–7 hours of sleep nightly
   D. Moderate daily alcohol intake

This patient is interested in bariatric surgery, and he is started in a bariatric surgery program. During his work-up, he is involved in a motor vehicle accident, suffering a traumatic brain injury and severe damage to his bilateral lower extremities. The neurologists expect him to recover fully from his head injury, but they note that he has sustained damage to his pituitary and hypothalamus. He undergoes several orthopedic surgeries to stabilize his lower-extremity fractures. He returns to you several months later during his rehabilitation. His cognitive function seems normal, and he requires a walker to ambulate, but he notes that he is getting stronger. You note that his BMI has increased to 49 kg/m^2 and his Hgb A1c is 7.8%. He would like to continue with bariatric surgery.

3. **When considering surgery for this patient, which of the following is true?**
   A. He is no longer a candidate because of hyperphagia.
   B. Vagal stimulator therapy shows promising results.
   C. His pituitary injury may contribute to his worsening diabetes mellitus.
   D. Acquired hypothalamus dysfunction has better obesity outcomes than does congenital ones like Prader–Willi syndrome (PWS).

The patient develops an infection in his orthopedic repairs, which require several more procedures and eventually result in bilateral amputations below the knee. He again returns to your office with even more increased BMI and Hgb A1c readings.

4. **Which of the following is true regarding weight loss surgery with this patient?**
   A. Amputation increases the risk of developing metabolic syndrome.
   B. Only lower-extremity amputees are at increased risk of developing obesity.
   C. Amputation is an absolute contraindication to bariatric surgery.
   D. The development of obesity in amputees takes several years to acquire.

ANSWERS

1. **A.** All of the answers can contribute to the development of obesity, but race has the strongest influence. This is true even if gender, socioeconomic status, and education is taken into account.[1] Combined data for 2015 through 2017 found that non-Hispanic black adults had the highest prevalence of obesity (38.4%) overall, followed by Hispanic adults (32.6%) and non-Hispanic white adults (28.6%); and similar rates apply to women and children within these races (Table 7-1).[2] Asian races tended to have the lowest rates of obesity.

   Using the level of education to determine its effect on the incidence of obesity is less clear because education does not reflect socioeconomic status equally across races. However, it appears that obesity rates have increased much more across non-Hispanic blacks than other races at all socioeconomic levels.[1] Logistic regression analysis evaluated the role of income, marital status, and obesity among black and white males and found that married, middle-income black males had the highest rates of obesity, while never-married, low-income while males had the lowest rates.[3]

   In addition, it has been well established that black Americans who are obese have a higher mortality rate than their counterparts. Therefore, this needs to be included in the discussion of the risks versus the benefits of surgery with the patient.[4] As shown in Table 7-2, stroke mortality rates for black individuals in 1997 were in the order of 81.6 as compared to 60.3 for non-Hispanic white individuals.

2. **C.** Several factors contribute to the development of obesity. While there are several factors that negatively affect the development of obesity, like genetics, environment, and culture, that are beyond the patient's control, there are several others that can be controlled. Those include activity, diet, and sleep patterns.

   Over a 10-year period, people who engaged in less than 30 minutes of daily activity had a higher risk of gaining weight; but those who performed 11–20 minutes per day had less weight gain than those who did none.[5] The subsequent weight gain associated with a sedentary lifestyle contributes to decreased muscle strength and cardiovascular fitness and may eventually result in difficulties with physical functions such as walking several blocks or climbing a flight of stairs.[6,7]

   Nutrition also plays an important role, but it can be confusing. For instance, not all dietary fat contributes to weight gain. Increased intake of monounsaturated or polyunsaturated fats is not associated with weight gain, but intake of animal, saturated, and trans fats is.[8] Increased carbohydrate intake seems to cause weight gain, but intake of whole grain or dietary fiber has a much lower risk of causing obesity than intake of refined grains.[9] Alcohol has also been implicated in weight gain, but more likely it is

Table 7-2 CORONARY HEART DISEASE (CHD) AND STROKE MORTALITY RATES BY RACE AND ETHNICITY IN THE UNITED STATES IN 1997

	CHD	Stroke
Non-Hispanic white	182.8	60.3
Black	186.8	81.6
Native American	112.7	39.2
Asian	100.1	54.6
Hispanic	124.2	40.0

Data are expressed as mortality per 100,000.
Data from Bell CN, Thorpe RJ Jr. Income and marital status interact on obesity among black and white men. *Am J Mens Health.* 2019;13(1):1557988319829952.

Table 7-1 PREVALENCE OF OBESITY AMONG VARIOUS GROUPS

	Women (%)	Adolescent Girls (%)[1]	Girls (%)[1]	Men (%)	Adolescent Boys (%)[1]	Boys (%)[1]
Non-Hispanic white	30.1	12.4	11.6	27.3	12.8	12.0
African American	49.7	26.2	22.2	28.1	20.7	17.1
Mexican American	39.7	19.4	19.6	28.9	27.5	27.3

[1]From NHANES 1999–2000 data.
Data from Bell CN, Thorpe RJ Jr. Income and marital status interact on obesity among black and white men. *Am J Mens Health.* 2019;13(1):1557988319829952.

the sugary liquids that are added to alcoholic drinks. Light alcohol consumption is estimated at 30 g/day, and light drinkers are found to be less likely to gain weight than nondrinkers or heavy drinkers.[10]

Lack of adequate sleep is also a risk factor for the development of obesity. Over 16 years, women who slept less than 5 hours nightly and those who slept 6–7 hours/night were 32% and 12% more likely to gain 15 kg, respectively, than those who slept more than 7 hours.[11] Of the risk factors, his biggest one for the development of obesity is his lack of adequate sleep.

3. **B.** Dysfunction of the hypothalamus can result in severe obesity due to alterations in the hunger and satisfaction pathways. Congenital disorders like PWS are hallmarked by hyperphagia, resulting in morbid obesity. Traumatic injuries to the hypothalamus more typically occur after surgery for craniopharyngiomas, but they also can occur after traumatic head injuries.[12] In both acquired and congenital hypothalamic dysfunction, there is malaise, reduced energy expenditure, and increased insulin secretion, leading to adipogenesis.[12]

Injuries to the pituitary gland can also have effects on metabolic disorders. Adrenocorticotropic hormone (ACTH) levels are often decreased after injury to the anterior pituitary gland, and while this effect is mostly transient, it can persist for longer than 12 months after the accident.[13] Decreased ACTH would most likely lead to low cortisol levels, which would suggest that blood glucose levels would also be lower. As such, his Hgb A1c levels would be expected to be under better control. However, if one factors in his increase in BMI, which may make his glucose more difficult to control, it is not clear if his type 2 diabetes would worsen. On the other hand, he may develop diabetes insipidus due to an injury of his posterior pituitary gland.[12]

The rate of developing obesity from hypothalamic dysfunction is very high, at 96.5% in one registry.[14] Regardless of the cause of the hypothalamic dysfunction, the development of obesity is similarly high, as is the risk for early cardiovascular disease (CVD) and mortality.[15] Surgery is the most effective means for treating this type of obesity, and methods that have been described for the sleeve gastrectomy (SG), Roux-en-Y gastric bypass (RYGB), adjustable gastric band (AGB), and the vagal stimulator. Long-term outcomes from these procedures are not known, but surgery is much more effective than medications and lifestyle modification.[13] Despite the hyperphagia that may occur in hypothalamic disorders, surgery should still be considered.

4. **A.** Amputees represent a unique and at-risk population for the development of obesity and obesity-related diseases. Bilateral lower-limb amputees have approximately 2.4 times greater increase in general mortality and a 4 times greater increase in cardiovascular mortality.[16] Moreover, a cross-sectional study after the Iran-Iraq war shows that 62% of lower-leg amputees developed metabolic syndrome.[17] A retrospective review of 978 patients who sustained combat-related amputees showed that their BMIs increased from 25.6 to 31.4 kg/m^2 within 8 years of the injury, and most of the patients who developed obesity did so within 16 months of the injury.[18] These patients were also more likely to develop type 2 diabetes, hypertension, and hyperlipidemia.[17] Finally, the development of these diseases occurred even in patients with only upper-extremity amputations.[17]

The exact reasons for this are unknown, but they could be related to metabolic changes, limited physical activity, or perhaps an undiagnosed hypothalamus injury. Weight loss surgery has been described in this population, but only in a single care report, so the data are weak.[15] However, no other therapy has been successfully described.

In summary, race, behavior, functional status, congenital disorders, and amputation status are all factors in the development of obesity, and these factors should all be taken into account when evaluating a patient as a suitable candidate for weight loss surgery.

REFERENCES

1. Wang Y, Beydoun M. The obesity epidemic in the United States—gender, age, socioeconomic, racial/ethnic, and geographic characteristics: a systematic review and meta-regression analysis. *Epid Reviews*. 2007;29:6-28.
2. Petersen R, Pan L, Blanck HM. Racial and ethnic disparities in adult obesity in the United States: CDC's tracking to inform state and local action. *Prev Chronic Dis.* 2019;16:E46.
3. Bell CN, Thorpe RJ. Income and marital status interact on obesity among black and white men. *Am J Mens Health.* 2019;13(1):1-9.
4. Cossrow N, Falkner B. Race/ethnic issues in obesity and obesity-related comorbidities. *J Clinical Endo Metab.* 2004;89(6):2590-2594.
5. Mekary RA, Feskanic D, Malspeis S, Hu FB, Willett WC, Field AE. Physical activity patterns and prevention

of weight gain in premenopausal women. *Int J Obes.* 2009;33(9):1039-1047.

6. Jenkins KR. Obesity's effects on the onset of functional impairment among older adults. *The Gerontologist.* 2004;44(2):206-216.
7. Himes CL. Obesity, disease, and functional limitation in later life. *Demography.* 2000;37:73-82. https://doi.org/10.2307/2648097.
8. Field AE, Willett WC, Lissner L, Colditz GA. Dietary fat and weight gain among women in the Nurses' Health Study. *Obesity.* 2007;15(4):967-976.
9. Liu S, Willett WC, Manson JE, Hu FB, Rosner B, Colditz G. Relation between changes in intakes of dietary fiber and grain products and changes in weight and development of obesity among middle-aged women. *Am J Clin Nutr.* 2003;78(5):920-927.
10. Wannamethee SG, Field AE, Colditz GA, Rimm EB. Alcohol intake and 8-year weight gain in women: a prospective study. *Obes Res.* 2004;12(9):1386-1396.
11. Patel SR, Hu FB. Short sleep duration and weight gain: a systematic review. *Obesity.* 2008;16(3):643-653.
12. Lustig RH. Hypothalamic obesity after craniopharyngioma: mechanisms, diagnosis, and treatment. *Front Endocrinol.* 2011;2(60).
13. Tan CL, Alavi SA, Baldeweg SE, et al. The screening and management of pituitary dysfunction following traumatic brain injury in adults: British neurotrauma group guidance. *J Neurol Neurosurg Psych.* 2017;88(11):971-981.
14. Rose SR, Honre VE, Bingham N, et al. Hypothalamic obesity: 4 years of the International Registry of Hypothalamic Obesity Disorders. *Obesity.* 2018;26(11):1727-1732.
15. Deepak D, Furlong NJ, Wilding JP, MacFarlane IA. Cardiovascular disease, hypertension, dyslipidaemia and obesity in patients with hypothalamic-pituitary disease. *Postgrad Med J.* 2007;83(978):277–280.
16. Zafar A, Rajeswaran C, Jameel JKA. Laparoscopic sleeve gastrectomy in a bilateral lower limb amputee: why is it worth doing? *SOARD.* 2014;10:e11-e12.
17. Ejtahed HS, Soroush MR, Hasani-Ranjbar S, et al. Prevalence of metabolic syndrome and health-related quality of life in war-related bilateral lower limb amputees. *J Diabetes Metab Disord.* 2017;16(17).
18. Tavares KB, Russell DM, Conrad RJ, et al. Time to weigh in on obesity and associated comorbidities in combat-wounded amputees. *J Trauma Acute Care Surg.* 2021;90(2):325-330.

8

Insurance Requirements

Stephanie Therrien, BSc, and Juliana Simonetti, MD

INSURANCE

1. **A 56-year-old female presents for a weight-loss surgery consult. The patient notes that she has struggled with her weight most of her life and has tried several diets, with only short-term success prior to regaining most of her weight. Most recently, she has lost 20 kg over the last 1.5 years so that she could have a total replacement of her left knee. She notes that her weight loss has plateaued and she is unable to lose additional weight. She decided to go forward with bariatric surgery. Her current body mass index (BMI) is 36 kg/m^2, and she has a history of gestational diabetes. She also complains of increased fatigue. Her physical exam is unremarkable, except for mild edema of her right knee, acanthosis nigricans on her neck, and a waist circumference of 112 cm.**

   Will this patient's private insurance cover bariatric surgery, given her current history? If no, what other tests could you order to gather evidence that would strengthen the argument for surgery?

   A. Yes, the patient's insurance will cover this surgery; comorbidities are not required for a BMI over 35.
   B. Yes, the patient's insurance will cover this surgery because she has the required number of comorbidities.
   C. No, the patient's insurance will not cover this surgery, and there are no other tests you can order to appeal this decision.
   D. No, the patient's insurance will not cover this surgery without a minimum of two comorbidities. You would order a fasting glucose/hemoglobin A1c to determine if she has diabetes and a sleep study to determine if she has obstructive sleep apnea.

2. **A 29-year-old female with a history of Roux-en-Y gastric bypass (RYGB) at an out-of-state facility presents for evaluation for weight regain. The patient is now 8 years postsurgery. She had an initial weight loss of 43 kg but has since gained back 34 kg. She tells you that she is exercising regularly but finds herself hungry and often has cravings for carbohydrates. She notes that she can only eat a maximum of 1 cup of food at one sitting. The patient has no other significant medical history. She is interested in exploring a "band over bypass." This patient reports that she is unable to pay out of pocket for surgery and will be relying on her insurance.**

   How should you proceed with this patient?

   A. Offer her the surgery; she meets the requirements.
   B. Inform her that before you can offer her the surgery, you will have to submit a prior authorization to her insurance to ensure that the procedure is covered.
   C. Do not offer the patient surgery; she is asking for a procedure that is not covered by any kind of insurance.
   D. Prior to offering any kind of revision or conversion surgical intervention, this patient should be redirected to focus on her diet, exercise, and behavior, given her history.

ANSWERS

1. **D.** Most insurers require candidates for bariatric surgery to have either a BMI of 40 or greater (severe obesity) or a BMI of 35 with an obesity-related comorbid conditions. These comorbidities can include, but are not limited to, diabetes, hypertension, fatty liver, sleep apnea, or cardiovascular disease.

   This patient is at increased risk for diabetes given her past medical history of gestational diabetes. The probability of developing type 2 diabetes after gestational diabetes is 3.7% at 9 months after delivery and 18.9% at 9 years after delivery.[2] In addition, this patient has acanthosis nigricans on her neck, which is a symptom associated with insulin resistance. A large waist circumference (for men: >102 cm and women: >88 cm) is also associated with an increased risk for type 2 diabetes, dyslipidemia, hypertension, and cardiovascular disease (CVD) in patients with a BMI in a range between 25 and 34.9 kg/m^2. As such, ordering an Hgb A1c test will confirm the diagnosis of type 2 diabetes mellitus. Monitoring changes in waist circumference over time may be helpful in addition to measuring BMI, since it can provide an estimate of increased abdominal fat, even in the absence of a change in BMI. Furthermore, in obese patients with metabolic complications, changes in waist circumference are useful predictors of changes in CVD risk factors.[3] Her left knee disease may be due to osteoarthritis, and this would help the patient to obtain bariatric surgery, however, it is not clear from this description that this is why she requires a knee replacement.

2. **D.** Given this patient's history of weight regain and lack of recent behavioral or dietary interventions, the patient is unlikely to have this procedure approved. Even though she has restrictions, her nutrition and exercise plan is likely poor, leading to the weight gain. She may have an anatomical reason for her weight gain, and it should be investigated with an esophagogastroduodenoscopy (EGD) and a barium swallow study or a computed tomography (CT) scan of her abdomen with oral contrast to rule out an enlarged pouch (>8 cm), a wide anastomosis (>20 mm), and a gastogastric fistula, which would allow food to enter the normal enteric pathway, leading to more absorption. Even if these are present, most insurance companies would not approve a revision without evidence of behavior modification. The only procedures known to be routinely covered by insurance are RYGB and sleeve gastrectomy (SL).

   As in all chronic, progressive diseases, some people with obesity are refractory to intervention, even surgery. Options for treatment of weight regain following bariatric surgery include repair conversion into another operation, endoscopic therapies, reintroduction of lifestyle-management counseling, and pharmacological treatments.[1,5] It is well established that revision and conversion surgeries have higher complication rates than primary operations.[3,6,7] Thus, pharmacological approaches may provide a safer and also effective strategy to treat weight regain after bariatric surgery. Despite the lack of a unified protocol for medical treatment of weight regain after bariatric surgery, there is evidence based on the statistical models to show that phentermine and topiramate, used individually or in combination, can significantly reduce weight regain after RYGB.[4,8]

REFERENCES

1. Obesity Action Coalition. *Reviewing your insurance policy or employer sponsored medical benefits plan*. (2020). Retrieved June 15, 2020, from https://www.obesityaction.org/action-through-advocacy/access-to-care/access-to-care-resources/reviewing-your-insurance-policy-or-employer-sponsored-medical-benefits-plan/.
2. Feig DS, Zinman B, Wang X, Hux JE. Risk of development of diabetes mellitus after diagnosis of gestational diabetes. *CMAJ*. 2008;179(3):229-234. https://doi.org/10.1503/cmaj.080012.
3. National Heart, Lung, and Blood Institute. *The practical guide: identification, evaluation, and treatment of overweight and obesity in adults*. October 2000. https://www.nhlbi.nih.gov/health-pro/guidelines/current/obesity-guidelines/e_textbook/txgd/4142.htm.
4. American Society for Metabolic and Bariatric Surgery. *Bariatric surgery procedures*. Retrieved June 15, 2020, from https://asmbs.org/patients/bariatric-surgery-procedures.
5. Billy HT. (2012). "Band over Bypass". Retrieved June 15, 2020, from https://www.obesityaction.org/community/article-library/band-over-bypass/
6. Brethauer SA, Kothari S, Sudan R, et al. Systemic review on reoperative bariatric surgery: American Society for Metabolic and Bariatric Surgery Revision Task Force. *Surg Obes Relat Dis*. 2014;10:952-972.
7. Cohen RV, Cummings DE. Weight regain after bariatric/metabolic surgery: a wake-up call. *Obesity*. 2020;28:1004-1004. doi:10.1002/oby.22822.
8. Istfan NW, Anderson WA, Hess DT, Yu L, Carmine B, Apovian CM. The mitigating effect of phentermine and topiramate on weight regain after Roux-en-Y gastric bypass surgery. *Obesity*. 2020;28:1023-1030.

SECTION 2

Medical Treatment

9

Lifestyle: Nutrition, Exercise, and Sleep

Alex Myers, MD, and Eric Ahnfeldt, DO

A 33-year-old male with a body mass index (BMI) of 48 kg/m^2, obstructive sleep apnea (OSA), hypertension, type 2 diabetes mellitus, degenerative disk disease, and rheumatoid arthritis has completed the preoperative pathway for bariatric surgery and is still deciding on which procedure he would like. He inquires about what steps he should take prior to surgery to reduce the chance of any complications.

1. Which of the following is correct about optimal preoperative management for reduction of complication rates?

A. Patients who are exercise-naive preoperatively should not begin an exercise regimen until after their bariatric surgery.
B. Patients should perform light aerobic exercise for 20–30 minutes 3–4 times weekly prior to bariatric surgery.
C. Patients with a history of sleep apnea should not use their continuous positive airway pressure (CPAP) machine for at least a week prior to bariatric surgery.
D. Patients should continue to eat their regular diet up to the day prior to their bariatric surgery.

2. The same patient inquires about what he should be doing about his sleep apnea following his Roux-en-Y gastric bypass (RYGB). Which of the following is correct regarding postoperative care of OSA?

A. Most bariatric patients with OSA may be monitored with intermittent pulse oximetry, with continuous pulse oximetry reserved for high-risk individuals.
B. Bariatric surgery typically does not affect OSA long-term outcomes; thus, postbariatric patients should expect to continue using their CPAP machines indefinitely.
C. Hospital CPAP machines are superior to patients' home CPAP machines, so they should be used in the postoperative setting for bariatric patients with OSA.
D. High-risk bariatric patients with OSA have worse pulmonary and overall outcomes when not monitored in an intensive care unit (ICU) setting post-operatively.

3. This patient is strongly considering the laparoscopic sleeve gastrectomy (LSG) but is worried about the postoperative diet. Which of the following statements would be accurate to include in your counseling regarding diet after an LSG?

A. Patients are able to get all of their vitamin/mineral supplementation from diet alone.
B. Protein intake should be increased in a bariatric diet, either through dietary protein or protein supplementation.
C. Patients should expect to be able to eat a small-portion regular diet in the first week following surgery.
D. Dumping syndrome is a common complication after LSG.

4. The patient also asks about his medication usage in the perioperative period. Which of the following medication regimens should he stop in the immediate postoperative period?

A. Blood pressure medication, if he is a complex hypertensive patient on multiple medications
B. Metformin, if his type 2 diabetes was previously uncontrolled
C. Chronic celecoxib use, if he has lumbar degenerative disk disease
D. Chronic steroids, if he has rheumatoid arthritis

ANSWERS

1. B. The American Society for Metabolic and Bariatric Surgery (ASMBS) released a set of recommendations in 2007 that encourage patients to engage in light aerobic exercise for 20–30 minutes 3–4 times weekly in the preoperative period, both for weight loss and for aid in transitioning to an increased postoperative exercise regimen.[1] This recommendation is made for all bariatric preoperative patients, even the exercise-naive. The ASMBS also has made a number of recommendations for postoperative exercise regimens and promotes regimens put forth by other organizations such as the Centers for Disease Control and Prevention (CDC) and American Heart Association (AHA).[2]

For patients with a history of sleep apnea, it is recommended that they continue to use their CPAP machine up to the date of surgery. The recommended bariatric surgery preoperative diet varies by center and by surgeon, but it is widely recommended that patients lower their caloric intake prior to surgery and increase dietary protein. As with physical activity, this acts as a helpful transition to a successful bariatric postoperative diet.

2. A. Extensive research has been conducted on the relationship between OSA, obesity, and bariatric surgery. In 2012, the ASMBS put forth a series of evidence-based guidelines for the perioperative management of OSA. These guidelines suggest that continuous pulse oximetry monitoring is the best method of monitoring patients with OSA, but that intermittent pulse oximetry is generally regarded as safe.[3]

Despite continuous pulse oximetry being favored for postoperative bariatric surgery patients with OSA, pulmonary and overall outcomes are no different for postoperative patients monitored in a floor setting versus in an ICU.[3] OSA is commonly associated with obesity, meaning that patients who meet their weight loss goals may see improvement in their sleep apnea postoperatively. Patients are recommended to continue using their home CPAP postoperatively but may discuss titrating down their settings or even discontinuing their CPAP altogether. Patients are generally recommended to use their home CPAP in the hospital following surgery, or at least to relay their home settings to hospital staff. Hospital CPAP machines are equivalent to home CPAP machines in that regard.

3. B. After any bariatric surgery, hydration and increased protein supplementation are two of the biggest dietary concerns.[1] Protein intake can be strictly via the diet, but patients commonly use some sort of supplementation, such as protein shakes or protein powders.

Vitamin and mineral supplementation is a key part of a successful postoperative course, as well. This includes calcium, iron, vitamin B12, vitamin C, and vitamin D, as well as a host of micronutrients and trace minerals.[1] Multivitamins and prenatal vitamins typically meet most of these needs, depending on the formulation, but some, especially vitamin B12, usually require additional supplementation. While bariatric postoperative diet advancement does vary somewhat from surgeon to surgeon, patients typically consume a liquid diet for at least a week following surgery. While dumping syndrome from increased carbohydrate load following bariatric surgery is a real concern, this patient is having an LSG and therefore is at much lower risk of this occurring. Dumping syndrome is a native risk to the RYGB due to the bypassing of the pylorus of the stomach, causing significant insulin response after consumption of a high-carbohydrate meal going straight to the small intestine. The LSG maintains normal digestive anatomy, and thus dumping syndrome is unlikely.

4. C. Bariatric surgery offers the possibility of reducing, or even eliminating, the need for certain medications in various chronic health conditions. Nonsteroidal anti-inflammatory drugs (NSAIDs) in particular should be eliminated in the immediate postoperative period following bariatric surgery. They carry a significant risk of marginal ulcer formation, which, besides pain, carries a risk of leak, stricture, and other complications.[4] Other medications such as diuretics are typically discontinued immediately postoperatively on a case-by-case basis.

For chronic health conditions such as hypertension and diabetes, it is generally advisable that patients discuss these conditions and associated medications with their primary care providers postoperatively. Initial postoperative reductions in blood pressure and blood sugar are usually not substantial enough to warrant immediate discontinuation of antihypertensives or diabetes medications, although this may be decided on a patient-to-patient basis. Steroids carry significant perioperative risks, including marginal ulcer, poor anastomosis healing, and poor wound healing; however, chronic steroids may require a tapering off for a high-enough dosage, and thus may be continued perioperatively.

REFERENCES

1. American Society of Bariatric Surgery Public/Professional Education Committee. *Bariatric Surgery: Postoperative Concerns*. 2007.
2. King W, Bond D. The importance of pre and postoperative physical activity counseling in bariatric surgery. *Exerc Sport Sci Rev*. 2013;41(1):26-35.
3. American Society of Metabolic and Bariatric Surgeons Clinical Issues Committee. Peri-operative management of obstructive sleep apnea. *SOARD*. 2012;8:e27-e32.
4. Mechanick J, Apovian C, Brethauer S, et al. Clinical practice guidelines for the perioperative nutritional, metabolic and nonsurgical support of the bariatric surgery patient. *SOARD*. 2013;9:159-191.

10

Pharmacology: Types, Efficacy, Long-Term Outcomes, and Postoperative Assistance

Jesse Richards, DO, ABOM

A 33-year-old female is referred by her primary care physician to the bariatric surgery clinic for obesity and a 23-kg weight gain over the past 5 years. She has a past medical history of hypertension, gastroesophageal reflux disease (GERD), diabetes mellitus, anxiety, hyperlipidemia diabetic neuropathy with albuminuria, polycystic ovary syndrome, and asthma. Her current medications include once-daily combined ethinyl estradiol and norgestimate, metformin 100 mg b.i.d., insulin glargine 20 units q.h.s., atorvastatin 20 mg, fluoxetine 20 mg, glipizide 5 mg b.i.d., gabapentin 300 mg t.i.d., and losartan 25 mg.

The patient reports 300 minutes of exercise weekly by swimming and biking and "tries to eat well," but eats large meals and fast food regularly. She has tracked her food before and was previously eating 2,000 calories daily.

The patient's height is 163 cm and her weight is 105 kg, giving her a body mass index (BMI) of 39.5 kg/m^2. Her abdominal circumference is 102 cm. On examination, the patient has a normal cardiopulmonary exam, excess abdominal adiposity, and no abdominal tenderness. She also has decreased sensation to fine touch in bilateral feet to ankles.

The patient's A1c is 6.9%, creatinine 0.9, electrolytes normal. Other test results include aspartate aminotransferase (AST) 43, alanine transaminase (ALT) 58, high-density lipoprotein (HDL) 49, low-density lipoprotein (LDL) 133, and hemoglobin 12.0.

1. The patient isn't sure about bariatric surgery and wants to try the "strongest" medication to lose weight. Which of these medications will likely cause the largest decrease in weight?

A. Orlistat
B. Liraglutide
C. Phentermine/topiramate
D. Naltrexone/bupropion

2. She presents for follow-up 3 months after pharmacotherapy initiation. She has lost 9 kg and several days ago developed right flank pain and urinary frequency, for which she was seen in the emergency room (ER). A computed tomography (CT) scan demonstrated multiple renal stones. Which of the following is most likely to have caused her condition?

A. Phentermine/topiramate
B. Orlistat
C. Liraglutide
D. Naltrexone/bupropion

3. A patient presents for assessment and discouraged that her A1C had recently increased to 8.9. In addition, she had chest pain and was recently diagnosed with coronary artery disease (CAD) on a stress test, although she did not require stenting at the time. Which of the following is the best option for a weight loss medication at this time?

A. Liraglutide
B. Phentermine/topiramate
C. Orlistat
D. Naltrexone/bupropion

4. The next year, the patient undergoes a Roux-en-Y gastric bypass (RYGB), with remission of diabetes and a weight loss of 36 kg. She is compliant with all postoperative management and takes vitamins

appropriately. Then, 5 years later, she has regained 14 kg and comes to the clinic to discuss initiation of pharmacotherapy to help treat weight regain. What obesity medication is now contraindicated after her bypass?

A. Liraglutide
B. Phentermine/topiramate
C. Naltrexone/bupropion
D. Orlistat

5. **Stefanie brings her daughter, who is 16 years old and has a BMI of 35, nonalcoholic fatty liver disease (NAFLD), and hypertension, to the clinic. What medication is approved in pediatric patients?**

A. Phentermine
B. Liraglutide
C. Phentermine/topiramate
D. Naltrexone/bupropion

ANSWERS

1. **C.** Of the medications for obesity treatment currently approved by the Food and Drug Administration (FDA), phentermine/topiramate has been shown to have the highest average weight loss in clinical trials, with an average of 10.9% total body weight loss at 52 weeks,[1] compared to 6.1% with naltrexone/buproprion,[2] and 8.0% with liraglutide 3.0 mg.[3] Orlistat was found to produce 5.2% weight loss at 206 weeks.[4] The strongest current medication for weight loss is semaglutide 2.4 mg, with an average weight loss of 14.9% at 68 weeks;[5] but this is currently awaiting FDA approval.

   Phentermine assists in weight loss by decreasing hunger. Topiramate is an anticonvulsant medication that also decreases appetite and causes feelings of satiety. Naltrexone/buproprion, also known as Contrave, contains naltrexone, which is an opioid antagonist, and buproprion, which is an antidepressant. Together, they are an effective weight loss medication, but the mechanism of action is poorly understood. It is felt that it helps promote satiety.

2. **B.** Orlistat, also known as Alli and Xenical, can facilitate weight loss by preventing the absorption of dietary fat. Orlistat is known to cause oxalate nephropathy and renal stones as a potential side effect of increased intraluminal fatty acids, similar to inflammatory bowel disease and chronic pancreatitis[6] or secondary to gastric bypass.[7] Drug-induced kidney stones can be caused by topiramate[8] and are a contraindication to phentermine/topiramate usage. Phentermine, liraglutide, and naltrexone/bupropion are not associated with renal stones.

3. **A.** In the liraglutide and cardiovascular outcomes in diabetes trial (LEADER) trial, liraglutide, also known as Saxenda, was shown to decrease risk of major adverse cardiac events (cardiac death, nonfatal myocardial infarction, or nonfatal stroke) in patients with type 2 diabetes and increased risk of CAD.[9] It is specifically approved with a cardiovascular benefit in patients with diabetes. CAD is a contraindication to phentermine, as well as arrhythmias, hyperthyroidism, and glaucoma.[10]

   Liraglutide was originally prescribed to assist with glucose control as a glucagon-like peptide-1 (GLP-1) agonist in patients with type 2 diabetes mellitus. It also promotes hunger control as an appetite suppressant.

4. **D.** Orlistat is contraindicated after malabsorptive procedures such as RYGB due to increased risk of vitamin deficiency.[11] Liraglutide is contraindicated with a personal or family history of medullary thyroid cancer, MEN-2 syndrome, or pancreatitis. Phentermine/topiramate is contraindicated with CAD, glaucoma, or renal stones. Naltrexone/bupropion is contraindicated with a history of epilepsy and carries a black box warning for suicidal ideation. *All* antiobesity pharmacotherapy is contraindicated during pregnancy and breastfeeding.

   Ultimately, weight loss medications have a modest effect on weight loss, and patients are at risk for weight regain after the medications are stopped. However, they are a reasonable choice for patients who do not want surgery, may be too high risk for surgery, are overweight or have class I obesity, and finally, have undergone successful bariatric surgery but experience weight regain after several years.

5. **B.** The FDA approved liraglutide 3.0 mg (brand name Saxenda) for pediatric use in December 2020 based on a randomized controlled trial that showed weight loss efficacy of over 5%.[12] Orlistat was previously the only FDA-approved medication for pediatric obesity with patients 12 and up.[13]

REFERENCES

1. Allison DB, Gadde KM, Garvey WT, et al. Controlled-release phentermine/topiramate in severely obese adults: a randomized controlled trial (EQUIP). *Obesity (Silver Spring)*. 2012;20(2):330-342. doi:10.1038/oby.2011.330.
2. Apovian CM, Aronne L, Rubino D, et al. A randomized, phase 3 trial of naltrexone SR/bupropion SR on weight and obesity-related risk factors (COR-II). *Obesity (Silver Spring)*. 2013;21(5):935-943. doi:10.1002/oby.20309. PMID: 23408728; PMCID: PMC3739931.
3. Pi-Sunyer X, Astrup A, Fujioka K, et al. A randomized, controlled trial of 3.0 mg of liraglutide in weight management. *N Engl J Med*. 2015;373(1):11-22. doi:10.1056/NEJMoa1411892. PMID: 26132939.
4. Torgerson JS, Hauptman J, Boldrin MN, Sjöström L. XENical in the prevention of diabetes in obese subjects (XENDOS) study: a randomized study of orlistat as an adjunct to lifestyle changes for the prevention of type 2 diabetes in obese patients. *Diabetes Care*. 2004;27(1):155-161. doi:10.2337/diacare.27.1.155. Erratum in: Diabetes Care. 2004 Mar;27(3):856. PMID: 14693982.
5. Wilding JPH, Batterham RL, Calanna S, et al. Once-weekly semaglutide in adults with overweight or obesity. *N Engl J Med*. 2021. doi:10.1056/NEJMoa2032183. PMID: 33567185.
6. Buysschaert B, Aydin S, Morelle J, Hermans MP, Jadoul M, Demoulin N. Weight loss at a high cost: orlistat-induced late-onset severe kidney disease. *Diabetes Metab*. 2016;42(1):62-64. doi:10.1016/j.diabet.2015.08.006. Epub 2015 Oct 9. PMID: 26454353.
7. Nasr SH, D'Agati VD, Said SM, et al. Oxalate nephropathy complicating Roux-en-Y gastric bypass: an underrecognized cause of irreversible renal failure. *Clin J Am Soc Nephrol*. 2008;3(6):1676-1683. doi:10.2215/CJN.02940608. Epub 2008 Aug 13. PMID: 18701613; PMCID: PMC2572276.
8. Daudon M, Frochot V, Bazin D, Jungers P. Drug-induced kidney stones and crystalline nephropathy: pathophysiology, prevention and treatment. *Drugs*. 2018;78(2):163-201. doi:10.1007/s40265-017-0853-7. PMID: 29264783.
9. Marso SP, Daniels GH, Brown-Frandsen K, et al. Liraglutide and cardiovascular outcomes in type 2 diabetes. *N Engl J Med*. 2016;375(4):311-322. doi:10.1056/NEJMoa1603827. PMID: 27295427; PMCID: PMC4985288.
10. Federal Drug Administration. *Adipex-P prescribing Information Reference ID: 3115694* [Brochure]. Washington, DC: Author; 2012.
11. McDuffie JR, Calis KA, Booth SL, Uwaifo GI, Yanovski JA. Effects of orlistat on fat-soluble vitamins in obese adolescents. *Pharmacotherapy*. 2002;22(7):814-822. doi:10.1592/phco.22.11.814.33627. PMID: 12126214.
12. Kelly AS, Auerbach P, Barrientos-Perez M, et al. A randomized, controlled trial of liraglutide for adolescents with obesity. *N Engl J Med*. 2020;382(22):2117-2128.
13. Rogovik AL, Goldman RD. Pharmacologic treatment of pediatric obesity. *Can Fam Phys*. 2011;57(2):195-197.

11

Medication Complications

Rachel L. Moore, MD

Elaine is a 49-year-old female patient who presents to your weight management clinic for a follow-up on her progress with weight loss after you diagnosed her with night eating syndrome. She has a past medical history of type 2 diabetes mellitus, complicated with nonproliferative retinopathy, nephropathy, and peripheral neuropathy, hypertension, cirrhosis secondary to nonalcoholic fatty liver disease (NAFLD), iron-deficiency anemia, hyperlipidemia, mild depression, and osteoarthritis in bilateral knees. Medications include metformin 1,000 mg daily, amlodipine 5 mg daily, gabapentin 300 mg t.i.d., ferrous gluconate 325 mg t.i.d., phentermine/topiramate ER (Qysmia) 7.5–46 mg q.d., liraglutide (Saxenda) 1.8 mg, lorcaserin (Belviq) 10 mg b.i.d., rosuvastatin 40 mg q.h.s., and a monoamine oxidase inhibitor.

Her family history includes a father who passed away from a myocardial infarction at the age of 48 and a mother who has obesity, type 2 diabetes mellitus, and thyroid cancer treated with a thyroidectomy and chemotherapy.

On examination, the patient's height is 1.75 m, weight is 129 kg, body mass index (BMI) is 42 kg/m^2, and waist circumference is 109 cm. Her vital signs are blood pressure 115/81 mmHg and heart rate 78 bpm. Her physical exam is notable for acanthosis nigricans on her posterior neck and decreased pinprick sensation bilaterally distal to the ankles.

Lab results from 6 months ago and 3 days ago are reported here:

6 months ago	3 days ago
A1c 7.8 g/dL	A1c 9.1 g/dL ↑
Total cholesterol 261 mg/dL	Total cholesterol 228 mg/dL ↓
HDL 59 mg/dL	HDL 62 mg/dL ↑
LDL 159 mg/dL	LDL 138 mg/dL ↓
GFR 51 ml/min	GFR 47 ml/min ↓
Hb 11.0 g/dL	Hb 11.8 g/dL ↑
AST 32 u/L	AST 62 u/L ↑↑
ALT 34 u/L	ALT 78 u/L ↑↑

The remainder of her blood work is within normal limits. Electrocardiography shows sinus arrhythmia.

When you ask her for a 24-h diet and activity recall, she states that she walks to and from the parking lot to her office building 2 blocks away daily, as knee pain limits her activity. She consumes 1,500 calories a day, with a daily average intake of 200 g of carbohydrates. She states that she has had headaches, blurry vision, and recognized halos around light sources.

1. Which of the following medications is *most* likely responsible for her vision complaints?

A. Metformin
B. Phentermine/topiramate ER (Qsymia)
C. Gabapentin
D. Lorcaserin (Belviq)
E. Liraglutide (Saxenda)

2. The following month, the patient returns to your clinic complaining of 2 days of abdominal pain radiating to her back, associated with severe nausea and vomiting. She initially saw her hepatologist, who ruled out any liver pathology but found her lipase to be 337 U/L. On examination, her temperature is 39°C and she has epigastric tenderness without rebound.

Which of the following medications is *most* likely responsible for the acute symptoms that she is experiencing?

A. Metformin
B. Topiramate
C. Gabapentin
D. Liraglutide (Saxenda)
E. Lorcaserin (Belviq)

3. Elaine is now in the emergency room (ER) with nausea and vomiting. The intern on call places admission orders and stops all medications except metformin for glucose control. During morning rounds, the team notices the intravenous (IV) fluids have not been started and the labs have returned. Her morning labs are as follows:

Cr 1.6 ↑
GFR 29 ↓
Blood pH 6.91 ↓
HCO^3 14 ↓
CO^2 30 ↓
Glucose 110 ↑

The patient's physical exam is notable for dry, chapped lips and sallow skin. Which of the following is the *most* likely cause of the metabolic derangements in this patient?

A. Hyperglycemic, hyperosmolar nonketotic acidosis
B. Diabetic ketoacidosis
C. Lactic acidosis
D. Renal tubular acidosis

4. This patient now asks to be considered for another weight loss medication because of the previous side effects she experienced. Which would be contraindicated in this patient?

A. Metformin
B. Diethylpropion
C. Orlistat (Xenacal, Alli)
D. Bupropion/naltrexone (Contrave)

5. In trying to determine another weight loss medication for Elaine, you notice that she should not have started on liraglutide based on her medical history. Which of the following *most* likely contraindicates the use of liraglutide in her?

A. Her father's history of an early myocardial infarction
B. Her cirrhosis
C. Her mother's history of thyroid cancer
D. Her night eating syndrome

ANSWERS

1. **B.** Topiramate is often used alone or in combination with phentermine as an off-label medication for weight management. Side effects from Qsymia include increased heart rate, suicidal tendencies, metabolic acidosis, paresthesia, confusion, myopia, and angle-closure glaucoma.[1] The ocular side effect of glaucoma occurs from the topiramate element of Qsymia. Topiramate can cause ciliary body edema, displacing the iris forward to precipitate acute angle-closure glaucoma. Symptoms of angle-closure glaucoma are headaches, blurry vision, and halos around lights that can be exacerbated by dilation of the pupil. Dilation can occur when moving from light to dark rooms. On average, symptoms appear within 2 weeks of starting topiramate. Its prevalence is higher in females and those on selective serotonin reuptake inhibitors (SSRIs).

   Side effects attributed to topiramate include kidney stones, paresthesia, confusion, and myopia.[2] Topiramate can cause nephrolithiasis in some patients because it is a carbonic anhydrase inhibitor, which reduces urinary citrate excretion and increases urinary pH, leading to the formation of kidney stones. This risk is increased in patients with a history of Roux-en-Y gastric bypass (RYGB) or those who have diets high in red meat and poor water intake. Thus, topiramate is avoided in patients who are concomitantly taking medications that can cause metabolic acidosis. However, this patient was not. Generally, this can be avoided with adequate hydration to prevent formation of new stones.[2]

   Side effects attributed to phentermine include tachycardia, hypertension, insomnia, dry mouth, and headaches.[3] Phentermine is approved by the Food and Drug Administration (FDA) to be used on its own, while topiramate can be used in an off-label manner on its own.[2,3] Phentermine modulates hunger by inhibiting the reuptake of norepinephrine, dopamine, and serotonin. Possible side effects include tachycardia, uncontrolled hypertension, coronary artery disease, anxiety, and insomnia. If any of these symptoms emerge or become uncontrolled, phentermine should be stopped.

Metformin and lorcaserin do not cause ocular side effects. Gabapentin can rarely cause nystagmus and diplopia, but not angle closure glaucoma.[4]

2. **D.** The patient presents with symptoms consistent with a diagnosis of acute pancreatitis, a side effect of liraglutide with an incidence of 0.3%. Fatal, nonfatal hemorrhagic, and necrotizing pancreatitis have all been noted with the use of liraglutide. Once pancreatitis is suspected, liraglutide should be discontinued immediately and once confirmed, patients should not be restarted on liraglutide. Patients need a baseline lipase and amylase prior to initiating liraglutide. A previous history of pancreatitis is not an absolute contraindication to initiating liraglutide; however, physicians are recommended to use their clinical judgment.[5,6]

   While metformin is known for gastrointestinal side effects, such as diarrhea, abdominal pain, abdominal distention, and heartburn, it is not known to cause pancreatitis.[7] Topiramate can cause dysgeusia, abdominal pain, and anorexia, but not pancreatitis.[2] Gabapentin can cause gastroenteritis, abdominal pain, and vomiting, but not pancreatitis.[4] Please note: At present, another glucagon-like peptide-1 (GLP-1) agonist, semaglutide, is on the horizon of entering the market for chronic weight management. It has a similar benefit and side effect profile as liraglutide.

3. **C.** Metformin can precipitate lactic acidosis in patients with renal impairment or in situations of dehydration, sepsis, liver disease, or alcohol use. Symptoms of lactic acidosis include muscle cramping, shallow, fast breathing, and sleepiness. There has been no association between metformin and the incidence of hyperglycemic, hyperosmolar nonketotic acidosis, diabetic ketoacidosis, or renal tubular acidosis.[7]

4. **D.** The concurrent use of bupropion/naltrexone SR (Contrave) and monoamine oxidase inhibitors (MAOIs) can cause a hypertensive crisis. A hypertensive crisis is a severe increase in blood pressure to equal or greater than 180/120 mmHg, with symptoms such as headache, blurry vision, dizziness, and malaise. If end organ damage becomes apparent, then it has become a hypertensive emergency. Bupropion/naltrexone should not be used within 14 days of MAOI use.[8] Metformin and orlistat do not have any interactions with MAOIs.[5–7,9] As of February 2020, orlistat has been withdrawn from the market due to its reported increase in cancer development; however, prior to that, it was not contraindicated for use with MAOIs. Diethylpropion is an appetite suppressant that is also FDA-approved for short-term use; however, its efficacy is debated, and there are no trials demonstrating long-term superiority over placebo. It is not contraindicated in this patient, but one probably should not use it and phentermine/topiramate together.

5. **C.** Liraglutide is currently used to treat type 2 diabetes mellitus at the 1.8 mg dose and obesity at the 3.0 mg dose, and it has the same adverse effects at both doses. It has demonstrated a dose- and duration-dependent development of medullary thyroid carcinoma in test animals. It is unknown in humans if there is a causal relationship, but the current contraindication to both doses of liraglutide is a family history of multiple endocrine neoplasia type 2 (MEN2) neoplasia or medullary thyroid carcinoma. Prescreening methods such as a thyroid ultrasound or serum calcitonin levels hold little value, and thus are not recommended. Patients should be counseled about the possible risk of developing medullary thyroid cancer and to monitor symptoms such as dysphagia, new or enlarging neck mass, or hoarseness of the voice. There has been no association with liraglutide with other types of thyroid cancer, such as papillary, anaplastic, or follicular thyroid cancer.[5,6]

   Her cirrhosis and her father's myocardial infarction and death at a young age do not preclude her from using liraglutide. Night eating syndrome is defined as consuming >25% of one's total daily caloric intake after dinner and/or by two or more nocturnal awakenings to eat food each week. For these patients, a combination of cognitive behavioral therapy and pharmacologic therapy is likely the best option and should be considered for her.

REFERENCES

1. Vivus, Inc. *Qsymia (phentermine/topiramate)* [FDA package insert]. Retrieved February 15, 2020, from

https://www.accessdata.fda.gov/drugsatfda_docs/label/2012/022580s000lbl.pdf.
2. Janssen Pharmaceutical Companies. *Topamax (topiramate)* [FDA package insert]. Retrieved January 17, 2020, from https://www.accessdata.fda.gov/drugsatfda_docs/label/2012/020844s041lbl.pdf.
3. Vivus, Inc. *Phentermine* [FDA package insert]. Retrieved January 17, 2020, from https://www.accessdata.fda.gov/drugsatfda_docs/label/2012/022580s000lbl.pdf.
4. Pfizer Inc. *Neurontin (gabapentin)* [FDA package insert]. Retrieved February 16, 2020, from https://www.accessdata.fda.gov/drugsatfda_docs/label/2017/020235s064_020882s047_021129s046lbl.pdf.
5. Novo Nordisk. *Liraglutide (Victoza)* [FDA package insert]. Retrieved February 16, 2020, from https://www.accessdata.fda.gov/drugsatfda_docs/label/2017/022341s027lbl.pdf.
6. Novo Nordisk. *Liraglutide (Saxenda)* [FDA package insert]. Retrieved February 16, 2020, from https://www.accessdata.fda.gov/drugsatfda_docs/label/2014/206321Orig1s000lbl.pdf.
7. Bristol-Myers Squibb Company. *Glucophage (metformin)* [FDA package insert]. Retrieved February 16, 2020, from https://www.accessdata.fda.gov/drugsatfda_docs/label/2017/020357s037s039,021202s021s023lbl.pdf.
8. Takeda Pharmaceutical America, Inc. *Contrave (buprenorphine/naltrexone)* [FDA package insert]. Retrieved February 16, 2020, from https://www.accessdata.fda.gov/drugsatfda_docs/label/2014/200063s000lbl.pdf.
9. Roche Laboratories Inc. *Xenical (Orlistat)* [FDA package insert]. Retrieved February 16, 2020, from https://www.accessdata.fda.gov/drugsatfda_docs/label/2009/020766s026lbl.pdf.

12

Preoperative Psychiatry

Ashley E. Walker, MD, Tessa L. Manning, MD, Sarah McClanahan, DO, and Ondria C. Gleason, MD

The patient is a 39-year-old, 162-cm small-framed female with a current weight of 100 kg. She has read that bariatric surgery can lead to large amounts of weight loss. She tells you that her goal is to lose enough weight to take her to her previous teenage weight of 52 kg, which she adds is her "ideal body weight." She uses "medical" marijuana regularly, but she has no history of problematic alcohol or drug use. She has recently completed law school and passed her state bar exam. She is hoping that she will now have more time to devote to improving her health. She has been diagnosed with bipolar disorder, posttraumatic stress disorder (PTSD) related to childhood abuse, and binge eating disorder, and she has a history of psychiatric hospitalization for a suicide attempt several years ago. She is prescribed bupropion 150 mg extended-release daily and sertraline 100 mg daily.

1. **When is the best time to conduct the pre–bariatric surgery psychosocial evaluation?**
   A. Immediately prior to surgery, before or after the anesthesiology evaluation
   B. Two months prior to surgery in order to help the patient lose weight
   C. After an internal medicine consultation has been completed
   D. After the patient receives information about the procedure to provide informed consent

2. **Which of the following provides the greatest potential contraindication for a candidate to undergo weight loss surgery?**
   A. Bipolar or other mood disorder
   B. PTSD from childhood trauma
   C. History of suicide attempt and psychiatric hospitalization
   D. Current use of compensatory behaviors, such as self-induced vomiting

3. **With regard to substance use, which of the following represents the greatest risk when evaluating a patient for weight loss surgery?**
   A. Any lifetime history of substance use
   B. Illicit substance use 4 months ago
   C. Participation in a methadone maintenance program
   D. Current use of medical marijuana

4. **Which of the following personality traits has been shown to predict postoperative weight loss success?**
   A. Persistence
   B. Novelty seeking
   C. Impulsivity
   D. Cooperativeness

5. **Following weight loss surgery, for which of the following will it be most important for this patient to receive counseling?**
   A. Negative changes to body image that may result from excess skin
   B. The amount of weight that she will realistically lose if following postsurgical guidelines
   C. Loss of subjective benefits of obesity resulting from significant weight loss

D. Increased alcohol absorption after Roux-en-Y gastric bypass surgery (RYGB)

6. Prior to surgery, which medication change would be advised for this patient?

A. Increase the dose of bupropion extended-release form
B. Switch bupropion extended-release to bupropion immediate-release
C. Continue bupropion extended-release form and decrease the dose of sertraline
D. Discontinue sertraline to avoid serotonin syndrome

ANSWERS

1. D. A formal preoperative psychosocial-behavioral evaluation performed by a qualified behavioral health professional is a requirement of the vast majority of bariatric surgery programs, as well as third-party payers.[1,2] Despite this prerequisite, as well as the existence of multiple guidelines to direct the assessment, there is no single gold standard for this type of evaluation.

The prebariatric psychosocial evaluation should be completed early in the process, but only after the patient has received enough information to provide informed consent for the procedure. In addition to obtaining a psychosocial history, including current and prior psychiatric disorders, social support, eating habits, and weight history, the psychiatrist or other evaluator will seek to confirm whether the patient can demonstrate the capacity to participate in informed consent for the surgery. For example, the patient needs to demonstrate an understanding of the reasons for the surgery and the risks, benefits, and alternatives to it; demonstrate an ability to rationally consider the information necessary to make the decision; and be able to communicate a consistent choice for treatment. Therefore, it is imperative that the patient has been provided the necessary education about the surgery, including potential risks, realistic benefits, and life changes that will be necessary postoperatively prior to presenting for the psychosocial evaluation.[1]

2. D. A history of mental health treatment and comorbid conditions is common among individuals seeking weight loss surgery, and can affect postsurgical outcomes. Depressive and anxiety disorders are the most common psychiatric conditions among people seeking weight loss surgery; personality disorders and, unsurprisingly, a history of trauma or adversity are also frequently reported in this population.[1,3] However, no single piece of historical psychiatric treatment or particular diagnosis presents an absolute contraindication to weight loss surgery. Of more importance are the individual's current symptoms and their severity, as well as the impact any symptoms or diagnoses may have on postsurgical adherence and self-care. Most guidelines agree that current severe, untreated psychopathology is a contraindication for weight loss surgery, not just a history of severe symptoms (such as suicide attempts or hospitalization). However, there is no clear consensus on any specific time frame to wait after psychiatric hospitalization before proceeding with surgery.[3]

With regard to eating disorders, binge eating disorder is most commonly observed in patients presenting for weight loss surgery with the experience of loss of control while eating (as opposed to volume consumed) the most important prognostic factor. There is very limited evidence implicating anorexia nervosa with surgery outcomes. However, ongoing use of compensatory behaviors, such as self-induced vomiting, is generally considered a contraindication to weight loss surgery.[3]

3. B. It is a general consensus among bariatric surgeons that an untreated and active substance use disorder is a contraindication to surgery, but a lifetime history of substance addiction is not considered a contraindication if an adequate period of abstinence has been maintained. The highest risk of relapse occurs in the first year postoperatively, and many programs require 1 year of sobriety immediately prior to surgery.[1,3] During the preoperative psychological evaluation, patients should be screened for a history of substance use disorders. Psychological evaluation should make sure to also gather information regarding current use patterns because substance use that does not meet the criteria for a formal diagnosis of a substance use disorder may interfere with postoperative recovery.[3] There is a lack of consensus in the guidelines regarding patients who are in methadone maintenance programs or using medical marijuana and these cases should be handled on a case-by-case basis. The evaluator should take into account abstinence from other drugs and the effect of the prescribed methadone or medical marijuana on the individual's cognitive and organizational abilities.[1] Individuals should also be counseled that there is an increase for problematic substance use (specifically alcohol) and other compulsive behaviors following weight loss surgery that is independent of prior history of substance use disorders.[3]

Those at highest risk for substance use following weight loss surgery are male gender, younger age, nicotine use, frequent or problematic alcohol use at time of surgery, and recreational drug use.[3]

4. **A.** Several studies have investigated the potential influence of preoperative psychological factors on weight loss surgery outcomes. This patient displays the trait of persistence, the ability to maintain a behavior in favor of valued goals despite the lack of immediate reward, as evidenced by her ability to complete a postgraduate degree. High scores on persistence have been shown to be associated with greater weight loss at 1-year follow-up, likely relating to a greater ability to adapt to postsurgical guidelines. High levels of cooperativeness, the ability to successfully get along with others, have also been associated with better outcomes, which likely reflects an individual's ability to turn to others and benefit from their support. Personality traits that have shown negative correlations with postoperative weight loss include impulsivity and novelty seeking. Several studies of patients with obesity show that impulsivity, depression, and pathological eating behavior are closely connected. However, to date, there have been no studies showing that personality disorder diagnoses have correlations with postsurgical weight loss.[4]

5. **B.** Prior to surgery, it is important that patients have an adequate understanding of typical results for weight loss. Specifically, the average patient can expect to lose and maintain loss of 50% to 70% of their excess body weight according to studies beyond 10 years after surgery.[5] For most patients who are obese, this means that they may remain overweight even after a successful surgery. In this scenario, the patient has unrealistic expectations of weight loss, as most patients will not be able to achieve "ideal body weight." Research has established that most patients hold unrealistic expectations about how much weight they will lose and that these beliefs tend to be resistant to change, even with adequate education.[3] It will be important for the bariatric surgery team to educate the patient regarding adequate expectations of her weight loss, as this may have an impact on her motivation to undergo the surgery and her willingness to accept a greater degree of surgical risk than if weight loss was expected to be lower, adhere to postsurgical dietary recommendations, and be satisfied with postsurgery weight loss.[6] Patients should also be counseled about the likelihood of weight loss surgery leading to excess skin. This can be distressing emotionally and exacerbate presurgical problems with negative body image. A psychological evaluation prior to bariatric surgery should also take into account the possible loss of subjective benefits of being obese. For some patients, excess weight can lead to help responses from others, a rationalization for social and vocational failings, avoidance of physical activity, and protection from fear of unwanted sex.[7] A previous history of sexual trauma is common in bariatric surgery candidates, ranging from 17% to 32%.[6] It is important for patients undergoing RYGB to understand that alcohol absorption will be increased, which can in turn lead to more robust intoxicating effects.[8]

6. **B.** The anatomical changes following bariatric surgery affect the absorption of many oral medications. The small intestine is primarily responsible for drug absorption. Surgical procedures that bypass the small intestine reduce the drug's contact with the mucosal surface, resulting in reduced absorption. This effect is pronounced with delayed release forms of medications.[9] A medication administered in a delayed-release formulation will pass through the gastrointestinal tract quickly, before all the drug can be released. Bariatric surgery candidates taking delayed release oral medications (such as bupropion extended-release form) should be switched to the immediate-release form when possible, preferably before the surgery to assess tolerability. Furthermore, selective serotonin reuptake inhibitors (SSRIs), such as sertraline, have shown reduced absorption following RYGB procedures.[10] Monitoring therapeutic drug levels, when available, is helpful.

REFERENCES

1. Shenouda R. Psychosocial evaluation and management of weight loss surgery patients: a guide to behavioral healthcare for the surgical patient. In: *Perioperative Psychiatry*. Cham, Switzerland: Springer; 2019: 195-221.

2. Mechanick JI, Youdim A, Jones DB, et al. Clinical practice guidelines for the perioperative nutritional, metabolic, and nonsurgical support of the bariatric surgery patient—2013 update: cosponsored by American Association of Clinical Endocrinologists, the Obesity Society, and American Society for Metabolic & Bariatric Surgery. *Obesity*. 2013;21(S1):S1-S27.
3. Sogg S, Lauretti J, West-Smith L. Recommendations for the presurgical psychosocial evaluation of bariatric surgery patients. ASMBS Guidelines/Statements. *Surg Obes Related Dis*. 2016;12:731-749.
4. Generali I, De Panfilis C. Personality traits and weight loss surgery outcome. *Curr Obes Rep*. 2018;7:227-234.
5. O'Brien PE, Hindle A, Brennan L, et al. Long-term outcomes after bariatric surgery: A systematic review and meta-analysis of weight loss at 10 or more years for all bariatric procedures and a single-centre review of 20-year outcomes after adjustable gastric banding. *Obes Surg*. 2019;29:3-14.
6. Sogg S, Mori D. The Boston Interview for Gastric Bypass: Determining the psychological suitability of surgical candidates. *Obes Surg*. 2004;14:370-380.
7. Benotti PN. *Patient Preparation for Bariatric Surgery*. New York: Springer New York; 2014.
8. Steffen KJ, Engel SG, Pollert GA, Li C, Mitchell JE. Blood alcohol concentrations rise rapidly and dramatically after Roux-en-Y gastric bypass. *Surg Obes Relat Dis*. 2013;9(3):470-473.
9. Padwal R, Brocks D, Sharma AM. A systematic review of drug absorption following bariatric surgery and its theoretical implications. *Obes Rev*. 2010;11:41-50.
10. Roerig JL, Steffen K, Zimmerman C, et al. Preliminary comparison of sertraline levels in postbariatric surgery patients versus matched nonsurgical cohort. *Surg Obes Rel Dis*. 2012;8(1):62-66.

SECTION 3

Endoscopic

13

Intragastric Balloons

Oleg Ryabinin, MD, Kyle Checchi, MD, and Gordon G. Wisbach, MD, MBA

A 27-year-old woman with a past medical history of long-term obesity, obstructive sleep apnea (OSA), hypertension, and hyperlipidemia desires assistance with weight loss. She has attempted multiple low-calorie diet regimens, including a 6-month supervised weight loss program with only temporary results. In clinic, her body mass index (BMI) is 32 kg/m^2 and her waist circumference is 85 cm. She is frustrated with her seesawing weight and would like to discuss her options regarding potential interventions.

1. Which of the following statements accurately describes the patient's eligibility for bariatric surgery versus the intragastric balloon?

A. The patient is eligible for bariatric surgery, but she does not meet indications for an intragastric balloon.
B. The patient is eligible for an intragastric balloon, but she does meet indications for bariatric surgery.
C. The patient is eligible for the intragastric balloon or bariatric surgery.
D. The patient is not eligible for either the intragastric balloon or for bariatric surgery.

2. If the patient were offered an intragastric balloon to aid her with weight loss, what risks are important to include in counseling?

A. Balloon migration can occur up to 28% of the time.
B. Pancreatitis and ischemic kidney injury occur in up to 5% of cases.
C. The risk of postprocedural adverse effects is low, occurring less than 1% of the time.
D. The risk of a small bowel obstruction is 2% to 5%.

3. Which of the following answers best describes the typical weight loss experienced by patients following treatment with an intragastric balloon?

A. Approximately 10% *total* body weight loss.
B. Approximately 10% *excess* body weight loss.
C. Following removal of the balloon, patients have minimal weight regain.
D. Most of the patients regain all their lost weight after removal.

4. Which of the following statements is true regarding the response of weight-related comorbidities for patients that participate in an intragastric balloon program?

A. The intragastric balloon has proved to be most effective in treating hypertension.
B. It is most effective in diabetes management with a modest effect on hypertension and hyperlipidemia.
C. The current literature suggests a moderate effect on most obesity-related comorbidities.
D. The intragastric balloon has shown to have little effect on obesity-related comorbidities.

5. The patient is interested in the intragastric balloon procedure. She asks you to describe the procedure. What would you tell her would be the key initial

step to make sure that the intragastric balloon can be inserted safely?

A. The patient should be on a proton pump inhibitor (PPI) for 2 weeks prior to insertion.
B. The patient needs a cardiac and pulmonary workup prior to insertion.
C. The patient should be typed and crossed.
D. A diagnostic endoscopy should be performed.

ANSWERS

1. **B.** Obesity is considered to be a global health crisis. In the United States alone, over 1/3 of the population is obese. It is recommended that primary care physicians, as well as obstetrics/gynecology (OB-GYN) physicians, intervene early in the disease process with behavioral counseling.[1] Pharmacologic therapy in conjunction with lifestyle and behavior modifications can be initiated at a BMI of 30 kg/m^2 alone or 27 kg/m^2 with one or more obesity-related comorbidities.[2] The National Institutes of Health (NIH) guidelines recommend bariatric surgery as an obesity treatment option for any patient with a BMI of 40 kg/m^2 and greater or 35 kg/m^2 and greater with one or more obesity-related comorbidities.[3] Both the Society of American Gastrointestinal Endoscopic Surgeons and the American Society of Metabolic and Bariatric Surgery concluded that bariatric surgery may be considered for a patient with a BMI 30 to 35 kg/m^2 with specific comorbidities (namely, difficult-to-control type 2 diabetes mellitus and dysmetabolic syndrome X).[4] In the United States, the intragastric balloon currently is approved for use in adult patients with a BMI of 30 to 40 kg/m^2. [5,6]

2. **A.** Mild to moderate nausea and vomiting are the most common adverse effects following intragastric balloon insertion. Trang and colleagues performed a meta-analysis on the most common balloon systems and showed that the rate of postinsertion nausea and vomiting was over 50%, with one of the studies that they reviewed reporting a 98% rate of post-insertion nausea and vomiting (see **Table 13-1**). The ORBERA balloon, currently the most common in use, had the highest rate of nausea and vomiting.[7] Balloon migration is not an infrequent phenomenon. In one study, the rate of migration was reported to be as high as 28%. However, almost all migration happened after the recommended therapeutic interval (6 months). This speaks to the importance of postprocedural follow-up in these patients. Migration leading to small bowel and large bowel obstruction is extremely rare but has been reported.[8] The highest rate of severe adverse effects came from literature on the ORBERA balloon reviewed by the U.S. Food and Drug Administration showing a 10% rate.[9] Newer studies describe a lower severe adverse effect rate, with some showing a rate of less than 1%.[10] We hypothesize that this could partially be due to growing experience with intragastric balloon leading to safer techniques, as well as newer, air-filled systems that report a less than 1% rate of adverse effects. To quote to the patient a rate of severe adverse effects of up to 10% would be appropriate. There have also been case reports of pancreatitis and kidney injury that occur very rarely (<about 1%); the mechanism of injury is believed to be related to direct compression of the parenchyma itself or the vascular supplies.[11]

3. **A.** Intragastric balloons are most effective for short-term weight loss. Most systems are placed for a period of 6 months; some studies show placement for as long as 12 months. Current FDA approval for intragastric balloons is 6 months.[5] Most of the current studies focus on short-term follow-up for as long to 6 months following balloon removal. At 6 months postremoval, most patients regain about 50% of the lost weight.[8,9,12] Although a few studies have longer follow-up periods, there is not enough literature to predict weight loss past the 6-month postremoval period. The amount of weight loss that occurs has been a difficult question to answer. This is primarily due to lack of consistency in how researchers report their weight-loss outcomes. A large-scale review by Chinara Tate and colleagues showed a 10.5% total body weight loss after a 6-month balloon insertion period (see **Table 13-2**).[9] A meta-analysis by Yiyuan Zheng and colleagues reported a 21% excess body weight loss.[12,13] It is important to note that the weight loss achieved is significantly increased over lifestyle modification alone. For instance, while Chinara et al. reported 10.5% total body weight loss with the intragastric balloon in conjunction with lifestyle modifications, the weight loss in the control group (lifestyle modifications only) was a more modest 5.5%.

4. **B.** Intragastric balloons are most effective for short-term weight loss. They have not been well studied in their effects past the initial 12 to 18 months in either weight loss or obesity-related comorbidities. Short-term trials show a good response in management of diabetes, but there is a relatively limited improvement in hypertension and hyperlipidemia.[14] More research is required to understand the effect that the intragastric balloons on other obesity-related comorbidities such as OSA.

Overall, other than diabetes, the effect of the intragastric balloon on obesity-related comorbidities is limited.

5. **D.** The procedural steps for any of the intragastric balloons can be obtained from the manufacturer's website. Most steps are similar between systems, with appropriate adjustments for positioning and fill volumes depending the balloon used. We do not endorse any one brand of intragastric balloon, but for this question, we have used the ORBERA system, as it is the most common in the United States and the rest of the world.[15] It is important to note that a preprocedure diagnostic endoscopy is always performed to exclude any contraindications to the procedure. These include a large hiatal hernia, a structural abnormality such as an esophageal diverticulum, an esophageal/gastric stenosis, an esophageal/gastric mass, large esophageal/gastric varices, esophagitis, or gastric ulcers.

Table 13-1. SUMMARY OF RATES OF NAUSEA, VOMITING, ABDOMINAL PAIN, GERD, MILD OR MODERATE ADVERSE EVENTS, AND SERIOUS ADVERSE EVENTS POST–INTRAGASTRIC BALLOON PLACEMENT

Study	IGB Subgroup	Treatment Sample Size	SAE* Sample Size	Nausea N	Nausea %	Vomiting N	Vomiting %	Abdominal Pain N	Abdominal Pain %
Machytka (2017)[16]	Elipse	34	34	15	44.12	18	52.94	7	20.50
Machytka (2016)[17]	Elipse	8	8	6	75.00	5	62.50	3	37.50
FDA, SMART (2016)[18]	Obalon	198	336	261	77.68	58	17.26	244	72.62
Nobili (2015)[19]	Obalon	10	10	5	50.00	5	50.00	5	50.00
Mion (2013)[20]	Obalon	17	17	7	41.18	3	17.65	13	76.47
FDA IB-005 (2015)[21]	ORBERA	125	160	139	86.88	121	75.63	92	57.50
Mitura (2015)[22]	ORBERA	57	57	33	57.89	33	57.89	13	22.81
Fuller (2013)[23]	ORBERA	31	31	23	74.19	24	77.42	0	0
FDA, REDUCE (2015)[24]	ReShape	187	264	64	24.24	229	86.74	144	54.55
Ponce (2013)[25]	ReShape	21	21	11	52.38	11	52.38	0	0
Total		688	938	564		507		521	
Meta-analytic average (95% CI)				63.33% (61.49%–65.16%)		55.29% (53.59%–56.99%)		58.55% (56.41%–60.68%)	

*SAE, Serious Adverse Events

Reproduced with permission from Trang J, Lee S, Miller A, et al. Incidence of nausea and vomiting after intra-gastric balloon placement in bariatric patients – A systematic review and meta analysis. *Int J Surg.* 2018; 57: 22-29.

Table 13-2. SUMMARY OF INTRAGASTRIC BALLOON STUDY CHARACTERISTICS, SAFETY, AND EFFICACY

Author	Year	Study Type	Location & Duration	Intervention & Control Groups	# of Subjects Randomized	Completers + Attrition Rate (%)
Included in Meta-Analysis						
Farina et al.[26]	2012	RCT (BIB vs Pharma) (Unblinded)	Italy: 12 Mo	Interv: BIB/ Pharma (6 Mo/ 6 Mo) or BIB/Lifestyle (6 Mo/ 6 Mo) Control: Pharma (12 Mo)	50 Subjects (20 Pharma vs 15 BIB/ Pharm vs 15 BIB/Lifestyle)	12 Mo Completers: 12/20 Pharma, 9/15 BIB/Pharma & 12/15 BIB/Lifestyle = 33 Attrition: 34%
Mohammed et al.[27]	2014	RCT (Unblinded)	Egypt: 9 Mo	Interv: BIB (6 Mo) Control: Diet + Excercise Alone (6 Mo)	128 Ss (84 BIB vs 44 Contol)	6 & 9 Mo Completers: 80 BIB & 40 Contol = 120 Attrition: 6.25%
Dayyeh et al.[28] (ORBERA: FDA Reviewed)	2015	Multi-Center RCT (Unblinded)	USA: 52 Wk	Interv: ORBERA + BMP (6 Mo) Control: BMP Only (6 Mo)	273 Ss (137 Orbera vs 136 Control)	9 Mo Completers: 98 ORBERA & 93 Control = 191 Attrition: 30.1%
Ponce et al.[24] (ReShape: FDA Reviewed)	2015	Multi-Center RCT (Double blinded)	USA: 48 Wk: Endpoint 1: 24 Wk	Interv: Reshape DUO (6 Mo) Control: Diet and Exercise only (6 Mo)	326 Ss (187 ReShape vs 139 Control)	24 Wk Completers: 167 DUO & 126 Control = 293 Attrition:10.2%
Included in Review						
Genco et al.[29]	2006	RCT Crosso-ver (Double Blinded)	Italy; 6 Mo (3 Mo BIB, 3 Mo Sham)	Interv; BIB (3 Mo) Control; Sham (3Mo)	32 Se (16 BIB vs 16 Control)	6 Mo Completers; 32 Attrition: 0%

Initial Wt (Kg)	Wt Loss (Kg)	% Total Body Weight Loss (%TBWL)	Contol-Subtracted %TBWL	S ig Wt Loss (IGB)	Risk of Bias	# of AEs	# of SAEs
Interv:115.1 ± 18.1 SD Control: 108.7 ± 12.9	6 Mo: Not reported 12 Mo: 8.9 ± 7.6 SD (Pharma) vs 17.6 ± 8.9 (BIB/Pharma) vs 7.4 ± 13.2 (BIB/Lifestyle)	6 Mo: 14.5% ± 6.6 SD (BIB) vs 9.1% ± 6.7 (Pharma) 12 Mo: 8.0% ± 6.3 SD (Pharma/Pharma) vs 15.8 % ± 8.9 (BIB/Pharma) vs 14.3 % ± 10.4 (BIB/Lifestyle)	6 Mo: 5.4% ± 9.4 SD	Yes	A = 1; B = 1; C = 1; D = 1 E = 1; F = 0 G = 1; H = 0 TOTAL: 6	36	0
Interv: 36.9 ± 7.8 SD Control: 137.80 ± 9.8	6 Mo: 14.3 ± 14.9 SD (BIB) vs 6.39 ± 13.0 (Control) 9 Mo: 18.1 ± 13.5 SD (BIB) vs 6 ± 12.5 (Control)	6 Mo: 10.4% ± 1.0 SD (BIB) vs 4.6% ± 2.0 (Control) 9 Mo: 13.2% ± 0.7 SD (BIB) vs 4.3% ± 2.1 (Control)	6 Mo: 5.8% ± 2.2 SD 9 Mo: 8.9% ±2.2	Yes	A = 0; B = 0; C = 1; D = 1; E = 0; F = 0; G = 0; H = 1 TOTAL: 3	Not reported	3
Not reported	6 Mo: 9.9 ± 6.6 SD (ORBERA) vs 3.2 ± 4.8 (Control) 9 Mo: 8.8 ± 7.1SD (ORBERA) vs 3.2 ± 0.6 (Control)	6 Mo: 10.2% ± 6.6 SD (ORBERA) vs 3.3% ± 5.0 (Control) 9 Mo: 9.1% ± 6.9 SD (ORBERA) vs 3.4% ± 5.3 Control: 12 Mo: 7.6% ± 7.5 SD (ORBERA) vs 3.1 ± 5.9 (Control)	6 Mo: 6.9% ± 8.4 SD 9 Mo: 5.7% ± 8.7 12 Mo: 4.5% ± 9.5	Yes	A = 0; B = 0; C = 1; D = 1; E = 0; F = 0; G = 0; H = 0 TOTAL: 2	Not reported	17
Interv: 95.1 ± 11.7 SD Control: 96.8 ± 11.6	6 Mo: 7.2 ± 5.4 SD (DUO) vs 3.5 ± 6.4 (Control)	6 Mo: 7.6% ± 5.5 SD (DUO) vs 3.6% ± 6.3 (Control)	6 Mo: 4% ± 8.4 SD	Yes	A = 0; B = 0; C = 1; D = 1; E = 1; F = 1; G = 0; H = 1 TOTAL: 5	4	28
Not Reported	3 Mo; 15 ± 6 SD (BIB) vs 3 ± 1 (Control)	Not reported	Could not be calculated	Yes	A = 0; B = 0; C = 1; D = 1; E = 1; F = 1; G = 1; H = 0 TOTAL: 5	0	0

Table 13-2. SUMMARY OF INTRAGASTRIC BALLOON STUDY CHARACTERISTICS, SAFETY, AND EFFICACY (Continued)

Author	Year	Study Type	Location & Duration	Intervention & Control Groups	# of Subjects Randomized	Completers + Attrition Rate (%)
Martinez et al.[30]	2007	RCT (Double Blinded)	Spain; 4 Mo	Interv; BIB (4 Mo) Control; Sham (4 Mo)	22 Ss (11 BIB vs 11 Control)	4 Mo Completers; 10 BIB & 11 Control = 21 Attrition; 4.6 %
Fuller et al.[23] (ORBERA: FDA Reviewed)	2013	RCT (Unblinded)	Australia;52 Wk	Interv; ORBERA (6 Mo) Mo + BMP then 6 Mo BMP only) Control; BMP only (12 Mo)	66 Ss (31 Orbera vs 36 Control)	6 Mo Completers; 29 ORBERA & 30 Control = 59 Attrition; 10.7% 12 Mo Completers; 23 ORBERA and 22 Control = 45 Attrition: 31.8 %
Mathus-Vllegen et al.[31]	2014	RCT (Double blinded)	Amsterdam: 26 Wk	Interv: BIB (6.5 Mo) Control: Sham (6.5 Mo)	40 Ss (19 BIB vs 21 Control)	13 Wk Completers; 21 Sham/BIB &19 BIB/BIB = 40 Attrition; 0% 26 Wk Completers; 12 Sham/BIB & 7 BIB/BIB = 19 Attrition: 52.5 %

Initial Wt (Kg)	Wt Loss (Kg)	% Total Body Weight Loss (%TBWL)	Contol-Subtracted %TBWL	S ig Wt Loss (IGB)	Risk of Bias	# of AEs	# of SAEs
Interv;143.8 kg ± 31.2 SD Control; 138.8 kg ± 24.5	4 Mo; 12.7 ± 5.6 SD (BIB) vs 8.9 ± 9.2 (Sham)	4 Mo: 8.8% ± 3.5 SD (BIB) vs 6.4% ± 4.0 (Sham)	4 Mo: 2.47% ± 5.3 SD	No	A = 1; B = 1; C = 0; D = 0; E = 1; F = 1; G = 1; H = 1 TOTAL: 6	Not reported	1
Interv;104.0 ± 14.8 SD Control; 103.4 + 13.9	6 Mo; 14.4 (ORBERA) vs 5.1 (Control) 12 Mo; 9.4 (ORBERA) vs 5.3 (control) SDs not provided	6 Mo; 14.2% ORBERA vs 4.8% Control 12 MO: 9.2% ORBERA vs 5.2% Control SDs not provided	6 Mo: 9.4% 12 Mo: 4.0% SDs not provided	Yes	A = 0; B = 0; C = 1; D = 1; E = 1; F = 0; G = 0; H = 1 TOTAL: 4	0	3
BIB/BIB; 124.0 ± 21.1 SD Sham/BIB; 122.5 ± 19.0	13 Wk: 10.6 ± 5.8 SD (sham/BIB) vs 13.1 ± 5.2 (BIB/BIB) 26 Wk: 18.0 ± 6.5 SD (sham/BIB) vs 16.4 ± 10.2 (BIB/BIB)	13 Wk: 8.8% ± 4.9 SD (Sham/BIB) vs 10.6% ± 3.8 (BIB/BIB) 26 Wk: 15.8% ± 5.7 SD (Sham/BIB) vs 14.2% ± 8.4 (BIB/BIB)	26 Wk: 1.6% ± 10.2 SD 13 Wk: 1.8% ± 6.2	No	A = 1; B = 1; C = 1; D = 1; E = 1; F = 0; G = 1; H = 1 TOTAL: 7	2	0

In general, PPIs are not needed prior to placement, but they are beneficial after placement to reduce the symptoms of reflux. While obese patients should be screened for cardiopulmonary risk prior to surgery, most do not require a cardiac and pulmonary workup prior to proceeding to placement. The risk of bleeding from the procedure is minimal, and as such, there is no requirement to type and crossmatch every patient who undergoes a procedure.

REFERENCES

1. Kahan S, Winston G. Addressing obesity in clinical gynecology practice. *Clin Obst Gynecol.* 2018;61(1):10-26.
2. Jensen M, Ryan D, MD, Apovian C, et al. 2013 AHA/ACC/TOS guideline for the management of overweight and obesity in adults. *Circulation.* 2014;129(25):s102-s138.
3. NIH Conference Consensus Development Conference Panel. Gastrointestinal surgery for severe obesity. *Ann Intern Med.* 1991;115:956-961.
4. SAGES Guidelines Committee. *Guidelines for clinical application of laparoscopic bariatric surgery.* SAGES, March 25, 2008, www.sages.org/publications/guidelines/guidelines-for-clinical-application-of-laparoscopic-bariatric-surgery/.
5. U.S. Food and Drug Administration (FDA). *Weight-loss and weight-management devices.* www.fda.gov/medical-devices/products-and-medical-procedures/weight-loss-and-weight-management-devices.
6. VA DoD *Clinical Practice Guidelines: Management of Overweight and Obesity.* U.S. Department of Defense, July 2020. https://www.healthquality.va.gov/guidelines/CD/obesity/VADoDObesityCPGFinal5087242020.pdf
7. Trang J, Lee S, Miller A, et al. Incidence of nausea and vomiting after intra-gastric balloon placement in bariatric patients—a systematic review and meta analysis. *Intl J Surg.* 2018;57:22-29.
8. Gaur S, Levy S, Mathus-Vliegen L, et al. Balancing risk and reward: a critical review of the intra-gastric balloon for weight loss. *Gastro Endosc.* 2015;81(6):1330-1336.
9. Tate C, Geliebter A. Intra-gastric balloon treatment for obesity: review of recent studies. *Adv Ther.* 2017;34:1859-1875.
10. Sullivan S, Swain J, Woodman G, et al. Randomized sham-controlled trial of the 6-month gas-filled intragastric balloon system for weight loss. *Surg Obes Rel Dis.* 2018;14:1876-1889.
11. Aljahdi E. Ischemic renal injury complicating intra-gastric balloon insertion. *ACG Case Rep J.* 2018;5:e16.
12. Zheng Y, Wang M, He S, Ji G. Short-term effects of intra-gastric balloon in association with conservative therapy on weight loss: a meta-analysis. *J Translat Med.* 2015;13:246-254.
13. Courcoulas A, Dayyeh BK, Eaton L, et al. Intra-gastric balloon as an adjunct to lifestyle intervention: a randomized trial. *Intl J Obes.* 2017;41:427-433.
14. Popov V, Ou A, Schulman A, et al. The impact of intragastric balloons on obesity-related co-morbidities: a systematic review and meta-analysis. *Am J Gastroenterol.* 2017;112:429-439.
15. Bazerbachi F, Vargas E, Abu Dayyeh B. Endoscopic bariatric therapy: a guide to the intra-gastric balloon. *Am J Gastroenterol.* 2019;114:1421-1431.
16. Machytka E, Gaur S, Chuttani R, et al. Elipse, the first procedureless gastric balloon for weight loss: a prospective, observational, open-label, multicenter study. *Endoscopy.* 2017;49(2):154-160.
17. Machytka E, Chuttani R, Bojkova M, et al. Elipse™, a procedureless gastric balloon for weight loss: a proof-of-concept pilot study. *Obes Surg.* 2016;26(3):512-516.
18. The Six-Month Adjunctive Weight Reduction Therapy (SMART) Trial. https://clinicaltrials.gov/ct2/show/NCT02235870
19. Nobili V, Corte CD, Liccardo D, et al. Obalonintragastric balloon in the treatment of paediatric obesity: a pilot study. *Pediatr Spanish Ed.* 10(5):e1-4. doi:10.1111/ijpo.268
20. Mion F, Ibrahim M, Marjoux S, et al. Current status of intragastric balloon for obesity treatment. *Obes Surg.* 2013;23(5):730-733.
21. A Study of BioEnterics® Intragastric Balloon (BIB®) System to Assist in the Weight Management of Obese Subjects. https://clinicaltrials.gov/ct2/show/NCT00730327
22. Mitura K, Garnysz K. Tolerance of intragastric balloon and patient's satisfaction in obesity treatment. *WideochirInne Tech Maloinwazyjne.* 2015;10(3):445-449.
23. Fuller NR, Pearson S, Lau NS, et al. An intragastric balloon in the treatment of obese individuals with metabolic syndrome: a randomized controlled study. *Obesity.* 2013;21(8):1561-1570.
24. Ponce J, Woodman G, Swain J, et al. The REDUCE pivotal trial: a prospective, randomized controlled pivotal trial of a dual intragastric balloon for the treatment of obesity. *Obes Surg.* 2015;11(4):874-871.
25. Ponce J. Prospective, randomized, multicenter study evaluating safety and efficacy of intragastric dual-balloon in obesity. *Surgery for obesity and related diseases.* 2013;9(2):290-295.
26. Farina MG, Baratta R, Nigro A, et al. Intragastric balloon in association with lifestyle and/or pharmacotherapy in the long-term management of obesity. *Obes Surg.* 2012;22(4):565-571.
27. Mohammed M. Effects of intragastric balloon versus conservative therapy on appetite regulatory hormones in obese subjects. *Trends Med Res.* 2014;1:1-5.
28. Abu Dayyeh BK, Eaton LL, Woodman G, et al. A randomized, multi-center study to evaluate the safety and effectiveness of an intragastric balloon as an adjunct to a behavioral modification program, in comparison with a behavioral modification program alone in the weight management of obese subject. *Gastrointest Endosc.* 2015;81(5):AB147.
29. Genco A, Cipriano M, Bacci V, et al. BioEnterics Intragastric Balloon (BIB): A short-term, double-double blind,

randomized, controlled, crossover study on weight reduction in morbidly obese patients. *Int J Obesity*. 2006;30(1): 129-133.

30. Martinez-Brocca MA, Belda O, Parejo J, et al. Intragastric balloon-induced satiety is not mediated by modification in fasting or postprandial plasma ghrelin levels in morbid obesity. *Obes Surg*. 2007;17(5):649-657.
31. Mathus-Vliegen EMH, Eichenberger RI. Fasting and meal-suppressed ghrelin levels before and after intragastric balloons and balloon-induced weight loss. *Obes Surg*. 2014;24(1):85-94.
32. Genco A, Maselli R, Casella G, Cipriano M, Redler A. Intragastricballoontreatment for obesity. *Obesity, bariatric and metabolic surgery*. 2016:485-492.

14

Gastric Plication

Katherine Aucoin, MD, MSc, FRCSC, and James Ellsmere, MD, MS, FRCSC, FACS

A 35-year-old African American female is referred from her family doctor for consideration of bariatric intervention. She is hesitant to proceed with surgery but would consider an endoscopic intervention. Her past medical history includes insulin-dependent type 2 diabetes, poorly controlled hypertension, history of deep vein thrombosis (DVT) 20 years ago after pregnancy, depression, nonalcoholic fatty liver disease (NAFLD), and a large hiatal hernia. She is concerned that her family doctor told her she is unlikely to be a surgical candidate. The patient's BMI is 42 kg/m^2.

1. What is the generally accepted indication for Endoscopic Sleeve Gastroplasty (ESG)?

A. Nonsurgical candidate with body mass index (BMI) >30 kg/m^2
B. Surgical candidate with BMI >45 kg/m^2
C. Bridge to surgical management with BMI >55 kg/m^2
D. BMI >30 kg/m^2 and failed noninvasive weight loss measures
E. Surgical candidate with BMI <45 kg/m^2

2. Which of her medical conditions would most concern you when considering ESG?

A. Poorly controlled hypertension
B. History of DVT after pregnancy 20 years ago
C. NAFLD
D. Large hiatal hernia
E. Depression

3. Which of the following is a described complication of ESG?

A. Splenic injury
B. Gall bladder perforation
C. Death
D. Pancreatitis
E. Transverse colon injury

4. The mechanism for weight reduction by ESG is which of the following?

A. Increase in gut hormones glucagon-like peptide-1 (GLP-1) and peptide YY (PYY)
B. Delay in gastric emptying of solids
C. Decrease in the gut hormone ghrelin
D. Permanently remodeling anatomy and limiting stomach capacity
E. Reduced satiety

5. Compared to other bariatric procedures, the efficacy of ESG has been described as which of the following?

A. Percent total weight loss at 6 months predicts weight loss at 24 months.
B. Parallels LSG in percent total weight loss at 24 months.
C. Approximates intragastric balloon therapy at 12 months.
D. Supersedes percent estimated weight loss by vertical banded gastroplasty (VBG) at 18 months.
E. Is superior to endoscopic aspiration therapy at 6 months for patients with class I obesity.

6. There is a lot of variation in the literature on ESG technique, and it is not standardized. What has been described as increasing the efficacy of ESG?

A. Ensuring suturing technique includes only mucosa and submucosa

B. An additional reinforcement layer of sutures
C. Including the fundus as part of the gastroplasty
D. A *U*-shaped suturing pattern
E. Preprocedure endoscopy

ANSWERS

1. **D.** The 2019 American Society for Metabolic and Bariatric Surgery (ASMBS) guidelines endorse ESG and primary obesity surgery endoluminal (such as the POSE procedure that involves endoscopic plication of the fundus and/or the stomach proximal to the antrum to create restriction and early satiety) as endoscopic procedures; however, indications are variable and debated.[1,2] ESG is cited as a bridge between medical and surgical therapies.[1,3] Other indications include consideration for patients who are nonsurgical candidates (portal hypertension, cirrhosis, uncontrolled inflammatory bowel disease, and severe disease that would contraindicate surgery[4] and patients who do not otherwise qualify for bariatric surgery.[5] Current research literature demonstrates that increasing BMI is a predictor of increased percent total weight loss in patients who have undergone ESG.[6]

ESG is a plausible bridge to bariatric surgery for patients who require revision of prior bariatric surgery due to insufficient weight loss or procedure-related adverse events. In a study where 20 patients underwent revision to laparoscopic sleeve gastrectomy (LSG) after ESG, they reported no adverse events, reoperations, and no mortality after revision.[7]

Most current studies on ESG in North America have an inclusion criterion of BMI >30 kg/m^2 with failed noninvasive weight loss measures.[8–10] One study from Australia includes patients with BMI >27 kg/m^2 with failed lifestyle modifications.[11] Another multicenter study out of Brazil included patients who had BMI >25 kg/m^2 and less than 30 kg/m^2, with failed diet and lifestyle modifications. While this study included 3 patients from the United States, they note that most guidelines do not recommend interventions in this population; however, ESG and intragastric balloon interventions are performed on this population in Brazilian centers.[6] Current North American guidelines state that patients with BMI >25 kg/m^2 and Asian ethnicity can be considered for bariatric intervention, but it is a grade D recommendation (grade A = very strong; B = strong; C = not strong; D = primarily based on expert opinion).[2]

2. **D.** While ideally the patient's blood pressure would be under control for the procedure, poorly controlled hypertension is an indication for bariatric intervention, as is NAFLD.[5] One of the principal goals of bariatric intervention is to help manage the comorbidities associated with obesity, including type 2 diabetes mellitus, hypertension, hypercholesterolemia, and NAFLD.[12]

Patients on therapeutic anticoagulation are excluded from most American studies.[5,8,9] In this case, the DVT was 20 years earlier, and the patient is unlikely to be on continued anticoagulation for more than 6 months.[13] Current guidelines report that patients with a history of DVT should undergo assessment prior to consideration of bariatric surgery.[2] While pulmonary embolism has been described as an adverse outcome in ESG, a history of provoked DVT is not currently described as an exclusion criterion in current studies.[5,9] A large hiatal hernia is an exclusion criteria in North American studies; one study specified hiatal hernia >5 cm.[5,9] Other exclusion criteria include gastric cancer, pregnancy, gastroesophageal motility disorders, and gastric ulcerations.[5]

Patients with BMI >40 kg/m^2 can be considered for this procedure.[8]

3. **B.** Two recent meta-analyses demonstrate the most common complications from ESG are gastrointestinal bleeding and perigastric fluid collection.[3,5] ESG complications were classified as mild, moderate, and severe as per the ASGE Quality Task Force recommendations.[3,14] De Miranda Neto et al reported that the total adverse event rate was 2.3%, with 1.5% for mild, 1.7% for moderate, and 0.8% for severe. In contrast, Singh et al reported a serious adverse event rate of 2.3%.[5] Importantly, no procedure-related mortalities were reported in either meta-analysis.

Less common complications include pulmonary embolism, pneumothorax, and gallbladder perforation during anchoring of the helix.[9,15]. Furthermore, an overtube is advocated in the literature to protect the esophagus from injury from the suturing device.[5]

4. **B.** LSG, Roux-en-Y gastric bypass (RYGB), and laparoscopic adjustable banded gastroplasty (LABG) have been shown to increase the gut hormones GLP-1 and PYY.[16] GLP-1, PYY, and leptin (LEP) did not change significantly 3 months after ESG, but insulin sensitivity did.[9] LSG and RYGB have

been demonstrated to have a significant decrease in active fasting and postprandial ghrelin after bariatric intervention.[17]

In one study, ESG caused a delay in gastric emptying of solids 3 months postprocedure, with an increase in time of 50% for emptying of solids, at 90 minutes.[9] ESG had no impact on gastric emptying of liquids. In the same study, it led to significantly increased satiation, causing earlier termination of a meal and decreased caloric intake.

While ESG may result in remodeling of the stomach, it does not significantly alter the stomach's anatomy permanently, in contrast to LSG.[3] One study assessing ESG by endoscopy at 12 months found 58.5% of sutures were fully intact, while 17% were partially intact.[18]

5. **A.** At 6 months postintervention, one study reported weight loss achieved by LSG was higher than ESG (23.6% versus 17.1%).[19] One of the problems with ESG is that long-term follow-up is lacking. Currently, only one study reports ESG outcomes at 24 months.[3,20] Studies comparing laparoscopic gastric plication with LSG show a significantly lower percentage of excess weight loss at 24 months in the laparoscopic gastric plication group than the LSG group (42.4% versus 78.9%, respectively, $p < 0.01$).[21]

In a systematic review and meta-analysis, the percentage of total weight loss at 6 months post-ESG approximates intragastric balloon therapy (14.9% versus 13.2%); however, current guidelines state that the maximal time for a balloon to remain intragastric is 6 months, at which time patients often experience weight recidivism.[5] Weight loss after ESG appears to plateau at 12 months.[3]

Currently, endoscopic aspiration therapy is approved by the Food and Drug Administration (FDA) only for class II and III obesity.[22] There are no studies comparing endoscopic aspiration therapy or VBG to ESG. Of note, VBG is no longer performed due to high complication rates and high failure rate (less than 10% of patients maintain weight loss of 16%+/−11% at 10 years).[23]

In the initial multicenter trial of ESG, weight loss at 24 months was predicted by weight at 6 months; if patients did not achieve >10% total body weight loss at 6 months, they had only an 18% chance of achieving it at 24 months.[20] Early weight loss after RYGB has been shown to be a predictor of long-term outcomes.[24]

6. **B.** While the results of ESG are reproducible, there is no standardization in technique.[5] In two recent meta-analyses, full thickness suturing and an additional layer of sutures for reinforcement are common practices and likely to result in better efficacy.[3,5] In these studies, the most common variations between techniques involve the suturing patterns. The variations include *Z*-shape, *U*-shape, and a triangular pattern. Furthermore, there is no consensus on the number of sutures that need placing.

Currently, the recommendation is a preprocedure endoscopy to rule out abnormalities that would be a contraindication or limit ESG, such as ulcerations, gastric cancer, or hiatal hernia, but this has not been evaluated for impact on outcomes. The correlation between preprocedure endoscopy and postoperative complications for bariatric surgery is unclear at present.[25]

Anatomically, the goal is to narrow the diameter and vertical length of the stomach.[20] This is described technically by performing a gastroplasty from the cardia to the level of the incisura, sparing the fundus.[22,26] Early descriptions of the procedure included the fundus, as does the POSE procedure.[10,12]

REFERENCES

1. Gys B, Plaeke P, Lamme B, et al. Endoscopic gastric plication for morbid obesity: a systematic review and meta-analysis of published data over time. *Obes Surg*. 2019;29(9): 3021-3029. https://doi.org/10.1007/s11695-019-04010-3.
2. Mechanick JI, Apovian C, Brethauer S, et al. Clinical practice guidelines for the perioperative nutrition, metabolic, and nonsurgical support of patients undergoing bariatric procedures—2019 update: cosponsored by American Association of Clinical Endocrinologists/ American College of Endocrinology, The Obesity Society, American Society for Metabolic & Bariatric Surgery, Obesity Medicine Association, and American Society of Anesthesiologists. *Endocr Pract*. 2019;25(12):1346-1359. doi:10.4158/GL-2019-0406.
3. de Miranda Neto AA, Hourneaux de Moura DT, Braga Ribeiro I, et al. Efficacy and safety of endoscopic sleeve gastroplasty at mid term in the management of overweight and obese patients: a systematic review and meta-analysis. *Obes Surg*. 2020;30(5):1971-1987. https://doi.org/10.1007/s11695-020-04449-9.
4. Zentner A. Clinical assessment to determine a patient's suitability for bariatric surgery. *BCMJ*. 2018;60(3):151-155.
5. Singh S, Turani Hourneaux de Moura, DT, Khan A, et al. Safety and efficacy of endoscopic sleeve gastroplasty worldwide for treatment of obesity: a systematic review and meta-analysis. *Surg Obes Rel Dis*. 2020;16(2): 340-351. https://doi.org/10.1016/j.soard.2019.11.012.

6. Barrichello B, Hourneaux de Moura, DT, Hourneaux de Moura, DG, et al. Endoscopic sleeve gastroplasty in the management of overweight and obesity: an international multicenter study. *Gastrointest Endosc.* 2019;90(5): 770-780. https://doi.org/10.1016/j.gie.2019.06.013.
7. Alqahtani AR, Elahmedi M, Alqahtani YA, Al-Darwish A. Laparoscopic sleeve gastrectomy after endoscopic sleeve gastroplasty: technical aspects and short-term outcomes. *Obes Surg.* 2019;29(11):3547-3552. https://doi.org/10.1007/s11695-019-04024-x.
8. Saumoy M, Schneider Y, Zhou XK, et al. A single-operator learning curve analysis for the endoscopic sleeve gastroplasty. *Gastrointestl Endosc.* 2018;87(2):442-447. https://doi.org/10.1016/j.gie.2017.08.014.
9. Abu Dayyeh BK, Acosta A, Camilleri M, et al. Endoscopic sleeve gastroplasty alters gastric physiology and induces loss of body weight in obese individuals. *Clin Gastroenterol Hepatol.* 2017;5(1):37-43.e1. https://doi.org/10.1016/j.cgh.2015.12.030.
10. Kumar N, Abu Dayyeh BK, Lopez-Nava Breviere G, Galvao Neto MP, et al. Endoscopic sutured gastroplasty: procedure evolution from first-in-man cases through current technique. *Surg Endosc.* 2018;32(4):2159-2164. https://doi.org/10.1007/s00464-017-5869-2.
11. Sartoretto A, Sui Z, Hill C, et al. Endoscopic sleeve gastroplasty (ESG) is a reproducible and effective endoscopic bariatric therapy suitable for widespread clinical adoption: a large, international multicenter study. *Obes Surg.* 2018;28(7):1812-1821. https://doi.org/10.1007/s11695-018-3135-x.
12. Abu Dayyeh BK, Edmundowicz SA, Sullivan S, et al. Endoscopic bariatric therapies. *Gastrointest Endosc.* 2015;81(5):1073-1086. https://doi.org/10.1016/j.gie.2015.02.023.
13. Kearon C, Kahn SR. Long-term treatment of venous thromboembolism. *Blood.* 2020;135(5):317-325. https://doi.org/10.1182/blood.2019002364.
14. Cotton PB, Eisen GM, Aabaken L, et al. A lexicon for endoscopic adverse events: report of an ASGE workshop. *Gastrointest Endosc.* 2010;71(3):446-454. https://doi.org/10.1016/j.gie.2009.10.027.
15. Asokkumar R, Pappu Babu M, Bautista I, Lopez-Nava G. The use of the OverStitch for bariatric weight loss in Europe. *Gastrointest Endosc Clin.* 2020;30(1):129-145. https://doi.org/10.1016/j.giec.2019.08.007.
16. Jirapinyo P, Thompson CC. Endoscopic bariatric and metabolic therapies: surgical analogues and mechanisms of action. *Clin Gastroenterol Hepatol.* 2017;15(5):619-630. https://doi.org/10.1016/j.cgh.2016.10.021.
17. Cummings DE, Weigle DS, Frayo RS, et al. Plasma ghrelin levels after diet-induced weight loss or gastric bypass surgery. *N Eng J Med.* 2002;346(21):1623-1630. https://doi.org/10.1056/NEJMoa012908;StavrosN,Karamanakos SN, Vagenas K, Kalfarentzos F, Alexandrides TK. Weight loss, appetite suppression, and changes in fasting and postprandial ghrelin and peptide-Yy levels after Roux-en-Y gastric bypass and sleeve gastrectomy: a prospective, double blind study. *Ann Surg.* 2008;247(3):401-407. https://doi.org/10.1097/SLA.0b013e318156f012.
18. Pizzicannella M, Lapergola A, Fiorillo C, et al. Does endoscopic sleeve gastroplasty stand the test of time? Objective assessment of endoscopic ESG appearance and its relation to weight loss in a large group of consecutive patients. *Surg Endosc.* 2020;34(8):3696-3705. https://doi.org/10.1007/s00464-019-07329-1.
19. Fayad L, Adam A, Schweitzer M, et al. Endoscopic sleeve gastroplasty versus laparoscopic sleeve gastrectomy: a case-matched study. *Gastrointest Endosc.* 2019;89(4): 782-788. https://doi.org/10.1016/j.gie.2018.08.030.
20. Lopez-Nava G, et al. Endoscopic Sleeve Gastroplasty for Obesity: A Multicenter Study of 248 Patients with 24 Months Follow-Up. *Obesity Surgery.* October 2017;27(10):2649–55. https://doi.org/10.1007/s11695-017-2693-7.
21. Grubnik VV, Ospanov OB, Namaeva KA, Medvedev OV, Kresyun MS. Randomized controlled trial comparing laparoscopic greater curvature plication versus laparoscopic sleeve gastrectomy. *Surg Endosc.* 2016;30(6): 2186-2191. https://doi.org/10.1007/s00464-015-4373-9.
22. Carrano FM, Peev MP, Saunders JK, et al. The role of minimally invasive and endoscopic technologies in morbid obesity treatment: review and critical appraisal of the current clinical practice. *Obes Surg.* 2019;30(2):736-752. https://doi.org/10.1007/s11695-019-04302-8.
23. Sjöström L, Narbro K, Sjöström CD, et al. "Swedish Obese Subjects Study. Effects of bariatric surgery on mortality in Swedish obese subjects." *New England Journal of Medicine.* 2007 Aug 23;357(8):741-52. doi:10.1056/NEJMoa066254. PMID: 17715408.
24. Mor A, Sharp L, Portenier D, Sudan R, Torquati A. Weight loss at the first postoperative visit predicts long term outcome of Roux-en-Y gastric bypass using the Duke weight loss surgery chart. *Surg Obes Rel Dis.* 2012;8(5):556-560. https://doi.org/10.1016/j.soard.2012.06.014.
25. Wolter S, Dupree A, Miro J, et al. Upper gastrointestinal endoscopy prior to bariatric surgery-mandatory or expendable? An analysis of 801 cases. *Obes Surg.* 2017;27(8): 1938-1943. https://doi.org/10.1007/s11695-017-2622-9.
26. Lopez-Nava G, Asokkumar R, Turró Arau R, Galvao Neto M, Abu Dayyeh B. Modified primary obesity surgery endoluminal (POSE-2) procedure for the treatment of obesity. *VideoGIE.* 2020;5(3):91-93. https://doi.org/10.1016/j.vgie.2019.11.010.

15

Gastric Aspiration as a Bariatric Procedure

Geoffrey S. Chow, MD

A 48-year-old male with a history of hypertension and a body mass index (BMI) of 39 kg/m^2 is referred for surgical consultation regarding endoscopic treatment for morbid obesity. The patient has seen a dietician and internist, who assessed that the patient was an appropriate candidate for a bariatric intervention. The patient is most interested in gastric aspiration therapy using the AspireAssist®.

1. Regarding AspireAssist® therapy, which of the following is correct?

A. A majority of patients require hospitalization for one night.
B. Successful tube placement occurs in more than 95% of patients.
C. Periprocedural mortality rates are higher than for other bariatric interventions.
D. A large amount of tension on the tube is required to ensure proper positioning.

2. Regarding the outcomes of patients undergoing gastric aspiration therapy, which of the following is correct?

A. The average total body weight loss at 1 year is 10%.
B. 75% of patients will discontinue all diabetic medications.
C. Clinically significant electrolyte abnormalities are rare with supervised gastric aspiration therapy.
D. Dehydration requiring hospital admission occurs in 15% of patients.

3. Regarding the proper use of gastric aspiration therapy, which of the following is correct?

A. Aspiration therapy should be used once a day.
B. The aspiration function should start between 20 and 30 minutes after a meal.
C. The best patient outcomes are observed with 4 to 5 uses per day.
D. Optimal outcomes are achieved if the starting HbA1c is >9.5%.

4. Which of the following is a contraindication for gastric aspiration therapy?

A. Prior gastrostomy tube placement
B. Upcoming need for magnetic resonance imaging (MRI) testing
C. Prior Roux-en-Y gastric bypass (RYGB)
D. Gastroesophageal reflux disease

ANSWERS

1. B. The AspireAssist® was approved by the Food and Drug Administration (FDA) in 2016 for the treatment of obesity in patients aged 22 or older with a BMI of 35 to 55 kg/m^2. Data utilized at that point demonstrated greater body weight loss with combined device and lifestyle therapy than with lifestyle therapy alone. Both groups also demonstrated improvement in hypertension, diabetes, and quality of life. The device consists of a modified gastrostomy tube with a segment of tubing that extends into the gastric lumen beyond the internal bumper (Figure 15-1). The device is placed using an upper endoscope and pull gastrostomy tube placement technique. This is performed under sedation or general anesthesia, as deemed appropriate by the

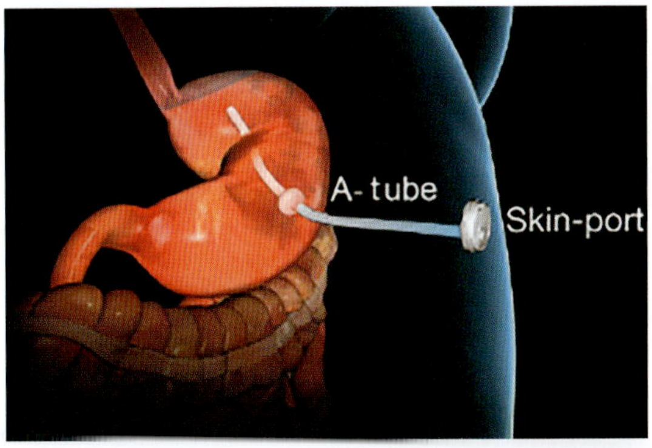

Figure 15-1 Gastric tube with extension into lumen.

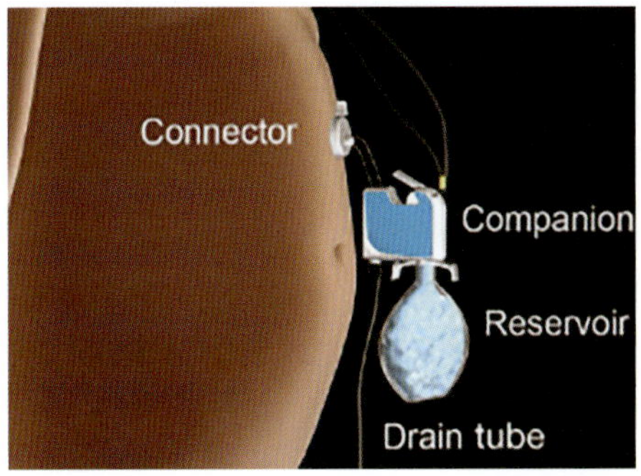

Figure 15-2 External reservoir to evacuate gastric contents.

surgeon, and almost all cases are performed on an outpatient basis.

Successful tube placement rates range from 95% to 97% success, and periprocedural complications include those associated with gastrostomy tube placement.[5] Precautions should be observed to avoid transcolonic puncture. Mortality rates are low, and multiple studies demonstrated 0% procedure-associated mortality.[2] In placement of the external bumper, care should be taken to ensure that there is no excess tension on the tubing, as this is associated with tube migration, malfunction, and risk of buried bumper syndrome. Early tube dislodgement can present with peritonitis that may require surgical intervention.

2. **C.** At a range of 1 to 4 years with intensive medical therapy, dietary consultation, and correct device usage, total excess body weight loss ranges from 14% to 21%.[1,3-5] In patients with diabetes, up to 60% of patients can have a decrease or eliminate medication for diabetes altogether at 1 year, and the average decrease in HbA1c is 1%.[3] The most common cause for postprocedural admission is peritonitis related to tube insertion, and this often presents in the first 2 weeks after tube placement. The rate of dehydration is reported to be low, and patients are instructed to empty gastric contents and then immediately instill drinking water into the stomach from the reservoir attached to the device (Figure 15-2). At 1-year follow-up, the majority of patients have normal electrolyte panel. If patients use this therapy more than recommended, hypokalemia can be observed. With continued monitoring and close follow up, clinically significant electrolyte abnormalities are rare.[5]

3. **B.** The trials evaluating outcomes of the device have utilized gastric aspiration in conjunction with intensive dietary and lifestyle modification, with a long-term goal of modifying eating habits and behavior. Patients are instructed to use the tube after each meal, and average initial daily use ranges from 2 to 3 times a day.[1,2] Increased use may be associated with maladaptive behavior and place patients at risk of increase psychological morbidity. The safety and efficacy of the device has not been tested in patients with HbA1c >9.5. Occlusion of the luminal portion of the tube with multiple side holes can occur, and patients are instructed to chew food to < 6 mm size and start aspiration therapy 20 to 30 minutes after completion of a meal.

4. **C.** Contraindications for device placement include situations where percutaneous gastrostomy is not safe or technically possible. Prior gastrostomy tube placement, along with gastroesophageal reflux, does not preclude placement. The device does not have any ferromagnetic materials and is MRI compatible. Device placement is contraindicated in patients with end-stage liver or renal disease, and it should not be placed in patients with bulimia or at risk of developing an eating disorder.[4,5] A detailed surgical history should be taken prior to device placement, and certain prior abdominal surgeries would not allow usage of this device. Patients who have undergone an RYGB would not be a candidate for placement of this device.

REFERENCES

1. Khan Z, Khan MA, Hajifathalian K, et al. Efficacy of endoscopic interventions for the management of obesity: a

meta-analysis to compare endoscopic sleeve gastroplasty, AspireAssist, and primary obesity surgery endolumenal. *Obes Surg*. 2019;29:2287-2298.

2. Norén E, Forssell H. Aspiration therapy for obesity; a safe and effective treatment. *BMC Obes*. 2016;3:56. https://doi.org/10.1186/s40608-016-0134-0.
3. Nyström M, Machytka E, Norén E, et al. Aspiration therapy as a tool to treat obesity: 1- to 4-year results in a 201-patient multi-center post-market European registry study. *Obes Surg*. 2018;28:1860-1868.
4. Sullivan S, Stein R, Jonnalagadda S, et al. Aspiration therapy leads to weight loss in obese subjects: a pilot study. *Gastroenterology*. 2013;145(6):1245-1252 e1-5.
5. Thompson CC, Abu Dayyeh BK, Kushner V, et al. Aspiration therapy for the treatment of obesity: 4-year results of a multicenter randomized controlled trial. *Surg Obes Relat Dis*. 2019;15(8):1348-1354.

16

Endobarrier

Zhamak Khorgami, MD

A 49-year-old male with obesity and a body mass index (BMI) of 43 kg/m^2 is interested in having an intervention for weight loss. He has hypertension and type 2 diabetes mellitus treated by metformin, and his last HbA1C was 8%. He has a history of a laparoscopic appendectomy and an open cholecystectomy. After a discussion about Roux-en-Y gastric bypass (RYGB) and sleeve gastrectomy (SG), he asks about recent research on less invasive options. He shows interest in the Endobarrier device, which is a duodenal-jejunal bypass liner (DJBL).

1. What is the best description of a DJBL?

A. A 60-cm sleeve anchored to the first portion of the duodenum
B. A 60-cm sleeve anchored to the pylorus
C. A 120-cm sleeve anchored to the gastroesophageal junction
D. A 120-cm sleeve anchored to the first portion of the duodenum

2. What is the direct mechanism of action of a DJBL?

A. Bypassing the upper part of the small intestine as a physical barrier
B. Modulation of enteric hormones
C. Changes in bile acids
D. Changing in the gut microbiota composition

3. How effective is DJBL in controlling diabetes mellitus?

A. Will decrease HbA1c significantly, but it will return to baseline within weeks after explantation
B. Will decrease HbA1c significantly, even after explantation
C. Will decrease HbA1c significantly, but it may increase close to the baseline level 1 year after explantation
D. Will cause significant weight loss, but with no significant effect on diabetes mellitus

4. What is the most common cause of the early removal of a DJBL?

A. Patient intolerance
B. Migration
C. Gastrointestinal bleeding
D. Perforation

5. What is the most common serious adverse event after the placement of a DJBL?

A. Liver abscess
B. Bleeding
C. Hypoglycemia
D. Acute pancreatitis
E. Migration

6. Which of the following is true regarding the DJBL as a weight loss option is this patient?

A. This is an approved alternative and can control his obesity and comorbidities.
B. This is a preferred option for this patient due to his prior abdominal surgeries.
C. Endobarrier is contraindicated in this patient due to his class III obesity.
D. Endobarrier is an investigational procedure in the US and can be done as part of a clinical trial.

ANSWERS

1. **A.** The DJBL is an intraluminal liner composed of a 60-cm thin, flexible, tube-shaped liner (Endobarrier, manufactured by GI Dynamics, Lexington, Massachusetts). This device has self-expanding metallic anchors with barbs (made of nitinol) and can be secured in the duodenal bulb (Figure 16-1). The Endobarrier is placed endoscopically. Its anchor has a drawstring to facilitate endoscopic removal of the device after the treatment period (Figure 16-2). This device should be considered in referral centers with an experienced and trained bariatric surgeon or gastroenterologist to perform the procedure, and with available surgical services.[1] This device is removed endoscopically, usually not later than 12 months after implantation.

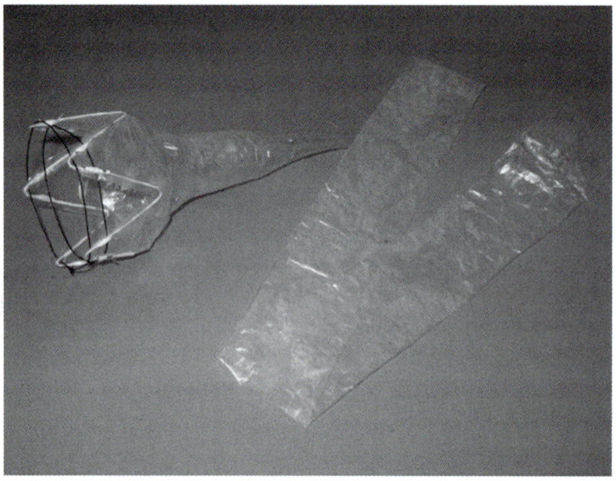

Figure 16-1 Endobarrier, a medical device for treatment of obesity and metabolic disorders, made of an impermeable fluoropolymer sleeve (60 cm), a nitinol anchor, and a drawstring for removal. (Reproduced with permission from Schouten R, Rijs CS, Bouvy ND, et al: A multicenter, randomized efficacy study of the EndoBarrier Gastrointestinal Liner for presurgical weight loss prior to bariatric surgery. *Ann Surg*. 2010;251(2):236-243.)

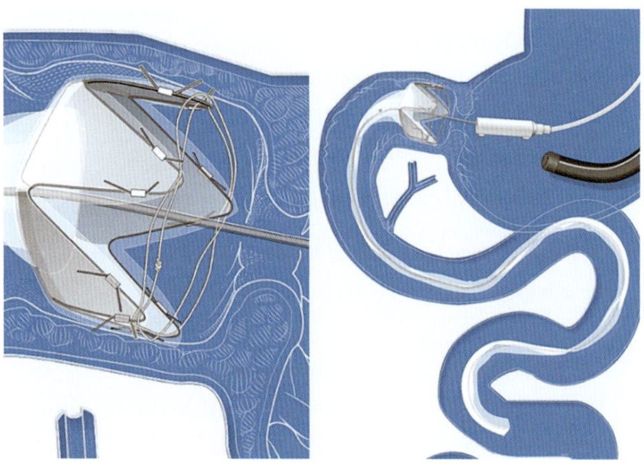

Figure 16-2 Endobarrier, placed endoscopically, and a nitinol anchor with barbs located in the duodenal bulb. EndoBarrier currently is for Investigational Use Only. (Reproduced with permission from GI Dynamics. Boston, MA.)

Another similar device is the gastro-duodeno-jejunal bypass sleeve (GJBS). This device (manufactured by ValenTx, Hopkins, Minnesota) is a 120-cm-long sleeve that is implanted in the gastroesophageal junction and bypasses the stomach, duodenum, and proximal jejunum). It is placed through a mixed endoscopic-laparoscopic technique and can be removed endoscopically. Sandler et al reported a prospective, single-center, 12-month trial showing a mean percentage excess weight loss of 54% at 1 year in 10 patients receiving a GJBS.[1,2]

Both DJBL and GJBS mimick the mechanisms of the RYGB by covering the proximal part of the small intestine and inducing hypoabsorption. There are limited data on these procedures, and they are still being investigated in the United States. These procedures may be considered for treating class I obesity, especially with diabetes mellitus that is difficult to control, in patients with morbid obesity and surgical contraindications, or for weight loss prior to bariatric surgery.[3]

2. **A.** Several potential mechanisms of action have been suggested for DJBL; however, bypassing the upper part of the small intestine by a sleeve barrier is the direct mechanism, and all other changes can be a result of this action. This device creates an internal barrier between the intestinal wall and the chyme. The pancreatic secretions and bile can run along the outside of the sleeve and are mixed with ingested food in the jejunum at the end of the sleeve. Other changes include modulation of enteric hormones, changes in bile and pancreatic secretions, and changes in the gut microbiota.[4] In one study, de Jonge et al looked at 17 obese patients with type 2 diabetes mellitus after DJBL. After 1 week, they showed decreased fasting and postprandial glucose levels, increased postprandial glucagon-like peptide-1 (GLP-1) level, and correction of abnormal glucagon peak following meal ingestion.[5] Evaluation of intestinal microbiota has shown an increase in typical small intestinal bacteria (*Proteobacteria, Veillonella,* and *Lactobacillus spp.*) following DJBL, and this changed back to baseline after removal of the device.[6] In another paper, van Nierop et al studied 17 obese diabetic patients after DJBL and found a significant profound increase in

unconjugated bile acid levels 24 weeks after DJBL placement, which is similar to effects of SG and RYGB.[7]

3. **C.** Multiple studies have evaluated the effect of DJBL on diabetes mellitus and showed significant improvement of diabetes mellitus markers. Jirapino et al performed a meta-analysis of 17 published studies assessing the outcomes of DJBL in obese patients with type 2 diabetes mellitus. At explantation, HbA1c was 1.3% lower and HOMA-IR was 4.6 lower than baseline. Six studies followed patients after the explantation of DJBL. Two studies with a total of 46 patients reported that the HgbA1c 3 months after explantation was significantly lower than the baseline by 2.2% ($P<0.001$). Four studies with a combined total of 120 patients followed patients for up to 6 months after the removal of DJBL and reported that HbA1c remained significantly lower than the baseline level (0.9%, $P<0.001$). By 1 year after explantation, there appears to be no difference in HgbA1c compared to the baseline level.[8] Based on this meta-analysis, control of HbA1c remains significantly lower after the explantation of DJBL for up to 6 months, but it may increase close to the baseline level 1 year after explantation.

4. **A.** Minor abdominal discomfort and nausea are the most common adverse events after the placement of DJBL. These are frequent in the first 2 weeks after implantation and can result in intolerance and early removal of the device. Betzel et al reported the early removal of DJBL due to intolerance in 18% of 185 patients with successful DJBL placement. This study also reported a number of serious device-related adverse events, which required hospitalization. Those included gastrointestinal bleeding, perforation of the anchor next to the pylorus into the stomach, the anchor being affixed in the duodenal bulb due to tissue overgrowth, ulceration and stenosis of the duodenal bulb by a distally migrated anchor, bowel obstruction, intussusception of the small intestine, acute pancreatitis, liver abscess, duodenitis, and esophageal perforation during explantation.[9]

5. **B.** Jirapino et al reported serious adverse events based on a meta-analysis of nine studies. Out of 350 DJBL cases, serious adverse events occurred in 55 patients (15.7%). The most common serious complication was gastrointestinal bleeding in 16 patients (4.6%). Other common serious adverse events included hypoglycemic events, acute pancreatitis, sleeve migration, severe abdominal pain, and liver abscesses.[8]

6. **D.** The DJBL is not approved for use in the United States. This device is on the market in Europe, Australia, and South America, but it is only being investigated in the United States and clinical trials are recruiting patients for the study.[10] This patient's prior abdominal surgeries (appendectomy and cholecystectomy) will not increase the risk of common bariatric surgery and not a reason for nonsurgical preference. The DJBLis being investigated in patients with BMI ≥ 30 kg/m^2 and ≤ 50 kg/m^2 and is not contraindicated in patients with class III obesity.

REFERENCES

1. Espinet-Coll E, Nebreda-Durán J, Gómez-Valero JA, et al. Current endoscopic techniques in the treatment of obesity. *Rev Esp Enferm Dig*. 2012;104(2):72-87.
2. Sandler BJ, Rumbaut R, Swain CP, et al. One-year human experience with a novel endoluminal, endoscopic gastric bypass sleeve for morbid obesity. *Surg Endosc*. 2015;29(11):3298-3303.
3. Schouten R, Rijs CS, Bouvy ND, et al. A multicenter, randomized efficacy study of the EndoBarrier gastrointestinal liner for presurgical weight loss prior to bariatric surgery. *Ann Surg*. 2010;251(2):236-243.
4. Ruban A, Ashrafian H, Teare JP. The EndoBarrier: Duodenal-jejunal bypass liner for diabetes and weight loss. *Gastroenterol Res Pract*. 2018;2018:7823182.
5. de Jonge C, Rensen SS, Verdam FJ, et al. Endoscopic duodenal-jejunal bypass liner rapidly improves type 2 diabetes. *Obes Surg*. 2013;23(9):1354-1360.
6. de Jonge C, Fuentes S, Zoetendal EG, et al. Metabolic improvement in obese patients after duodenal-jejunal exclusion is associated with intestinal microbiota composition changes. *Int J Obes (Lond)*. 2019;43(12):2509-2517.
7. van Nierop FS, de Jonge C, Kulik W, et al. Duodenal-jejunal lining increases postprandial unconjugated bile acid responses and disrupts the bile acid-FXR-FGF19 axis in humans. *Metabolism*. 2019;93:25-32.
8. Jirapinyo P, Haas AV, Thompson CC. Effect of the duodenal-jejunal bypass liner on glycemic control in patients with type 2 diabetes with obesity: a meta-analysis with secondary analysis on weight loss and hormonal changes. *Diabetes Care*. 2018;41(5):1106-1115.
9. Betzel B, Homan J, Aarts EO, et al. Weight reduction and improvement in diabetes by the duodenal-jejunal bypass liner: a 198 patient cohort study. *Surg Endosc*. 2017;31(7):2881-2891.
10. The American Society for Metabolic and Bariatric Surgery. GI Dynamics Endobarrier. Accessed March 26, 2020, from https://asmbs.org/emerging-technologies-inventory/gi-dynamics-endobarrier.

SECTION 4

Surgical

17

Indications for Surgical Management of Obesity: Metabolic and Bariatric Surgery Examination and Board Review

Jordan D. Bohnen, MD, MBA, and Ozanan R. Meireles, MD

A 37-year-old female with class II obesity, obstructive sleep apnea (OSA), gastroesophageal reflux disease (GERD), and diabetes mellitus presents for surgical evaluation at your hospital's weight loss center. She is 165 cm tall and weighs 102 kg. Her body mass index (BMI) is 37.4 kg/m^2. She has struggled with her weight since college, losing up to 7 to 9 kg on several prior occasions with diet and exercise but regaining it each time. She admits periods of depression related to her weight and is eager to discuss weight loss surgery options. She is interested in sleeve gastrectomy (SG) and adjustable gastric banding (AGB), but opposes the Roux-en-Y gastric bypass (RYGB) due to its perceived higher complication rate.

1. **Which of the following is required to be considered for surgery?**
   A. At least class II obesity
   B. Documented attempts of physician-supervised medical weight loss
   C. Endoscopy
   D. Evaluation by a bariatrician
   E. No psychiatric illness

2. **Regarding the medical and surgical management of obesity, which of the following statements is most accurate?**
   A. Sustained weight loss can be expected at least 10 years following bariatric surgery.
   B. In patients with type 2 diabetes mellitus, expected postoperative weight loss is equivalent between RYGB and SG.
   C. Long-term complication rates are higher after RYGB compared to AGB.
   D. Prior foregut surgery is a contraindication to bariatric surgery.
   E. End-stage heart failure is a contraindication to bariatric surgery.

3. **Your patient enquires about her 17-year-old daughter, who also suffers from obesity (BMI 41.3 kg/m^2) and OSA, and has seen an inability to lose weight despite several prior attempts. Which of the following is correct regarding the surgical management of adolescent patients (i.e., ages 10–19) with obesity?**
   A. Bariatric surgery is contraindicated.
   B. Bariatric surgery should be considered only in adolescents who have gone through puberty.
   C. Adolescents with BMI $\geq$40 kg/m^2 must try a course of weight loss medication prior to being considered for bariatric surgery.
   D. BMI $\geq$40 kg/m^2 is an indication for bariatric surgery in adolescent patients.
   E. Bariatric surgery is indicated only in "super obese" (i.e. BMI $\geq$50 kg/m^2) adolescent patients.

4. Regarding the pros and cons of RYGB versus SG, which of the following statements is true?

A. Internal hernia rates are similar over 10 years.
B. SG is superior for treating long-term remission of type 2 diabetes mellitus.
C. RYGB is superior for remission of GERD.
D. The risk of developing gallstones is less after SG.
E. Postoperative bleeding following SG tends to require more reoperations.

ANSWERS

1. B. It is generally accepted that patients in the United States must meet the following criteria to be eligible for bariatric surgery: BMI $\geq$ 40 kg/m^2 or >45 kg overweight, *or* BMI $\geq$ 35 kg/m^2 with one or more obesity-related medical comorbidities, such as type 2 diabetes mellitus, hypertension, hyperlipidemia, OSA or other respiratory disorders, nonalcoholic fatty liver disease (NAFLD), osteoarthritis, gastrointestinal disorders, and/or heart disease. Patients with BMI of 30 to 35 kg/m^2 with difficult-to-control type 2 diabetes mellitus or dysmetabolic syndrome X are also considered candidates for surgery. In addition, patients must demonstrate an inability to achieve sustained weight loss with previous physician-supervised weight loss attempts. While this is recommended, it is also loosely defined. Documentation in the patient's medical record by referring physicians will suffice. These criteria are endorsed by the American Society for Metabolic and Bariatric Surgery (ASMBS),[1] as well as the National Institute of Diabetes and Digestive and Kidney Diseases (NIDDK), a part of the National Institutes of Health (NIH).[2] Several other societies, including the American Heart Association (AHA), American College of Cardiology, and The Obesity Society (TOS) endorse referral to a bariatric surgeon for patients who meet these criteria and are motivated to lose weight.[3] While surgeons should always exercise their best judgment before taking a patient to the operating room, patients who fail to meet these criteria are unlikely to be candidates for bariatric surgery or to obtain insurance approval for weight loss procedures. Medical comorbidities are common in the bariatric patient population, as listed here. Note that there are many other conditions that are caused by obesity, such as polycystic ovarian syndrome and stress urinary incontinence, or worsened by it, such as abdominal wall hernias, GERD, and venous stasis disease. While these comorbidities often increase the risk profile of a patient undergoing surgery, they are not contraindications. In many cases, obesity-related comorbidities can be expected to improve after bariatric surgery.[4,5]

Patients being considered for bariatric surgery must be motivated to lose weight and must undergo preoperative assessment by a multidisciplinary team, ideally within a center that meets ASMBS-approved quality standards as outlined by the Metabolic and Bariatric Surgery Accreditation and Quality Improvement Program (MBSAQIP).[1,6] Preoperative clearance typically requires a detailed assessment by a mental health professional to ensure that the patient is psychologically stable to undergo surgery and can manage the lifestyle changes required in the perioperative setting. Having an Axis I or Axis II psychologic disorder by itself, however, is not a contraindication to surgery. In addition, assessment by a registered dietician ensures that the patient understands and can manage the significant dietary changes required of bariatric surgery patients.[7] It is noteworthy that mental health conditions including clinically significant depression and anxiety and disordered eating are common in obese patients, and therefore they must be properly addressed as part of a comprehensive bariatric surgery workup. Some patients may be seen by an obesity medicine specialist (i.e., an internist or a bariatrician) for preoperative discussion and/or consideration of nonsurgical weight loss options including lifestyle modifications and pharmacotherapy; however, this is not a requirement. Similarly, preoperative endoscopy is not mandatory for routine bariatric surgery patients.

2. A. Bariatric surgery has been repeatedly shown to produce sustained weight loss beyond 10 years after surgery. In contrast, fewer than 5% of patients with a BMI >40 kg/m^2, are able to achieve sustained weight loss to a BMI <35 kg/m^2 with medical management alone.[7–9] The landmark Swedish Obese Subjects (SOS) study compared long-term outcomes of medical versus surgical management for morbid obesity in a cohort of >4,000 morbidly obese patients with diabetes; in this trial, patients undergoing bariatric surgery sustained an average weight loss of 18% body weight 15 years after surgery, while patients in the medical control group averaged 1% sustained weight loss.[9] This trial also highlighted the superior efficacy of bariatric surgery versus medical management in reducing mortality and cardiovascular event rates.

SG and RYGB are the most common weight loss operations performed today, and both procedures result in substantial and sustained weight loss.[10,11] This observation remains true in patients with obesity and type 2 diabetes mellitus.[12,13] A recent study by McTigue et al. demonstrated 5-year total weight loss of 24.1% following RYGB versus 16.1% following SG for patients with obesity and type 2 diabetes, a difference of 10.2 kg (95% CI: 8.3–12.1 kg, $p < 0.001$) between procedure groups.[13] Laparoscopic adjustable gastric band procedures (LAGB), which were common in the 2000s and early 2010s, have demonstrated unsatisfactory long-term complication rates, including higher complication rates than RYGB without the same benefits.[5] One study with long-term (>12-year follow-up) outcomes of LAGB demonstrated a 39% rate of long-term major complications (e.g., pouch dilation, band erosion), 60% rate of reoperation (i.e., for complications or weight issues), and 50% rate of band removal.[14] Neither prior foregut surgery nor end-stage heart failure is an absolute contraindication to bariatric surgery. Prior foregut surgery may increase the intraoperative risk during a bariatric procedure and should be managed by an experienced surgeon. In patients with end-stage heart failure, BMI ≥35 is often considered a contraindication to heart transplant; bariatric surgery has been used successfully alongside ventricular assist device (VAD) placement as a bridge to heart transplant in appropriately selected patients.[15,16] It is important to note that patients with heart failure should be appropriately optimized prior to consideration of bariatric surgery.

3. **D.** Obesity is common among adolescents (i.e., age 10–19), and some adolescents with obesity may qualify for bariatric surgery. Guidelines for bariatric surgery in adolescent patient populations have been developed by the ASMBS and endorsed by the Society of American Gastrointestinal and Endoscopic Surgeons. An adolescent patient must meet one of the following two criteria to be eligible for bariatric surgery:
   a. *BMI ≥35 kg/m² or 120% of the 95th percentile of BMI for age* ***and*** *one or more clinically significant obesity-related comorbidities* [e.g., OSA, type 2 diabetes mellitus, idiopathic intracranial hypertension, nonalcoholic steatohepatitis, Blount's disease, slipped capital femoral epiphysis (SCFE), GERD, hypertension].
   b. *BMI ≥40 kg/m² or 140% of the 95th percentile of BMI for age.*[17]

   Puberty status and physical maturation alone does not determine one's candidacy either for or against bariatric surgery in this patient population. Note that diseases like slipped capital femoral epiphysis (SCFE) will likely not improve without bariatric surgery. If the patient otherwise meets this criterion and does not have any significant medical, behavioral, or cognitive contraindications to surgery, they can be considered candidates regardless of their physical development. Patients who meet this criterion are not obligated to try a course of weight loss medication before pursuing bariatric surgery. Adolescents undergoing bariatric surgery should receive their care at an MBSAQIP-accredited center meeting prespecified "Adolescent Qualifications," including case volume thresholds, multidisciplinary representation by clinical specialists with expertise in the care of pediatric and adolescent patients with obesity, and a successful performance during a site visit.[6] The behavioral component can often be the most challenging aspect because it involves the family's attitudes toward weight loss as well.

4. **C.** RYGB is superior to SG for management of GERD. Specifically, remission of GERD occurs more frequently after RYGB and GERD worsens more commonly after SG.[18]

   Internal hernia is generally considered a complication of RYGB, but not SG; this is a function of the intestinal rearrangement in RYGB with resulting mesenteric defects that increase the risk of internal hernia formation any time after RYGB. Several studies have investigated remission rates for type 2 diabetes mellitus following SG and RYGB. On the whole, SG is at least as good as RYGB for remission of type 2 diabetes, and in many studies, RYGB significantly outperforms SG for patients with type 2 diabetes. The risk of developing gallstones is known to increase after RYGB and SG.[19] Rapid weight loss during the first 6 to 12 months after surgery has been proposed as a key risk factor for development of gallstones after bariatric surgery, although there are conflicting data regarding the underlying mechanism. One procedure is not superior over the other for gallstone development. Postoperative bleeding following both SG and RYGB usually occurs at the staple lines and is self-limited. Patients should be monitored closely with serial labs and transfusion as necessary. In rare circumstances, postoperative bleeding after SG or RYGB requires reoperation.

REFERENCES

1. American Society for Metabolic and Bariatric Surgery (ASMBS). Who is a candidate for bariatric surgery? Accessed June 27, 2020, from https://asmbs.org/patients/who-is-a-candidate-for-bariatric-surgery#:~:text=BMI%20%E2%89%A5%2040%2C%20or%20more,gastrointestinal%20disorders%2C%20or%20heart%20disease.
2. National Institute of Diabetes and Digestive and Kidney Diseases (NIDDK). Potential candidates for bariatric surgery. Accessed June 27, 2020, from https://www.niddk.nih.gov/health-information/weight-management/bariatric-surgery/potential-candidates.
3. Jensen MD, Ryan DH, Apovian CM, et al. 2013 AHA/ACC/TOS guideline for the management of overweight and obesity in adults: a report of the American College of Cardiology/American Heart Association Task Force on Practice Guidelines and The Obesity Society. *Circulation.* 2014;129:S102-S138.
4. Schauer PR, Bhatt DL, Kirwan JP, et al. Bariatric surgery versus intensive medical therapy for diabetes—3-year outcomes. *N Engl J Med.* 2014;370(21):2002-2013.
5. Puzziferri N, Roshek TB, Mayo HG, et al. Long-term follow-up after bariatric surgery: a systematic review. *JAMA.* 2014;312(9):934-942.
6. Metabolic and Bariatric Surgery Accreditation and Quality Improvement Program (MBSAQIP). *Standards Manual.* Accessed June 30, 2020, from https://www.facs.org/-/media/files/quality-programs/bariatric/2019_mbsaqip_standards_manual.ashx.
7. Richards WO. "Morbid Obesity." In: David Sabiston, ed. *Textbook of Surgery, 20th ed.* Elsevier; 2017:1160-1187.
8. O'Brien PE, Hindle A, Brennan L, et al. Long-term outcomes after bariatric surgery: a systematic review and meta-analysis of weight loss at 10 or more years for all bariatric procedures and a single-centre review of 20-year outcomes after adjustable gastric banding. *Obes Surg.* 2019;29(1):3-14.
9. Sjöström L, Narbro K, Sjöström CD, et al. Effects of bariatric surgery on mortality in Swedish obese subjects. *N Engl J Med.* 2007;357:741-752.
10. Li J, Lai D, Wu D. Laparoscopic Roux-en-Y gastric bypass versus laparoscopic sleeve gastrectomy to treat morbid obesity-related comorbidities: a systematic review and meta-analysis. *Obes Surg.* 2016;26(2):429-442.
11. Salminen P, Helmiö M, Ovaska J, et al. Effect of laparoscopic sleeve gastrectomy vs laparoscopic Roux-en-Y gastric bypass on weight loss at 5 years among patients with morbid obesity: the SLEEVEPASS randomized clinical trial. *JAMA.* 2018;319(3):241-254.
12. Schauer PR, Bhatt DL, Kirwan JP, et al. Bariatric surgery versus intensive medical therapy for diabetes—5-year outcomes. *N Engl J Med.* 2017;376(7):641-651.
13. McTigue KM, Wellman R, Nauman E, et al. Comparing the 5-year diabetes outcomes of sleeve gastrectomy and gastric bypass: the National Patient-Centered Clinical Research Network (PCORNet) bariatric study. *JAMA Surg.* 2020. [Epub ahead of print]
14. Himpens J, Cadière GB, Bazi M, et al. Long-term outcomes of laparoscopic adjustable gastric banding. *Arch Surg.* 2011;146(7):802-807.
15. Shah SK, Gregoric ID, Nathan SS, et al. Simultaneous left ventricular assist device placement and laparoscopic sleeve gastrectomy as a bridge to transplant for morbidly obese patients with severe heart failure. *J Heart Lung Transplant.* 2015;34(11):1489-1491.
16. Hawkins RB, Go K, Raymond SL, et al. Laparoscopic sleeve gastrectomy in patients with heart failure and left ventricular assist devices as a bridge to transplant. *Surg Obes Relat Dis.* 2018;14(9):1269-1273.
17. Pratt JSA, Browne A, Browne NT, et al. ASMBS pediatric metabolic and bariatric surgery guidelines, 2018. *Surg Obes Relat Dis.* 2018;14(7):882-901.
18. Peterli R, Wölnerhanssen BK, Peters T, et al. Effect of laparoscopic sleeve gastrectomy vs laparoscopic Roux-en-Y gastric bypass on weight loss in patients with morbid obesity: The SM-BOSS randomized clinical trial. *JAMA.* 2018;319(3):255-265.
19. Coupaye M, Castel B, Sami O, et al. Comparison of the incidence of cholelithiasis after sleeve gastrectomy and Roux-en-Y gastric bypass in obese patients: a prospective study. *Surg Obes Relat Dis.* 2015;11(4):779-784.

18

Bariatric Surgery in Pediatric Patients

Janey S. A. Pratt, MD, FACS, FASMBS

You are seeing an 11-year-old boy with severe pediatric obesity. His body mass index (BMI) is 39.5 kg/m^2 or 160% of the 95th percentile. He has sleep apnea with an apnea hypopnea index (AHI) of 26 and has already undergone a tonsil and adenoidectomy, with mild improvement to an AHI of 15. He has significant difficulty tolerating the continuous positive airway pressure (CPAP) mask. He has attention deficit hyperactivity disorder (ADHD) and autism spectrum disorder (ASD). He was bullied at school so much that just this year, he started homeschooling instead. He comes with his mother for consideration of metabolic and bariatric surgery.

1. **The patient's mother reports a history of him being overweight since 2 years old. Which findings might suggest a syndromic obesity like Prader-Willi syndrome (PWS) or Bardet-Biedl syndrome (BBS)?**
   A. Very high IQ reading at a level above his grade.
   B. Hyperphagia
   C. Height at the 95th percentile for his age.
   D. Morning headaches
   E. Dark skin around his neck

2. **On a physical exam, you find acanthosis nigrans on the patient's neck and near his umbilicus. Which of the following comorbidities would you be most concerned about?**
   A. Slipped capital femoral epiphysis (SCFE)
   B. Idiopathic intracranial hypertension (pseudotumor cerebri)
   C. Insulin resistance and/or type 2 diabetes
   D. Hypothyroidism
   E. Obstructive sleep apnea (OSA)

3. **In your preoperative evaluation, which laboratory tests are most important to look at?**
   A. Hemoglobin A1c, thyroid, liver function tests
   B. Prealbumin, calcium, parathyroid hormone, albumin
   C. HLA B27, hepatitis screen, celiac panel
   D. Genetic testing
   E. Zinc, copper, and selenium levels

4. **In discussing surgery with the patient, he seems to understand that you are planning surgery, but he is very distractible during your conversation, and it is unclear if he understands the reason. Before scheduling surgery, ideally, who would you have this child evaluated by?**
   A. Child Life specialist
   B. Pulmonologist
   C. Occupational Therapist
   D. Ethics committee
   E. Endocrinologist

5. **Before surgery, you see the patient and his mother every month for 6 months. Over that time, he has stopped drinking soda, skipping meals, and snacking. He is eating smaller portions. His weight had dropped to a BMI of 32, or 134% of the 95th percentile, but it has been stable for the last few months. He is asking when he can get the surgery.**
   A. You decide not to operate because he no longer qualifies for surgery.
   B. With this patient, 134% of the 95th percentile is considered class II obesity in his age group, and

therefore you proceed with a sleeve gastrectomy (SG) as planned.

C. You continue to follow him for another 3 months to see if he will continue to lose weight.
D. You offer weight loss medications instead of surgery, as he no longer qualifies for surgery.
E. You tell him that he is now at a safe weight and should come back only if he gains weight again.

6. You perform an uncomplicated SG. In the postanestheisa care unit (PACU), the patient complains of worsening abdominal pain. He is tachycardic to 110, and his blood pressure is 180/90. You give him pain and antianxiety medications, and you bolus 1 liter. An hour later, his heart rate is 145 and his blood pressure is 100/65. He is very tender in the entire abdomen and very pale on exam. What is the next step in the management of this patient?

A. Send the patient to the floor.
B. Take an abdominal computed tomography (CT) scan with oral and intravenous (IV) contrast.
C. Bolus him with heparin and take a chest CT scan.
D. Take him back to the operating room.
E. Check upper gastrointestinal (UGI) swallow.

7. Six weeks after SG, your patient reports lethargy, nausea, vomiting, unstable gait, and double vision. Which of the following is the next best step in management?

A. Consult neuro-ophthalmology to rule out idiopathic intracranial hypertension (IIH)
B. Tell him to drink more and eat more salt, as his condition is likely due to low blood pressure from dehydration.
C. Test vitamin B6 and B12 and iron levels.
D. Test vitamin B1, start thiamine IV, and consult neurology.
E. Send for a repeat sleep study to see if his sleep apnea has resolved.

ANSWERS

1. B. Hyperphagia, secondary to persistent hunger, is very common in monogenic obesity like PWS.[1] Patients with syndromic obesity typically have intellectual delay and short stature, in addition to hyperphagia. Morning headache is a symptom associated with untreated sleep apnea or IIH (pseudotumor cerebri). Dark skin around the neck is acanthosis nigrans. Any child presenting with early-onset obesity should be considered for genetic testing to assess for syndromic or monogenic obesity. Metabolic and bariatric surgery may play a role in treating these patients, although early studies on gastric bypass had high complication rates and weight loss may not be as robust as in patients without genetic obesity. Complication rates are low and weight loss is significant using the SG in these patients.[2,3]

2. C. Acanthosis nigrans is a thickening and brown/black hyperpigmentation of the skin, usually around the posterior neck and in skin folds. It is associated with insulin resistance and type 2 diabetes. It is a direct result of high blood insulin levels, so it also can be caused by medications that increase circulating insulin. Many children presenting for obesity treatment have not been fully evaluated for complications of obesity. Pediatric bariatric programs should screen for sleep apnea, diabetes and thyroid disorders before proceeding to surgery. It is important to ask about visual changes and headaches and consult a neuro-opthamologist to assess for IIH. If diagnosed, it is one of the few indications for emergency metabolic and bariatric surgery and can save a patient's vision.[4] Slipped capital femoral epiphysis (SCFE) and Blount's disease are associated with obesity. These are both orthopedic complications caused by excess weight on growth plates. Metabolic and bariatric surgery should be considered early on in these patients as well. If patients complain of hip or knee pain or show signs of leg bowing, it is important to involve orthopedic surgery early.[5]

3. A. Assessing for diabetes, thyroid disease, and fatty liver disease is important in every patient, as often these conditions are undiagnosed. Significant abnormalities may require intervention preoperatively to ensure that the patient has a safe surgery. It is also possible that treatment for one of these underlying conditions might be adequate to treat this patient's obesity.[6] While many patients with obesity also suffer from malnutrition, prealbumin is not routinely required. Screening for arthritis, hepatitis, or celiac disease should be pursued only based on patient symptoms. Genetic testing should be performed if there is a history of obesity since early childhood, short stature, intellectual delay, family history, or other risk factors for monogenic obesity. While this may not change treatment plans, new targeted therapies are being developed, so knowing about a genetic cause may lead to important opportunities for novel therapies. Mineral deficiencies are very uncommon preoperatively, but they can develop over time after surgery. Checking zinc, copper, and selenium a year or two postoperatively may identify the need for improved supplementation, but there is no need to screen for these deficiencies in the preoperative period.[7]

4. **D.** An ethics committee consultation is recommended in cases where the child is unable to assent to surgery. The committee will consider the medical necessity of the operation and help define the risk versus benefit for this child and his family. The preoperative psychological evaluation should be completed first, to determine the patient's cognitive level and ability to understand the procedure. Often, ethics committees may recommend resources like child life professional, physical therapy, occupational therapy, or other hospital resources that can ease the inpatient stay and possibly improve outcomes.[8] Child Life professionals are people who specialize in making the child comfortable in the hospital. They may use toys, games, movies, animals and other tricks to help the child relax and feel at home. Physical therapists and behavior specialists can help children with obesity develop healthy habits related to sleep, eating and physical activity prior to metabolic and bariatric surgery. Pulmonology and endocrine consults should be considered based on physical findings, history, and test results. Obesity is a life-threatening disease, and metabolic and bariatric surgeries are the most effective treatments available today. Denial of treatment based on age or cognitive functioning should never occur. It is important to make sure that a child will be able to stay on a liquid diet for 2 weeks after surgery and also has the ability to drink adequate fluids and eat adequate protein. Having an understanding of the operation is no more important than it is for a patient who needs a tonsillectomy or a transplantation. However, when operating on children, it is important to take into consideration the readiness of the parents to create a supportive environment and provide the foods and vitamins that the child will need.

5. **B.** Recent changes in the definition of obesity and the criteria for pediatric metabolic and bariatric surgery have led experts to use the standard Centers for Disease Control and Prevention (CDC) growth curves both to define obesity and to determine a patient's eligibility for metabolic and bariatric surgery. The current guideline is any child with class II obesity (a BMI of 120% above the 95th percentile) and a comorbidity or class III obesity (a BMI of 140% above the 95th percentile). This patient could actually have a BMI of 29 kg/m^2 (120% above the 95th percentile) and still benefit from surgery due to his OSA.[9] The use of medications in class II–III obesity is usually recommended only for the treatment of inadequate weight loss after surgery; however, it may play a role in the treatment of patients with class I obesity (a BMI above the 95th percentile but less than 120% of the 95th percentile) and overweight (BMI ranging from the 85th to less than the 95th percentile), as well as in the treatment of patients with extreme obesity as a preoperative intervention.[10]

6. **D.** This is a case of acute postoperative bleeding; a return to the operating room should occur immediately. Most postop bleeds are from the staple line; postop hypertension may also lead to bleeding from the short gastric vessels. While many patients will stop bleeding spontaneously, in this case, returning to the operating room immediately is the best option. Postoperative leaks are exceedingly uncommon after SG before 1–2 weeks postop and usually do not present as acutely as this patient. If the patient were hemodynamically stable but reported severe abdominal pain and persistent tachycardia, then a CT through the lungs and upper abdomen with oral and IV contrast can assess for bleeding from a trocar site, short gastric vessels, or the staple line, as well as evaluate for a pulmonary embolism and a leak. Any patient following SG with persistent tachycardia should not be sent to the floor without a diagnosis.[11]

7. **D.** Symptoms described are consistent with Wernike's encephalopathy as a result of vitamin B1 (thiamine) deficiency. Other symptoms include memory loss and mental status changes. All bariatric surgery patients presenting with acute vomiting should have a thorough neurologic exam. Wernicke's encephalopathy can happen after any bariatric procedure, and as early at 4–6 weeks postop. Checking a preoperative vitamin B1 level and treating if it is low, as

well as supplementing with 50 mg of vitamin B1 daily for 6 months postoperatively, can decrease the risk of deficiency.[12] Treatment consists of vitamin B1 100 mg IV 3 times a day for the first few days then intramuscularly for a few weeks, followed by oral administration. It is important in the emergency setting to give thiamine early before administering IV glucose, which can induce acute Wernike's symptoms. As one repletes thiamine, sometimes magnesium levels can drop, so the patient should be followed and treated for the first few days.[13] It would be unlikely to see IIH develop after an SG. Patients with IIH usually present with headaches and visual changes before surgery and are significantly improved by 3 months postop. Patients with recurrent symptoms of postural hypotension may improve with increased salt intake. Anemia due to B12, B6, and/or iron deficiency is common after bariatric surgery, and it is more common in menstruating females. OSA may resolve 3 months after surgery in about 50% of cases, but resolves in over 80% of them at 6 months after surgery.[14]

REFERENCES

1. Huvenne H, Dubern B, Clément K, Poitou C. Rare genetic forms of obesity: clinical approach and current treatments in 2016. *Obes Facts*. 2016;9:158-173.
2. Iossa A, De Peppo F, Caccamo R, et al. Laparoscopic sleeve gastrectomy in adolescents with or without syndromic obesity: two years follow-up. *Eat Weight Disord.* 2018;23(4):479-486.
3. Alqahtani AR, Elahmedi M, Alqahtani YA. Bariatric surgery in monogenic and syndromic forms of obesity. *Semin Pediatr Surg*. 2014;23(1):37-42.
4. Sun WYL, Switzer NJ, Dang IT, et al. Idiopathic intracranial hypertension and bariatric surgery: a systematic review. *Can J Surg*. 2020;63(2):E123-E128.
5. Griggs CL, Perez NP, Chan MC, Pratt JS. Slipped capital femoral epiphysis and Blount disease as indicators for early metabolic surgical intervention. *Surg Obes Relat Dis*. 2019;15(10):1836-1841.
6. Pratt JSA, Roque SS, Valera R, Czepiel KS, Tsao DD, Stanford FC. Preoperative considerations for the pediatric patient undergoing metabolic and bariatric surgery. *Semin Pediatr Surg*. 2020;29(1):150890.
7. Pratt JSA, Browne A, Browne NT, et al. ASMBS pediatric metabolic and bariatric surgery guidelines, 2018. *Surg Obes Relat Dis*. 2018;14(7):882-901.
8. Pratt JSA, Browne A, Browne NT, et al. ASMBS pediatric metabolic and bariatric surgery guidelines, 2018. *Surg Obes Relat Dis*. 2018;14(7):882-901.
9. Armstrong SC, Bolling CF, Michalsky MP, Reichard KW, SECTION ON OBESITY, SECTION ON SURGERY. Pediatric metabolic and bariatric surgery: evidence, barriers, and best practices. *Pediatrics*. 2019;144(6):e20193223. https://doi.org/10.1542/peds.2019-3223.
10. Srivastava G, Fox CK, Kelly AS, et al. Clinical considerations regarding the use of obesity pharmacotherapy in adolescents with obesity. *Obesity*. 2019;27(2):190-204.
11. Mocanu V, Dang J, Ladak F, Switzer N, Birch DW, Karmali S. Predictors and outcomes of bleed after sleeve gastrectomy: an analysis of the MBSAQIP data registry. *Surg Obes Relat Dis*. 2019;15(10):1675-1681.
12. Armstrong-Javors A, Pratt J, Kharasch S. Wernicke encephalopathy in adolescents after bariatric surgery: case report and review. *Pediatrics*. 2016;138(6).
13. Sinha S, Kataria A, Kolla BP, Thusius N, Loukianova LL. Wernicke encephalopathy—clinical pearls. *Mayo Clin Proc*. 2019;94(6):1065-1072.
14. Alqahtani AR, Elahmedi MO, Al Qahtani A. Co-morbidity resolution in morbidly obese children and adolescents undergoing sleeve gastrectomy. *Surg Obes Relat Dis*. 2014;10(5):842-850.

19

Laparoscopic Sleeve Gastrectomy

Timothy Kelly, MD, and Marina Kurian, MD

A 35-year-old male presents to the bariatric surgery office for consultation. His body mass index (BMI) is 44 kg/m^2, and his comorbidities include hypertension, type II diabetes, and obstructive sleep apnea (OSA) treated with a continuous positive airway pressure (CPAP) machine. He is an active smoker. He is interested in the laparoscopic sleeve gastrectomy (LSG).

1. When comparing the LSG to the laparoscopic Roux-en-Y gastric bypass (RYGB), which of the following is correct?

A. Sleeve gastrectomy (SG) is more likely to resolve the patient's OSA.
B. SG is less likely to cause postoperative gastroesophageal reflux disease (GERD).
C. RYGB and SG show equivalent weight loss at 5 years.
D. RYGB has a higher diabetes remission rate with less relapse than SG.
E. SG has less 30-day mortality compared to RYGB.

2. With regard to the patient's comorbidities and the SG, which of the following is correct?

A. Hypertension predicts poor weight loss.
B. SG is likely to resolve hypertension at 5 years.
C. Dietary modification is equivalent for diabetes resolution.
D. Glucose levels no longer require monitoring after surgery.
E. Only gastric bypass is expected to improve the patient's OSA.

3. Which of the following statements is correct regarding management of the patient prior to undergoing SG?

A. All patients should be referred for an ultrasound screening to evaluate for liver disease.
B. The patient may proceed to SG without efforts at preprocedural glycemic control.
C. Surgery should be delayed in the event, a thyroid-stimulating hormone (TSH) screening that is positive for hypothyroidism .
D. The patient should be referred for an electrocardiogram (EKG) prior to undergoing surgery.
E. The patient should quit smoking 1 week prior to the procedure.

4. Regarding SG, when does maximum weight loss occur, on average?

A. 6 months
B. 1 year
C. 3 years
D. 5 years
E. 10 years

5. With regards to leaks after a SG, which of the following is true?

A. Leaks increase morbidity, but not mortality.
B. Most leaks occur in the first 48 hours after surgery.
C. Endoscopic interventions are useful in the initial management of leak.
D. The middle third of the stomach is the most common site of a leak.
E. RYGB leak rates are higher.

ANSWERS

1. **D.** In patients with diabetes, RYGB shows superior rates of diabetes remission and relapse.[1,2] Weight loss at 5 years is slightly better in patients undergoing RYGB.[3] SG may be more likely to lead to postoperative GERD. Also, 30-day mortality is similar between SG and RYGB. OSA is not more likely to resolve with SG.

2. **B.** SG has been demonstrated to improve the incidence of hypertension significantly. Most patients will see resolution or improvement of their hypertension after undergoing SG. There is no evidence that preoperative hypertension predicts poorer weight loss.[4] Dietary modification is inferior to bariatric surgery with regard to resolution of diabetes. Periopeative glucose levels should be monitored in patients with diabetes.[5] Both SG and RYGB will improve OSA.

3. **C.** A new diagnosis of hypothyroidism requires treatment prior to proceeding with bariatric surgery. All patients do not need to be routinely referred for liver ultrasound prior to surgery. Efforts should be made to optimize preoperative glycemic control prior to bariatric surgery.[5] Smoking should be stopped at least 8 weeks prior to surgery.

4. **B.** Multiple studies have shown that the maximum weight loss after SG occurs on average at about 1 year, with slow weight regain in subsequent years.[6,7]

5. **C.** Endoscopic interventions have shown promise in multiple studies for the initial management of leak.[10] Also, 50% of leaks occur more than 10 days postop. Most leaks occur in the proximal third of the stomach. A leak increases the patient's chance of mortality. Higher-BMI (>50 kg/m^2) patients have a higher risk of leak.[8,9] In general, the leak rate of RYGB is 0 to 1.7%, while that of SG is about 1% to 3%, making the overall rate of sleeve leaks equivalent to or greater than that of RYGB.

REFERENCES

1. McTigue KM, Wellman R, Nauman E, et al. Comparing the 5-year diabetes outcomes of sleeve gastrectomy and gastric bypass. *JAMA Surg*. 2020;155(5):e200087. doi:10.1001/jamasurg.2020.0087.
2. Shaor S, Saber AA. Long-term and midterm outcomes of laparoscopic sleeve gastrectomy versus Roux-en-Y gastric bypass: a systematic review and meta-analysis of comparative studies. *Surg Obes Relat Dis*. 2017;13(2):170-180.
3. Salminen P, Helmiö M, Ovaska J, et al. Effect of laparoscopic sleeve gastrectomy vs laparoscopic Roux-en-Y gastric bypass on weight loss at 5 years among patients with morbid obesity: the SLEEVEPASS randomized clinical trial. *JAMA*. 2018;319(3):241-254.
4. Graham C, Switzer N, Reso A, et al. Sleeve gastrectomy and hypertension: a systematic review of long-term outcomes. *Surg Endosc*. 2019;33(9):3001-3007.
5. Mechanick JI, Apovian C, Brethauer S, et al. Clinical practice guidelines for the perioperative nutrition, metabolic, and nonsurgical support of patients undergoing bariatric procedures—2019 update: cosponsored by American Association of Clinical Endocrinologists/American College of Endocrinology, The Obesity Society, American Society for Metabolic & Bariatric Surgery, Obesity Medicine Association, and American Society of Anesthesiologists—executive summary. *Surg Obes Relat Dis*. 2020;25(12):1346-1359.
6. Arterburn DE, Johnson E, Coleman KJ, et al. Weight outcomes of sleeve gastrectomy and gastric bypass compared to nonsurgical treatment. *Ann Surg*. 2020. doi:10.1097/SLA.0000000000003826.
7. Osland E, Yunus RM, Khan S, Memon B, Memon MA. Weight loss outcomes in laparoscopic vertical sleeve gastrectomy (LVSG) versus laparoscopic Roux-en-Y gastric bypass (LRYGB) procedures: a meta-analysis and systematic review of randomized controlled trials. *Surg Laparosc Endosc Percutan Tech*. 2017;27(1):8-18.
8. Hughes D, Hughes I, Khanna A. Management of staple line leaks following sleeve gastrectomy—a systematic review. *Obes Surg*. 2019;29(9):2759-2772.
9. Aurora AR, Khaitan L, Saber AA. Sleeve gastrectomy and the risk of leak: a systematic analysis of 4,888 patients. *Surg Endosc*. 2011;26(6):1509-1515.
10. Nedelcu M, Danan M, Noel P, et al. Surgical management for chronic leak following sleeve gastrectomy: review of literature. *Surg Obs Relat Dis*. 2019;15(10):1844-1849.

20

Laparoscopic Roux-En-Y Gastric Bypass

Kliment Bozhilov, MD, and Racquel Bueno, MD

A 38-year-old female with a body mass index (BMI) of 52 kg/m^2 suffered from weight-related comorbidities, including type 2 diabetes mellitus, hypertension, and hyperlipidemia. She has failed at multiple attempts to control her weight and comorbidities using nonsurgical modalities. She was evaluated by a comprehensive weight management program and determined to be an appropriate candidate for surgical management of her obesity. She opted for a laparoscopic Roux-en-Y gastric bypass (LRYGB).

1. **When constructing gastrojejunal anastomosis during a LRYGB, which operative technique has the lowest stricture rate?**

   A. A 25-mm circular stapled gastrojejunal anastomosis
   B. A linear stapled anastomosis
   C. A hand-sewn anastomosis
   D. Robot-assisted hand-sewn anastomosis

2. **Regarding LRGYB limb lengths, which of the following statements is correct?**

   A. The combined alimentary and biliopancreatic limb lengths should be >200 cm.
   B. Standard (130–150 cm) alimentary limb lengths (ALLs) are associated with greater EWL compared to shorter (40–100 cm) ALLs.
   C. An RYGB configuration with a common limb length of 100 cm and a variable ALL decreases the risk for postoperative nutritional deficiency.
   D. The biliopancreatic limb length should be 120 cm.

3. **Which of the following statements about the gastric pouch in an LRYGB is correct?**

   A. Larger gastric pouches have lower marginal ulcer rates.
   B. The optimal gastric pouch volume is 50 mL.
   C. The gastric pouch should be based vertically off the greater curvature.
   D. Larger gastric pouch sizes have poorer weight loss outcomes.

4. **One year after surgery, your patient reports to the emergency room (ER) with nausea, vomiting, and abdominal pain. A computed tomography (CT) scan suggests an internal hernia, and you take her to the operating room for an urgent exploration. Which of the following is true regarding internal hernias and LRYGB?**

   A. The antecolic orientation has a lower rate of internal hernia than the retrocolic orientation.
   B. The antecolic orientation has three mesenteric defects.
   C. The antecolic orientation has a mesocolic defect, which is not formed in the retrocolic orientation.
   D. Closure of the mesenteric defects does not affect internal hernia rates.

ANSWERS

1. **B.** An LRYGB gastrojejunostomy (GJ) can be created using either a circular or linear stapled technique, or it can be completely hand-sewn. A meta-analysis comparing a linear stapled GJ anastomosis to either a 21- or 25-mm circular stapled GJ anastomosis demonstrated a significantly decreased risk for GJ stricture when using a linear stapler (RR, 0.34; 95% CI, 0.12–0.93; $P = 0.04$)[1]

to construct a GJ anastomosis. A randomized control trial comparing a 45-mm linear stapled GJ anastomosis to a 21-mm circular stapled GJ anastomosis demonstrated stricture rates of 2.5% and 17% ($P < 0.05$), respectively.[2] Other retrospective studies reported GJ stricture rates ranging from 0 to 3%[3-5] when a linear stapler device is used for the GJ anastomosis.

The diameter of the circular stapling device also significantly affects postoperative GJ stricture rates. Smaller circular staple diameters are associated with higher stricture rates. A 15.9% GJ stricture rate is expected when using a 21-mm circular stapler diameter, compared to a 6.2% GJ stricture rate with a 25-mm circular stapler diameter ($P = 0.03$).[6]

The GJ anastomosis stricture rate when a hand-sewn technique is employed is highly variable (3% to 36.6%).[7,8] The linear stapling technique remains the superior option, yielding the lowest postoperative GJ stricture rates compared to either the circular stapled or hand-sewn technique. Even when using the robot platform, the robot-assisted hand-sewn anastomosis was not superior to the linear stapler, 25-mm EEA stapler, or traditional laparoscopic hand-sewn technique.

The treatment for GJ anastomotic stricture is endoscopic balloon dilation. The majority of patients will see resolution of symptoms after one session of balloon dilation.[9,10]

2. **B.** A meta-analysis of eight studies with a total of 1,714 patients suggests that the efficacy of LRYGB, measured by postoperative excess weight loss (EWL) achieved, is influenced by the ALL. This meta-analysis compared three ALLs used for Roux-en-Y construction: short (40–100 cm), standard (130–150 cm), and long (170–250 cm).[11] Standard ALL is associated with improved postoperative EWL outcomes compared to short ALL. Meanwhile, long ALL was found to have no statistical increase in EWL or BMI loss compared to standard ALL, but it was found to be associated with increased nutritional deficiencies.[12]

A randomized control trial examined the issue of optimal common channel length (CCL) and ALL.[13] Two groups were randomized to have either a Roux-en-Y configuration with a 100-cm CCL and variable ALL, or a configuration with variable CCL and a 150-cm ALL. The LRYGB patients with a 100-cm CLL and variable ALL were noted to have an increased risk for postoperative nutritional deficiencies, with significantly lower levels of calcium, iron, and vitamin D, compared to patients with variable CCL and a 150 cm ALL.[14]

A systemic review examined the outcomes of combined ALL and biliopancreatic limb length (BPL).[15] A short (<130 cm) combined ALL and BPL conferred decreased EWL. The standard (130–200 cm) and extended (>200 cm) groups had similar EWL rates, but there were increased rates of macronutrient deficiencies in the extended bypass group.

A long BPL is associated with greater vitamin deficiencies. A prospective randomized control trial comparing BPL of 70 cm to 120 cm with a constant, 150-cm ALL demonstrated no difference in weight loss or remission of comorbidities. Longer BPL lengths, however, had greater vitamin B12, vitamin A, and folic acid deficiencies.[16]

Taken all together, the optimal configuration of limb lengths in a LRYGB is a combined ALL and BPL between 130 and 200 cm, an ALL of 130–150 cm, and variable CCL. Shorter ALL is associated with less postoperative EWL. Longer ALL (beyond 150 cm) not only fails to significantly improve EWL, but it also increases the risk for nutrient deficiencies. Similarly, the BPL should be approximately 60–70 cm. The common channel consists of the distal jejunum and ileum, where most nutrients are absorbed and the enterohepatic circulation of bile salts and fat is maintained (see Figure 20-1). Consequently, preserving CCL reduces the risk of nutritional deficiencies.

3. **D.** The LRYGB is both a restrictive and malabsorptive procedure. Malabsorption may make only a small contribution to short-term weight loss.[17] LRYGB mediates hunger and satiety, and decreases caloric intake through several incompletely understood mechanisms. The size of the gastric pouch may influence these factors and has been implicated in weight loss outcomes. A systemic review of two randomized control trials demonstrated that larger gastric pouch sizes have poorer weight loss outcomes.[18-20] Due to the difference in gastric pouch size and measuring technique in the included studies, an exact size of gastric pouch that conferred the most efficacious EWL was not elucidated. Nonetheless, most studies performed a vertical, lesser curvature-based gastric pouch that was approximately <50 mL.

Larger gastric pouches have higher marginal ulcer rates.[18,21,22] The relative risk of marginal ulcers increased by 14% for each centimeter of stapler used for the gastric pouch.[20] A larger gastric pouch allows more acid-producing cells, which leaves the mucosa of the proximal roux limb more susceptible to gastric acid injury.

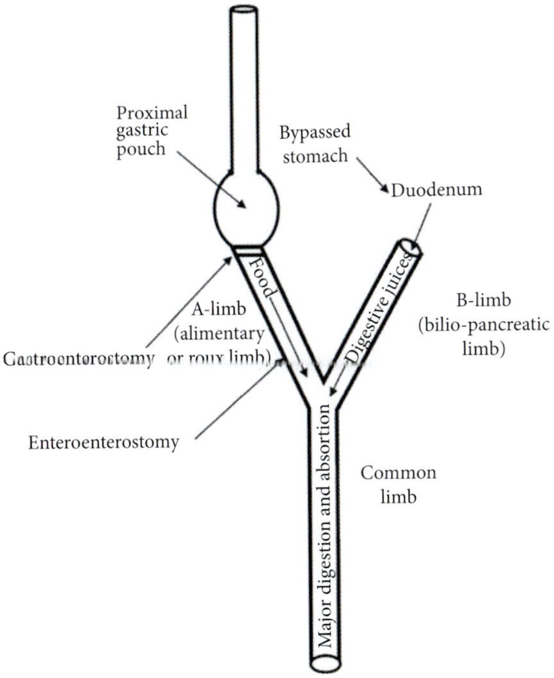

Figure 20-1 RYGB construction and names of the resultant limbs. (Reproduced with permission from Gadiot RP, Grotenhuis BA, Biter LU, et al: Study protocol of the DUCATI-study: a randomized controlled trial investigating the optimal common channel length in laparoscopic gastric bypass for morbid obese patients. *BMC Obes*. 2015;2:28.)

4. A. The LRYGB creates mesenteric defects in the peritoneal space, which are potential internal hernia sites. The orientation of the alimentary limb (retrocolic versus antecolic) and closure of the mesenteric defects affect internal hernia rates in LRYGB.[23]

In the antecolic antegastric technique, two mesenteric defects are created: Petersen's defect between the mesentery and of the alimentary limb and transverse mesocolon, and the mesomesenteric defect at the jejuno-jejunostomy between the mesenteries of the alimentary limb and the biliopancreatic limb and common channel.

In the retrocolic retrogastric technique, three mesenteric defects are created: Petersen's defect, the mesomesenteric defect, and the mesocolic defect, where the alimentary limb traverses the mesocolon into the lesser sac.

In a meta-analysis, internal hernia rates were significantly more frequent in patients undergoing LRYGB with a retrocolic than with an antecolic orientation (2.8% versus 1.2%; OR, 3.94; 95% CI, 1.49–7.98; $P = 0.004$).[24] The decrease in internal hernia rates in the antecolic orientation is primarily attributed to the absence of the mesocolic defect (see Figure 20-2).

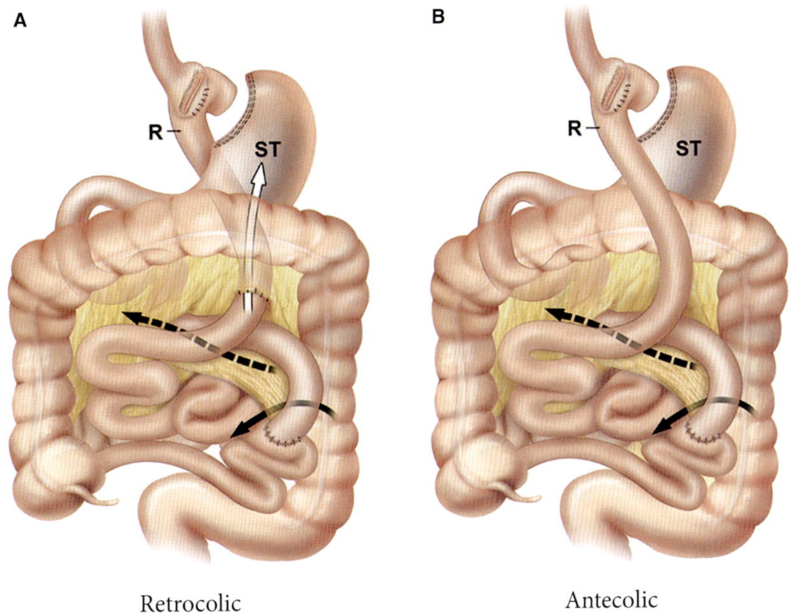

Figure 20-2 Arrows 1–3 indicate potential spaces for hernia formation: (1) Petersen's space, between the Roux limb mesentery and the transverse mesocolon; (2) the mesenteric opening at the biliopancreatic limb; (3) the opening through the transverse mesentery when the bypass is in retrocolic fashion. (Reproduced with permission from Huang CK: *Essentials and controversies in bariatric surgery*. London: IntechOpen; 2014.)

A multicenter randomized control trial comparing outcomes of open versus closed mesenteric defects discovered that closure of mesenteric defects with nonabsorbable running sutures significantly reduced the risk for reoperation for small bowel obstruction within 3 years (cumulative incidence 0.055 versus 0.102; HR, 0.56; 95% CI, 0.41–0.76; $P = 0.0002$).[25] However, closure of the mesenteric defect resulted in more early (<30 days) severe complications, which was mainly kinking of the jejuno-jejunostomy.

REFERENCES

1. Giordano S, Salminen P, Biancari F, Victorzon M. Linear stapler technique may be safer than circular in gastrojejunal anastomosis for laparoscopic Roux-en-Y gastric bypass: a meta-analysis of comparative studies. *Obes Surg*. 2011;21:1958-1964.
2. Leyba JL, Llopis SN, Isaac J, et al. Laparoscopic gastric bypass for morbid obesity—a randomized controlled trial comparing two gastrojejunal anastomosis techniques. *JSLS*. 2008;12:385-388.
3. Bohdjalian A, Langer FB, Kranner A, et al. Circular- vs. linear- stapled gastrojejunostomy in laparoscopic Roux-en-Y gastric bypass. *Obes Surg*. 2010;20:440-446.
4. Giordano S, Tolonen P, Victorzon M. Comparison of linear versus circular stapling techniques in laparoscopic gastric bypass surgery— a pilot study. *Scand J Surg*. 2010;99(3):127-131.
5. Abdel-Galil E, Sabry AA. Laparoscopic Roux-en-Y gastric bypass— evaluation of three different techniques. *Obes Surg*. 2002;12:639-642.
6. Gould JC, Garren M, Boll V, Starling J. The impact of circular stapler diameter on the incidence of gastrojejunostomy stenosis and weight loss following laparoscopic Roux-en-Y gastric bypass. *Surg Endosc*. 2006;20:1017-1020.
7. Gonzalez R, Lin E, Venkatesh KR, et al. Gastrojejunostomy during laparoscopic gastric bypass: analysis of 3 techniques. *Arch Surg*. 2003;138:181-184.
8. Bendewald FP, Choi JN, Blythe LS, et al. Comparison of hand-sewn, linear-stapled, and circular-stapled gastrojejunostomy in laparoscopic Roux-en-Y gastric bypass. *Obes Surg*. 2011;11:1671-1675.
9. Nguyen NT, Stevens CM, Wolfe BM. Incidence and outcome of anastomotic stricture after laparoscopic gastric bypass. *J Gastrointest Surg*. 2003;7:997-1003.
10. Rogula T, Koprivanac M, Janik MR, et al. Does robotic Roux-en-Y gastric bypass provide outcome advantages over standard laparoscopic approaches? *Obes Surg*. 2018; 28(9):2589-2596.
11. Gan J, Wang Y, Zhou X. Whether a short or long alimentary limb influences weight loss in gastric bypass: a systematic review and meta-analysis. *Obes Surg*. 2018;28(11):3701-3710.
12. Freeman JB, Kotlarewsky M, Phoenix C. Weight loss after extended gastric bypass. *Obes Surg*. 1997;7(4): 337-344.
13. Gadiot RP, Grotenhuis BA, Biter LU, et al. Study protocol of the DUCATI-study: a randomized controlled trial investigating the optimal common channel length in laparoscopic gastric bypass for morbid obese patients. *BMC Obes*. 2015;2:28. Published 2015 Jul 15. doi:10.1186/s40608-015-0059-z.
14. Leeman M, Gadiot RPM, Wijnand JMA, et al. Effects of standard versus very long Roux limb Roux-en-Y gastric bypass on nutrient status: a 1 year follow-up report from the DUCATI study. [published online ahead of print, 2020 Feb 20]. *Br J Nutr*. 2020;123(12):14341-1440–19.
15. Mahawar KK, Kumar P, Parmar C, et al. Small bowel limb lengths and Roux-en-Y gastric bypass: a systematic review. *Obes Surg*. 2016;26(3):660-671.
16. Ruiz-Tovar J, Vorwald P, Gonzalez-Ramirez G, et al. Impact of biliopancreatic limb length (70 cm vs 120 cm), with constant 150 cm alimentary limb, on long-term weight loss, remission of comorbidities and supplementation needs after Roux-en-Y gastric bypass: a prospective randomized clinical trial. *Obes Surg*. 2019;29(8):2367-2372.
17. Mahawar KK, Sharples AJ. Contribution of malabsorption to weight loss after Roux-en-Y gastric bypass: a systematic review. *Obes Surg*. 2017;27(8):2194-2206. doi:10.1007/s11695-017-2762-y.
18. Mahawar K, Sharples AJ, Graham Y. A systematic review of the effect of gastric pouch and/or gastrojejunostomy (stoma) size on weight loss outcomes with Roux-en-Y gastric bypass. *Surg Endosc*. 2020;34(3):1048-1060. doi:10.1007/s00464-019-07277-w.
19. Yi B, Jiang J, Zhu L, Li P, Im I, Zhu S. Comparison of the effects of Roux-en-Y gastrojejunostomy and LRYGB with small stomach pouch on type 2 diabetes mellitus in patients with BMI< 35 kg/m(2). *Surg Obes Relat Dis*. 2015;11(5):1061-1068. doi:10.1016/j.soard.2014.12.029.
20. Ren Y, Yang W, Yang J, Wang C. Effect of Roux-en-Y gastric bypass with different pouch size in Chinese T2DM patients with BMI 30-35 kg/m2. *Obes Surg*. 2015;25(3):457-463. doi:10.1007/s11695-014-1411-y.
21. Edholm D, Ottosson J, Sundbom M. Importance of pouch size in laparoscopic Roux-en-Y gastric bypass: a cohort study of 14,168 patients. *Surg Endosc*. 2016;30(5):2011-2015. doi:10.1007/s00464-015-4432-2.
22. Azagury DE, Abu Dayyeh BK, Greenwalt IT, Thompson CC. Marginal ulceration after Roux-en-Y gastric bypass surgery: characteristics, risk factors, treatment, and outcomes. *Endoscopy*. 2011;43(11):950-954. doi:10.1055/s-0030-1256951.
23. Marema RT, Perez M, Buffington CK. Comparison of the benefits and complications between laparoscopic and open Roux-en-Y gastric bypass surgeries. *Surg Endosc*. 2005;19(4):525-530. doi:10.1007/s00464-004-8907-9.
24. Rondelli F, Bugiantella W, Desio M, et al. Antecolic or retrocolic alimentary limb in laparoscopic Roux-en-Y gastric bypass? a meta-analysis. *Obes Surg*. 2016;26(1):182-195. doi:10.1007/s11695-015-1918-x.
25. Stenberg E, Szabo E, Ågren G, et al. Closure of mesenteric defects in laparoscopic gastric bypass: a multicentre, randomised, parallel, open-label trial. *Lancet*. 2016;387(10026):1397-1404.doi:10.1016/S0140-6736(15)01126-5.

21

Biliopancreatic Diversion with Duodenal Switch

Ben Schwab, MD, and Daniel M. Herron, MD, FACS, FASMBS

A 49-year-old man presents to the bariatric surgery clinic to discuss potential surgical options for management of his severe obesity. His current body mass index (BMI) is 53 kg/m^2. He has a past medical history that is significant for obstructive sleep apnea (OSA), hyperlipidemia, hypertension, and severe type 2 diabetes mellitus requiring insulin. Since his initial evaluation, he has completed a thorough preoperative clearance process, including psychological and nutritional evaluation, and is thought to be an excellent candidate for weight loss surgery. His primary care physician notes that glycemic control has been particularly difficult despite close titration of his insulin dosing; his last hemoglobin A1c level was 9.9%. He uses a continuous positive airway pressure (CPAP) machine at night and is currently on two antihypertensive medications to control his blood pressure. The patient asks whether a biliopancreatic diversion with duodenal switch (BPD-DS) would be a good option for him.

1. **When counseling this patient regarding the indications for bariatric surgery, which of the following statements is correct?**
   A. In superobese patients, the majority of patients remain significantly obese after surgery.
   B. Resolution of hypertension is superior in patients undergoing sleeve gastrectomy (SG) compared to BPD-DS.
   C. Approximately 15% of patients undergoing bariatric surgery in the United States are superobese.
   D. Patients undergoing BPD-DS or Roux-en-Y gastric bypass (RYGB) are at equal risk for severe nutritional complications.

2. **The patient asks about the details of how his operation will be performed. Which of the following technical considerations regarding laparoscopic BPD-DS is correct?**
   A. There is no significant difference in operation time for patients undergoing BPD-DS and RYGB.
   B. A larger bougie is typically utilized when performing the gastric resection than with a primary SG.
   C. Most surgeons would use a 200–250-cm common channel length (CCL) for optimal weight loss outcomes.
   D. Routine closure of mesenteric defects eliminates the risk of internal hernia.

3. **When discussing the expected impact of bariatric surgery, which of the following physiologic and metabolic considerations after BPD-DS is correct?**
   A. Micronutrient deficiencies occur in less than 30% of patients after BPD-DS.
   B. The CCL influences the risk for long-term, postoperative nutritional deficiencies.
   C. The proportion of patients with insulin-dependent diabetes who experience long-term clinical resolution is similar to RYGB.
   D. Most insurance policies cover the cost of postoperative vitamin supplementation for patients who undergo BPD-DS.

4. **The patient's partner asks about possible complications after bariatric surgery. Which of the following statements regarding complications after BPD-DS is correct?**

A. In patients after BPD-DS who present with severe nutritional deficiencies, the treatment is primarily medical.
B. Patients who present with small bowel obstruction are more likely to require operative intervention compared to those who undergo RYGB.
C. There is a lower risk of marginal ulceration compared to RYGB.
D. There is a lower risk of requiring cholecystectomy compared to RYGB.

5. **Which of the following statements regarding long-term metabolic and nutritional outcomes after BPD-DS is true?**
A. The risk of severe malnutrition requiring hospital admission is not significantly higher compared to RYGB.
B. The prevalence of weight recidivism after bariatric surgery is similar compared to RYGB.
C. Vitamin/mineral deficiencies and protein/calorie malnutrition are rare if patients can maintain normal meal consumption.
D. Patients are more likely to require additional surgical interventions compared to RYGB.

ANSWERS

1. **A.** The prevalence of severe obesity continues to increase in the United States and worldwide. From 1999 to 2018 in the United States, the prevalence of adult obesity increased from 31% to 42%, and that of severe obesity (BMI >40 kg/m^2) increased from 5% to 9%.[1] Approximately 25% of patients undergoing bariatric surgery in the United States are classified as superobese (BMI >50 kg/m^2). While bariatric surgery is known to be an effective weight loss strategy in the management of severely obese patients, some studies have demonstrated that bariatric surgery in superobese patients is less effective, with many patients unable to lower their BMI below 35 kg/m^2. While the exact cause for this is not known, possible reasons include alternative metabolic mechanisms for weight gain in superobese patients, technical difficulties during surgery (i.e., inappropriate pouch size during RYGB) secondary to excessive intra-abdominal adiposity, and various psychosocial factors, including diet and exercise in the postoperative period. BPD-DS has been shown to result in superior rates of excess weight loss (EWL), in addition to less weight recidivism and lower rate of failure.[2]

In a recent randomized controlled study comparing 5-year outcomes after laparoscopic Roux-en-Y gastric bypass (LRYGB) and BPD-DS, mean reductions in BMI were 13.6 and 22.1 kg/m^2 after RYGB and BPD-DS, respectively.[3]

Studies have shown that BPD-DS is associated with superior resolution of various comorbidities, including diabetes and hypertension, when compared to other bariatric procedures, including RYGB and SG.[4] While weight loss after BPD-DS has been consistently shown to be superior, there is an increased risk of hospital admission secondary to severe malnutrition within 5 years of the index operation.[3,5] The presence of severe gastroesophageal reflux or reflux esophagitis detected on preoperative endoscopy is considered a relative contraindication to BPD-DS due to the need to perform an SG, which is believed to exacerbate GERD in certain patients.

2. **B.** BPD-DS is considered a complex, technically challenging bariatric operation. Classically, BPD-DS has been performed using an open technique, but the laparoscopic approach is an acceptable option for experienced minimally invasive surgeons. The major steps of BPD-DS consist of SG, division of the proximal duodenum distal to the pylorus, closure of the duodenal stump, formation of an alimentary limb typically measured at 250 cm proximal to the ileocecal valve, and the creation of an antecolic duodenoileostomy and anastomosis of the long biliopancreatic limb to the distal ileum, which causes a very short CCL, and the common channel is typically 50–100 cm from the ileocecal valve.

In contrast to a primary SG, a larger bougie, typically 50 to 60 Fr, is commonly used in BPD-DS during the performance of the gastric resection. Like RYGB, the formation of an antecolic alimentary limb to create the duodenoileostomy results in a potential hernia space posterior to the mesentery that should be closed if technically feasible. In addition, the mesenteric defect at the distal anastomosis similarly requires closure when possible. However, closure of these mesenteric defects does not eliminate the risk of internal hernia. Given the complexity of the BPD-DS, operating times have been shown to be significantly longer than RYGB.[5]

More recently, single-anastomosis duodenal-ileal bypass with sleeve (SADI-S) has emerged as an alternative to BPD-DS. This operation differs from BPD-DS in that a loop of ileum is anastomosed to the divided duodenum, avoiding the creation of a second distal anastomosis. In addition, this operation creates a longer CCL (~300 cm), in an attempt to minimize the risk of severe malnutrition. Preliminary studies have demonstrated that patients undergoing SADI-S have significant resolution of metabolic comorbidities with a similar complication rate compared to established malabsorptive operations.[6]

3. **B.** In the classic description of BPD-DS, the CCL is typically 50–100 cm, as measured from the ileocecal valve to the biliopancreatic anastomosis. An important technical consideration with BPD-DS is an accurate measurement of the bowel length prior to creation of the anastomosis. If the common channel is too short, patients have an increased risk for the development of clinically significant protein or micronutrient deficiencies. In patients who present with significant malnutrition after BPD-DS, a potential surgical option involves lengthening of the common channel to allow an increased absorptive capacity. It is estimated that up to 90% of patients will show laboratory evidence of micronutrient deficiency within 3 years after BPD-DS, so careful preoperative counseling of patients is required to minimize their risk.[7] In addition, it is important for patients who are undergoing any malabsorptive operation, including RYGB and BPD-DS, to understand that insurance company policies often exclude coverage for nutritional supplements. Patients often spend $50 to $70 per month for appropriate vitamin and mineral supplements.

   BPD-DS has been shown to result in superior resolution of diabetes and hypertension when compared to RYGB. In a recent study assessing the long-term resolution of diabetes, all patients on medication preoperatively were able to discontinue their medication use after 10-year follow-up, as opposed to approximately 50% of patients who underwent RYGB.[8]

   Studies of long-term outcomes after BPD-DS have demonstrated a consistent increase in the rate of gastrointestinal side effects, including diarrhea, flatulence, abdominal bloating, and GERD. In a recent study comparing the prevalence of diarrhea in patients undergoing various bariatric operations, the prevalence of diarrhea after 5 years in RYGB, SG, and BPD-DS was 2.7%, 5.8%, and 11.3%, respectively. This represents a sixfold increase in patients undergoing BPD-DS.[9] The estimated reflux rate after BPD-DS has been reported to be as high as 43.8%.

4. **C.** In comparison to RYGB, the incidence of marginal ulcer in BPD-DS is significantly less. This is thought to be secondary to the technical differences between RYGB and BPD-DS. In BPD-DS, the creation of a duodenoileostomy limits the exposure of the small bowel mucosa to acidic gastric contents, in comparison to the gastrojejunostomy created during RYGB, which can lead to ulceration of the jejunal mucosa (the most common side effect) secondary to prolonged acid exposure.

   The risk of a postoperative leak has been shown to be consistently greater in BPD-DS than in RYGB. While the reasons for this are likely multifactorial, potential causative factors include additional staple lines, the presence of a duodenal stump, lengthier operative times, and an expanded operative field as a result of the distal anastomosis.[10] The risk of small bowel obstruction requiring operative intervention is similar in patients after RYGB or BPD-DS. Studies have demonstrated a higher rate of cholecystectomy after BPD-DS compared to RYGB, which is thought to be related to the increased weight loss seen in patients who undergo BPD-DS.[5] Despite this fact, routine prophylactic cholecystectomy in asymptomatic patients undergoing bariatric surgery, including RYGB or BPD-DS, is not currently recommended.[11]

5. **D.** Multiple studies have confirmed that the rate of severe malnutrition requiring hospital admission, parenteral nutrition, and possibly surgical revision for management of side effects is significantly higher for BPD-DS versus RYGB.[2,5] In a study comparing long-term weight loss and maintenance after RYGB versus BPD-DS, weight recidivism was significantly lower with BPD-DS as opposed to RYGB. In addition, patients undergoing RYGB were more likely to require surgical revision secondary to inadequate weight loss or weight regain in comparison to BPD-DS, where revision was more likely secondary to side effects, including severe malnutrition or chronic abdominal pain.[2] Overall, BPD-DS is associated with an increased risk for needing an additional abdominal operation, including cholecystectomy and incisional hernia, which likely reflects the proportionally larger number of cases performed utilizing an open approach.[5] While BPD-DS has been shown to be superior to RYGB in reducing the prevalence of diabetes and hypertension, the reduction in hyperlipidemia is similar between the two.[8]

As a result of the extreme malabsorptive nature of BPD-DS secondary to the short CCL, vitamin and mineral deficiencies are extremely common despite normal meal consumption. Aggressive nutritional supplementation is an absolute requirement for BPD-DS patients postoperatively. While patients are susceptible to any micronutrient deficiency after BPD-DS, they are especially at risk for deficiencies of vitamin A and D, calcium, and zinc. While lifelong vitamin and mineral supplementation is also required after RYGB, patients often require significantly higher dosing of these supplements after BPD-DS.[12] As a result of these considerations, BPD-DS should be offered only to highly compliant patients who demonstrate a psychological and financial commitment to the required nutritional supplement regimen.

REFERENCES

1. Hales CM, Carroll MD, Fryar CD, Ogden CL. *Prevalence of Obesity and Severe Obesity Among Adults: United States, 2017–2018*. NCHS Data Brief, no. 360. Hyattsville, MD: National Center for Health Statistics; 2020.
2. Topart P, Becouarn G, Ritz P. Weight loss is more sustained after biliopancreatic diversion with duodenal switch than Roux-en-Y gastric bypass in superobese patients. *Surg Obes Relat Dis*. 2013;9(4):526-530.
3. Risstad H, Søvik TT, Engström M, et al. Five-year outcomes after laparoscopic gastric bypass and laparoscopic duodenal switch in patients with body mass index of 50 to 60: a randomized clinical trial. *JAMA Surg*. 2015;150(4):352-361.
4. Prachand VN, Ward M, Alverdy JC. Duodenal switch provides superior resolution of metabolic comorbidities independent of weight loss in the super-obese (BMI > or = 50 kg/m2) compared with gastric bypass. *J Gastrointest Surg*. 2010;14(2):211-220.
5. Skogar ML, Sundbom M. Early complications, long-term adverse events, and quality of life after duodenal switch and gastric bypass in a matched national cohort. *Surg Obes Relat Dis*. 2020. pii: S1550-7289(20)30081-2.
6. Cottam D, Roslin M, Enochs P, et al. Single anastomosis duodenal switch: 1-year outcomes. *Obes Surg*. 2020;30(4):1506-1514.
7. Homan J, Berends FJ, Aarts EO, et al. Vitamin and mineral deficiencies after biliopancreatic diversion and biliopancreatic diversion with duodenal switch – the rule rather than the exception. *Obes Surg*. 2015;25(9):1626-1632.
8. Skogar M, Sundbom M. Weight loss and effect on comorbidities in the long-term after duodenal switch and gastric bypass: a population-based cohort study. *Surg Obes Relat Dis*. 2020;16(1):17-23.
9. Elias K, Hedberg J, Sundbom M. Prevalence and impact of acid-related symptoms and diarrhea in patients undergoing Roux-en-Y gastric bypass, sleeve gastrectomy, and biliopancreatic diversion with duodenal switch. *Surg Obes Relat Dis*. 2019;16(4):520-527. pii: S1550-7289(19)31158-X.
10. Hedberg J, Sundström J, Sundbom M. Duodenal switch versus gastric bypass for morbid obesity: systematic review and metaanalysis of weight results, diabetes resolution and early complications in single-centre comparisons. *Obes Rev*. 2014;15(7):555-563.
11. Leyva-Alvizo A, Arredondo-Saldaña G, Leal-Isla-Flores V, et al. Systematic review of management of gallbladder disease in patients undergoing minimally invasive bariatric surgery. *Surg Obes Relat Dis*. 2020;16(1):158-164.
12. Homan J, Schijins W, Aarts EO, et al. Treatment of vitamin and mineral deficiencies after biliopancreatic diversion with or without duodenal switch: a major challenge. *Obes Surg*. 2018;28(1):234-241.

22

Laparoscopic Adjustable Gastric Band

Jesse Bandle, MD, and Dan Eisenberg, MD, MS

A 41-year old female with a body mass index (BMI) of 41 kg/m^2 had a laparoscopic adjustable gastric band (LAGB) placed 12 years ago and presents to clinic for a band fill. Over the past year, she has had worsening nausea, vomiting, and retrosternal chest pain, which has progressed to food intolerance. Early in the post-operative period, she had good weight loss, but she is now gaining weight despite her symptoms. She has been receiving port adjustments intermittently, but she is unsure of the amount of her last fill or the total volume instilled in the band. She states that her previous doctor had "a very hard time filling my band, and used several different needles." Although concerned about her symptoms, she would like a band fill to curb her weight gain.

1. **What is the most appropriate initial diagnostic tool and intervention to address this patient's current symptoms?**
   A. Oral-contrast computed tomography (CT) scan and spinal needle aspiration of the access port
   B. Upper endoscopy and surgical refixation of the port
   C. Complete blood count (CBC)/chemistry labs and diagnostic laparoscopy
   D. Serum lactate and intravenous (IV) ondansetron
   E. Upright plain abdominal x-ray and noncoring needle aspiration of the access port

2. **What is the recommended timing and technique for LAGB adjustments?**
   A. Patient self-adjustment every 4–6 weeks
   B. Use of a syringeless spinal needle as needed, with timing based on patient desire
   C. Outpatient adjustment with a non-coring needle (with or without radiographic guidance) every 4–6 weeks during the first year
   D. Emptying of the port when patients have rapid satiety after small meals
   E. Fill the LAGB monthly to the point of patient inability to tolerate oral liquids

3. **During the physical exam, the physician sees several needle marks and mild erythema overlying the port site, which is tender when manipulated. What is the most concerning complication that could be associated with these findings?**
   A. Allergic reaction to the LAGB system components
   B. Improper port access technique, leading to superficial skin infection
   C. Infection of the access port
   D. Erosion of the LAGB system into the gastric/esophageal lumen
   E. Malpositioning of the fill port

4. **A patient with a recently placed LAGB has undergone several fills but feels no restriction. What is the most commonly reported complication associated with LAGB placement?**
   A. Slipped band
   B. Band erosion
   C. Band or port infection
   D. Mechanical malfunction of the access port or tubing
   E. Poor positioning of the band

5. A 32-year-old woman underwent a LAGB placement 5 years ago. She experienced 25% excess weight loss (EWL) to date, but she has plateaued for the past 2 years. She desires revisional surgery to achieve more weight loss; her current BMI is 41 kg/m^2. She reports feeling very little restriction over the past year, but notes worsening reflux and heartburn during the same time period, despite close follow-up with a bariatric dietician. Device-related complications were ruled out. Which is the best revisional surgical option for this patient?

A. Sleeve gastrectomy (SG)
B. Band replacement
C. Roux-en-Y gastric bypass (RYGB)
D. Single anastomosis duodenal-ileal bypass (SADI)
E. One anastomosis gastric bypass

ANSWERS

1. **E.** Several complications associated with LAGBs often share presenting symptoms. Symptoms of band slippage include nausea/vomiting, dysphagia, retrosternal chest pain, heartburn, and food intolerance. The same constellation of symptoms may occur from an overfilled band, which usually is not an emergency, or they may represent the initial warnings of band erosion and impending sepsis. The inability to secure the diagnosis based on history and clinical findings alone necessitates radiographic studies. Aspiration of the port should be done early for symptomatic relief and to help clarify the etiology of the patient's symptoms.

A slipped band can be a surgical emergency, as the slipped portion of the stomach can swell and cause obstruction at the band outlet, similar to a strangulated hernia. These patients often have severe abdominal pain, tachycardia, fever, and an elevated white blood cell count.[1] For the vast majority of stable patients, the first step in treating gastric band complications begins with accessing the fill port and aspirating fluid from the band. This office-based intervention can frequently relieve symptoms in cases that are not severe and can avoid the need for urgent surgical management.[2]

An upright upper-abdominal x-ray (Figure 22-1)[3] can demonstrate several features of a properly placed, well-seated band. The band should be placed just below the gastroesophageal junction and create a gastric pouch capacity of approximately 50–80 mL. The angle of the band should be close to 45°

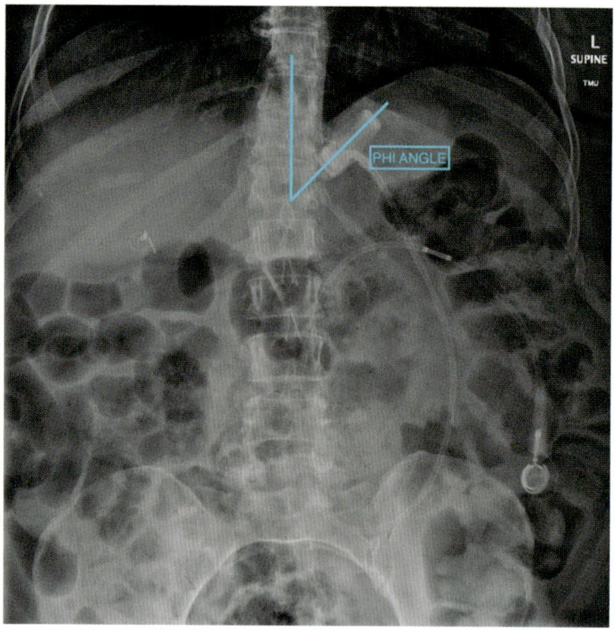

Figure 22-1 A properly positioned LAGB.

measured from the vertical line of the patient's spine (known as the phi angle) and oriented toward the left shoulder (normal can range from 4°–58°). In addition, the central lumen of the band is not visible from a properly oriented upright-abdominal film (the "O" sign shown in Figure 22-2).[4]

A phi angle greater than 58° is associated with a 91% to 95% sensitivity of band slippage, and an "O" sign has 97% specificity. Additional radiographic signs of band slippage include inferior displacement of the superolateral band margin by more than 2.4 cm from the diaphragm (95% sensitivity, 98% specificity) and the presence of any pouch air-fluid level (95% sensitivity, 100% specificity).[5] An esophagram is useful to evaluate the degree of slippage, especially if complete intolerance to oral intake is present. Failure of contrast to progress past the dilated pouch necessitates urgent surgical band removal due to the risk of gastric ischemia, necrosis, and perforation. Plain upright and supine x-rays often provide sufficient information to suggest a diagnosis, and additional imaging is rarely indicated.

Spinal needles should not be used to access the fill port because they may damage the diaphragm and lead to subcutaneous leak of fluid. Serum lactate is a general marker that may help assess for end-organ ischemia, but in the setting of foregut symptoms and

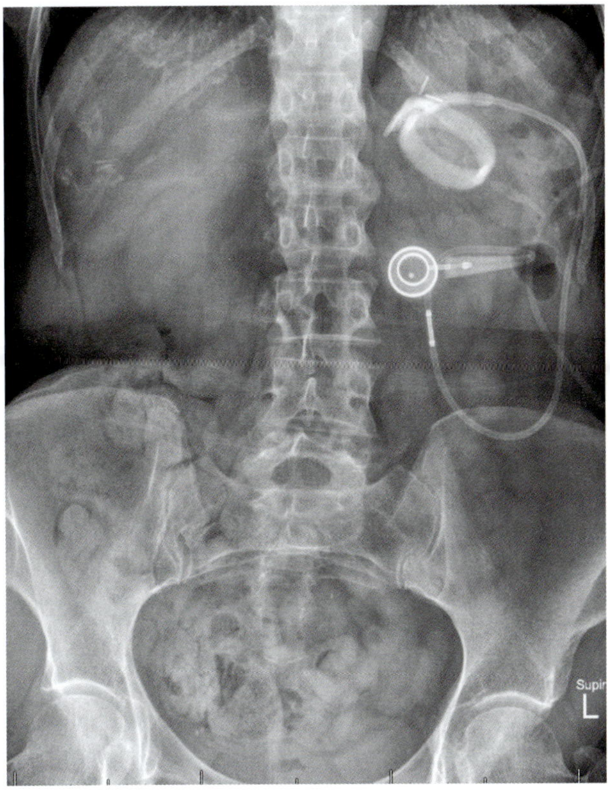

Figure 22-2 "O" sign is highly specific for band slippage.

history of a LAGB placement, it is necessary to assess the anatomy of the stomach and gastric band early in the diagnostic workup. Antiemetic medications, such as ondansetron, may ameliorate symptoms of nausea, but provide no diagnostic information and do not address the underlying pathology.

2. **C.** An advantage of the LAGB is its ability to be adjusted. Adjustments must be undertaken by a provider who is familiar with the band system, knows the appropriate technique, and has the proper equipment. During the initial placement of the band, it is recommended that no fluid be added to the system. A common protocol is the addition of 1 mL of sterile saline (or water) in the outpatient setting 4–6 weeks from the date of placement. The patient's progress and symptoms are then monitored every 4–6 weeks for up to 1 year, with instillation of no more than 0.5 mL per visit. When utilizing fluoroscopic guidance for band tightness, up to 1 mL can be used per visit.[6] Subjective indicators of the need for more frequent filling include inadequate weight loss, rapid loss of satiety after meals, and hunger between meals. Indications for removal of fluid include persistent food intolerance and regurgitation, vomiting, heartburn, reflux, coughing, choking, and difficulty digesting a wide variety of foods.[6]

   Guidelines from the Food and Drug Administration (FDA) and manufacturer instructions strongly recommend the use of a noncoring (Huber) needle to access the port.[7,8] Centers that do not frequently treat LAGB patients may not have the proper needle—especially the appropriate length of Huber needle—to access the port. Unless there is need for urgent deflation, these patients should be referred to a center/physician with the proper equipment and expertise. Damage to the dome/membrane of the fill port may lead to a slow leak and poor band performance. Even with strict adherence to the proper technique, there are reports of slow reduction in fluid volume in the band over time, presumably due to diffusion across the semipermeable silicone membrane.[9] Patients should be made aware of this effect and seek help if the band's effectiveness seems to be reduced.

3. **D.** Infection noted at the access port site should be considered evidence of band erosion until proven otherwise. Access port infections have been reported to occur in 0.3% to 9% of patients following LAGB.[10,11] Port site infections can occur by three major mechanisms: intraoperative contamination, contamination during transcutaneous fill-port access, or contamination as a result of band erosion into the gastrointestinal tract with ascending infection via the connector tubing. The correlation of events (e.g., chronologically close to the date of operation versus port fill) can help distinguish the cause of the infection and raise suspicion of a specific etiology. Most late occurrences of port site infection require removal of the port and/or band, as they do not typically resolve with nonsurgical management.

   Band erosion is a rare complication of LAGB placement, that ranges from 0.2% to 14% of cases[12,13] based on reports in the published literature. Several causes of band erosion have been postulated, including overdistention of the band with subsequent gastric ischemia, gastric ischemia due to aggressive dissection and inadvertent devascularization (inclusion of the ascending branch of the left gastric artery), and unobserved intraoperative injury to the stomach at the time of surgery.[14] Patients with erosion can present with a wide spectrum of symptoms, and mean time to presentation is 22 months after band placement. Some patients have mild abdominal pain and nausea or are even asymptomatic, with mild weight regain. They may present with a local port site infection chronologically remote from the index procedure or in frank sepsis from perforation and spillage of gastric contents. Upper endoscopy is the study of choice to secure the diagnosis when radiographic studies are equivocal.[15]

The timing and technique for band removal should be based on the severity of patient presentation and the capabilities of the institution. A laparoscopic or robot-assisted laparoscopic approach to band removal and suture repair of the gastric fistula/gastrostomy, with or without omental patch, is common. Occasionally, an anterior gastrotomy is required to remove a significantly eroded band that is inaccessible from the extraluminal space. Preoperative or intraoperative esophagogastroduodenoscopy (EGD) can be helpful in evaluating the extent of erosion and determining the band location when it is not apparent (Figure 22-3).[16] With appropriately experienced staff in select cases, endoscopic removal of the band may be possible, typically when more than 50% of the band has eroded through the stomach, thus avoiding performing surgery in an inflamed field.[17]

4. **D.** Access port or connector tube malfunctions are the most frequently reported complication[15] associated with the LAGB procedure, with rates ranging from 2.5% to 24% of cases.[18,19] Damage to the port and/or tubing may occur intraoperatively, be associated with trauma, or be secondary to improper port access. Mechanical failure of any part of the system typically presents with leakage of the filled volume of fluid and failure to provide restriction. An abdominal x-ray or fluoroscopy can be helpful to assess gross system failure of the intra-abdominal components (Figure 22-4).[15]

Smaller leaks can be detected via injection of dilute contrast into the fill port and localization of the leak via fluoroscopy. Intra-operatively, filling the port with dilute methylene blue can assist in locating occult leaks.[20]

The fill port itself may flip in the subcutaneous tissue (improper fixation to the anterior rectus fascia), making percutaneous access through the membrane of the device impossible. Fill-port rotation also may be the consequence of significant weight loss, resulting in changes in the contour of the abdominal wall.[20] This can usually be managed with local exploration, avoiding intra-abdominal intervention.[11]

Band erosion, slipped bands, and band infections are typically late-term complications. An improperly based band can be placed transgastrically or around the esophagus instead of the fundus. These events are rare, however.

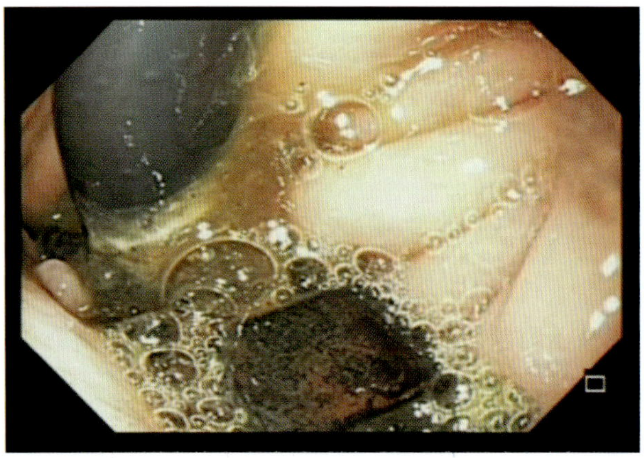

Figure 22-3 Endoscopic view of an eroded LAGB; note the discoloration of the band secondary to gastric acid exposure. (Reproduced with permission from Dr. Eric Pauli.)

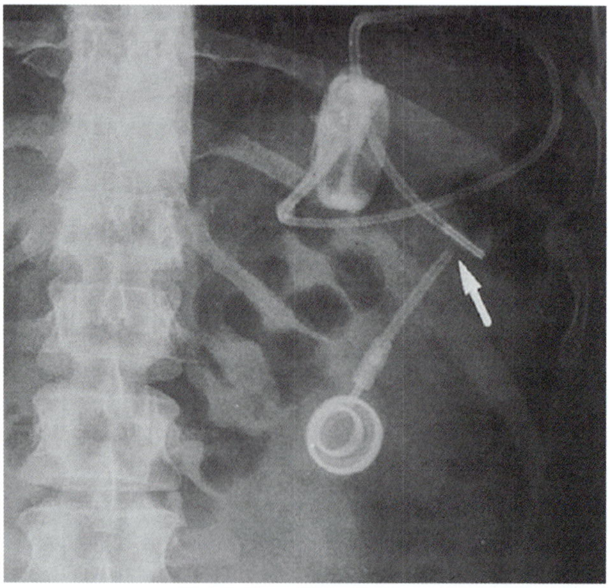

Figure 22-4 Disrupted LAGB due to trauma. Arrow demonstrates disruption of the tubing connecting the fill port and gastric band.

5. **A.** Several large studies have demonstrated high rates (20.2% to 40%)[21,22] of revisional surgery over the lifetime of a patient who has had prior placement of LAGB. Pouch enlargement with associated reflux is a common complication (14% to 18.3%),[23] leading to the need for LAGB removal or revision. Given the significant reflux that this patient is experiencing, along with the need for further weight loss, proceeding with revisional RYGB should be considered. Studies have demonstrated a significant decrease in esophagitis and increase in normal bolus transit on swallow studies following conversion from LAGB to RYGB.[24] A systematic review of reoperative bariatric surgery demonstrated collectively higher risks associated with revision versus primary surgery, but it also reported generally favorable outcomes, including comorbidity reduction and increased weight loss following the revisional procedure.[25] The decision on the type of revision and whether a one- or two-stage procedure should be pursued is based on the primary operation, patient anatomy/comorbidity, and surgeon experience.

REFERENCES

1. Lim R, Beekley A, Johnson D, Davis K. Early and late complications of bariatric operation. *Trauma Surg Acute Care Open.* 2018;3:e000219.
2. Kodner K, Hartman D. Complications of adjustable gastric banding surgery for obesity. *Am Fam Physician.* 2014;89(10):813-818.
3. Case courtesy of Dr. Grace Carpenter, Radiopaedia.org, rID: 74401 https://radiopaedia.org/articles/gastric-band.
4. Case courtesy of Dr. Jayanth Keshavamurthy, Radiopaedia.org, rID: 33405 https://radiopaedia.org/articles/gastric-band.
5. Swensson D, Pietryga J, Grand D, Chang K, Murphy B, Egglin T. Gastric band slippage: a case-controlled study comparing new and old radiographic signs of this important surgical complication. *Am J Roentgenol.* 2014;203:10-16.
6. Favretti F, O'Brien P, Dixon J. Patient management after LAP-BAND placement. *Am J Surg.* 2002;184:38S-41S.
7. *The Lap-Band® Adjustable Gastric Banding System Summary of Safety and Effectiveness Data.* June 5, 2001. https://www.accessdata.fda.gov/cdrh_docs/pdf/P000008b.pdf.
8. Lap-Band AP® *Adjustable Gastric Banding System with Rapid-Port® Ez and OMNIFORM™ Design.* http://apolloendo.com/wp-content/uploads/2016/07/GRF-00304-00_R01.pdf.
9. Dixon B, O'Brien P. Permeability of the silicone membrane in laparoscopic adjustable gastric bands has important clinical implications. *Obes Surg.* 2005;15:624-629.
10. Angrisani L, Furbetta F, Doldi SB, et al. Lap band adjustable gastric banding system: the Italian experience with 1863 patients operated on 6 years. *Surg Endosc.* 2003;17(3):409-412.
11. Keidar A, Carmon E, Szold A, Abu-Abeid S. Port complications following laparoscopic adjustable gastric banding for morbid obesity. *Obes Surg.* 2005;15(3):361-365.
12. Mozzi E, Lattuada E, Zappa MA, Granelli P, De Ruberto F, Armocida A, Roviaro G. Treatment of band erosion: feasibility and safety of endoscopic band removal. *Surg Endosc.* 2011;25:3918-3922.
13. Brown WA, Egberts KJ, Franke-Richard D, Thodiyil P, Anderson ML, O'Brien PE. Erosions after laparoscopic adjustable gastric banding: diagnosis and management. *Ann Surg.* 2013;257:1047-1052.
14. Chisholm J, Kitan N, Toouli J, Kow L. Gastric band erosion in 63 cases: endoscopic removal and rebanding evaluated. *Obes Surg.* 2011;21:1676-1681.
15. Eid I, Birch D, Sharma A, Sherman V, Karmali S. Complications associated with adjustable gasteic banding for morbid obesity: a surgeon's guide. *Can J Surg.* 2011;54(1):61-66.
16. Dogan U, Akin M, Yalaki S, Akova A, Yilmaz C. Endoscopic management of gastric band erosions: A 7-year series of 14 patients. *Canadian J Surg.* 2004;57:106-111.
17. Quadri P, Gonzalez-Heredia R, Masrur M, Sanchez-Johnsen L, Elli E. Management of laparoscopic adjustable gastric band erosion. *Surg Endosc.* 2017;31:1505-1512.
18. Szold A, Abu-Abeid S. Laparoscopic adjustable silicone gastric banding for morbid obesity—results and complications in 715 patients. *Surg Endosc.* 2000;16:230-233.
19. Busetto L, Segato G, De Marchi F, et al. Outcome predictors in morbid obesity: experience with 1,000 patients over 7 years. *Obes Surg.* 2003;12:83-92.
20. Lattuada E, Zappa M, Mozzi E, Antonini I, Boati P, Roviaro G. Injection port and connector tube complications after laparoscopic adjustable banding. *Obes Surg.* 2010;20:410-414.
21. Altieri MS, Yang J, Telem DA, et al. Lap band outcomes from 19,221 patients across centers and over a decade within the state of New York. *Surg Endosc.* 2016;30:1725-1732.
22. Lazzati A, De Antonio M, Paolino L, et al. Natural history of adjustable gastric banding: lifespan and revisional rate: a nationwide study on administrative data on 53,000 patients. *Ann Surg.* 2017;265:439-445.
23. Kowalewski P, Olszewski R, Kwiatkowski A, Paśnik K. Revisional bariatric surgery after failed laparoscopic adjustable gastric banding—a single-center, long-term retrospective study. *Videosurg Miniinv.* 2017;12(1):32-36.
24. Borovicka J, Krieger-Grübel C, Van der Weg B, et al. Effect of morbid obesity, gastric banding and gastric bypass on esophageal symptoms, mucosa and function. *Surg Endosc.* 2017;31:552-560.
25. Berthauer SA, Kothan S, Sudan R, et al. Systematic review on reoperative bariatric surgery (American Society for Metabolic and Bariatric Surgery Revision Task Force). *Surg Obes Relat Dis.* 2014;10(5):952-972.

23

One Anastomosis Gastric Bypass (OAGB)/Mini Gastric Bypass (MGB)

Souheil Adra, MD, FACS, FASMBS, ABOM

A 46-year-old female with a body mass index (BMI) of 48 kg/m^2 and comorbid conditions that include type 2 diabetes mellitus for 5 years, hypertension, and obstructive sleep apnea (OSA). After her preoperative evaluation and counseling, she cannot decide whether to have a Roux-en-Y gastric bypass (RYGB) or a laparoscopic sleeve gastrectomy (LSG). You had just added the one anastomosis gastric bypass/mini-gastric bypass (OAGB/MGB) to your surgical skill set but heretofore had been limiting it to class II obese patients. She is interested in the procedure, so she asks you what the impact of OAGB/MGB is on weight and her comorbidities compared to other two procedures.

1. Regarding weight loss, which of the following is true?

A. 5-year excess weight loss (EWL) is <60%.
B. The percent of EWL is equivalent to or greater than that of RYGB.
C. The percent of EWL is not as durable as that of RYGB.
D. Total body weight loss is inferior compared to RYGB.
E. The percent of EWL of MGB/OAGB is less than for LSG.

2. Which of the following statements about OAGB/MGB early complications is true?

A. They are higher than with RYGB.
B. Leaks may require reoperation in 50% of patients.
C. Symptomatic leaks occur in 0.2% of patients, usually in the third week.
D. Postoperative bleeding occurs in 5% of patients.
E. Postoperative bleeding requires reintervention in 25% of patients.

3. Which of the following is true regarding OAGB/MGB outcomes?

A. The marginal ulcer rate after OAGB/MGB is 10%.
B. Iron deficiency anemia occurs in 10% of patients.
C. Bile reflux is noted in 4% of patients.
D. Cancer of the esophagus and stomach occurs in ~2% of patients.
E. Malabsorption and diarrhea are rare.

ANSWERS

1. **B.** Recent randomized controlled trials confirmed the noninferiority of OAGB at 2 years versus RYGB with respect to weight loss,[1] while other studies showed superior outcomes.[2,3] The range of EWL at long-term (≥5 years) follow-up is between 68.6% and 85%,[4–11] while total weight loss for OAGB/MGB is about 36.18 ± 9.18%, as opposed to RYGB, 33.8 ± 8.75%.[12]

   Similarly, comparing weight loss with OAGB to LSG, OAGB provided superior,[7,13–15] or at least similar weight loss.[16]

2. **B.** The early complication rates of OAGB are in the 3.5% to 7.5% range, which is lower than the RYGB.[4,11,12,17–19]

Leaks are rare and may occur in 0.7% to 2% of cases. The site of the leak may be from staple lines in the gastric remnant, the gastric pouch, or the anastomosis. The majority of leaks occur within 2 weeks postoperatively, and up to half of leaks may require reoperation.[4,20–22]

Postoperative bleeding is usually self-limited. It occurs in <3% of patients and requires surgical intervention in a minority of cases.[20,23,24]

3. **C.** Marginal ulcer rates after OAGB/MGB range from 0.5% to 8.0%,[17,25] which is similar to the rates after RYGB. Iron deficiency anemia after OAGB varies from 5% to 10% without iron supplementation.[18,23,25] Iron supplementation is prudent for OAGB/MGB patients as well as yearly labs.

Bile reflux has been reported in 0.9% to 4.0% of patients.[4,5,12,23,24,26–28] This reflux could cause malignant changes in the stomach and esophagus.[27,28] There is an increased risk of reflux after OAGB/MGB compared to RYGB (3.55% vs. 0.70%);[12] the first case of OAGB causing gastric cancer was recently reported.[28] The controversy surrounding the risk of cancer development after an OAGB/MGB is based on the historical data regarding a Billroth II anastomosis. However, there is no direct evidence of OAGB/MGB increasing the risk of malignant degeneration.

Diarrhea and excess weight loss (EWL) can occur with a long biliopancreatic (BP) limb, which can be corrected by shortening the BP limb to increase the common limb length. Biliary limb length in a single anastomosis gastric bypass is important to prevent malnutrition. If the BP limb is longer than 250 cm, patients are more likely to develop protein calorie malnutrition with complications due to malabsorption. The common limb length should be ~200 to 220 cm.[1,4,17,18,23,25,30–32] However, more recent studies are challenging this finding in patients with shorter total intestinal length.[33] The data are mixed with respect to the impact of OAGB versus RYGB; a retrospective study described both higher rates of malnutrition and anemia[34] and no difference.[35] Furthermore, a more recent randomized controlled trial[1] reported a 21.4% rate of nutritional complications in OAGB/MGB with a relatively short (200 cm) afferent limb, as opposed to 0% in the RYGB group.

In summary, OAGB/MGB has clinical outcomes equivalent to that of RYGB and may be superior to LSG in terms of weight loss. It does have significantly more bile reflux, and the malignant potential of this is suspected to be significantly increased, but this is not truly known. Malnutrition seems to be more prevalent after OAGB/MGB, especially when BP limb lengths exceed 250 cm. The procedure is currently not endorsed by the American Society for Metabolic and Bariatric Surgery (ASMBS).

REFERENCES

1. Robert M, Espalieu P, Pelascini E, et al. Efficacy and safety of one anastomosis gastric bypass versus Roux-en-Y gastric bypass for obesity (YOMEGA): a multicentre, randomised, open-label, non-inferiority trial. *Lancet.* 2019;393(10178):1299-1309. doi:10.1016/S0140-6736(19)30475-1. [Published correction appears in *Lancet.* 2019; 393 (10178):1298.]
2. Ruiz-Tovar J, Carbajo MA, Jimenez JM, et al. Long-term follow-up after sleeve gastrectomy versus Roux-en-Y gastric bypass versus one-anastomosis gastric bypass: a prospective randomized comparative study of weight loss and remission of comorbidities. *Surg Endosc.* 2019;33(2): 401-410.
3. Shivakumar S, Tantia O, Goyal G, et al. LSG vs MGB-OAGB-3 year follow-up data: a randomised control trial. *Obes Surg.* 2018;28(9):2820-2828. doi:10.1007/s11695-018-3255-3.
4. Carbajo MA, Luque-de-León E, Jiménez JM, Ortiz-de-Solórzano J, Pérez-Miranda M, Castro-Alija MJ. Laparoscopic one-anastomosis gastric bypass: technique, results, and long-term follow-up in 1200 patients. *Obes Surg.* 2017;27(5):1153-1167.
5. Bruzzi M, Rau C, Voron T, Guenzi M, Berger A, Chevallier JM. Single anastomosis or mini-gastric bypass: long-term results and quality of life after a 5-year follow-up. *Surg Obes Relat Dis.* 2015;11(2):321-326.
6. Musella M, Susa A, Greco F, et al. The laparoscopic mini-gastric bypass: the Italian experience: outcomes from 974 consecutive cases in a multicenter review. *Surg Endosc.* 2014;28(1):156-163.
7. Lee WJ, Ser KH, Lee YC, Tsou JJ, Chen SC, Chen JC. Laparoscopic Roux-en-Y vs. mini-gastric bypass for the treatment of morbid obesity: a 10-year experience. *Obes Surg.* 2012;22(12):1827-1834.
8. Kular KS, Manchanda N, Rutledge R. A 6-year experience with 1,054 mini-gastric bypasses—first study from Indian subcontinent. *Obes Surg.* 2014;24(9):1430-1435.
9. Noun R, Skaff J, Riachi E, Daher R, Antoun NA, Nasr M. One thousand consecutive mini-gastric bypass: short- and long-term outcome. *Obes Surg.* 2012;22(5):697-703.
10. Peraglie C. Laparoscopic mini-gastric bypass in patients age 60 and older. *Surg Endosc.* 2016;30(1):38-43.
11. Lee WJ, Yu PJ, Wang W, Chen TC, Wei PL, Huang MT. Laparoscopic Roux-en-Y versus mini-gastric bypass for

the treatment of morbid obesity: a prospective randomized controlled trial. *Ann Surg*. 2005;242(1):20-28.
12. Rheinwalt KP, Plamper A, Rückbeil MV, Kroh A, Neumann UP, Ulmer TF. One anastomosis gastric bypass-mini-gastric bypass (OAGB-MGB) versus Roux-en-Y gastric bypass (RYGB)—a mid-term cohort study with 612 patients. *Obes Surg*. 2019;10:1230-1240.
13. Plamper A, Lingohr P, Nadal J, Rheinwalt KP. Comparison of mini–gastric bypass with sleeve gastrectomy in a mainly super-obese patient group: first results. *Surg Endosc*. 2017;31(3):1156-1162.
14. Madhok B, Mahawar KK, Boyle M, et al. Management of super-super obese patients: comparison between mini (one anastomosis) gastric bypass and sleeve gastrectomy. *Obes Surg*. 2016;26(7):1646-1649.
15. Magouliotis DE, Tasiopoulou VS, Svokos AA, Svokos KA, Sioka E, Zacharoulis D. One-anastomosis gastric bypass versus sleeve gastrectomy for morbid obesity: a systematic review and meta-analysis. *Obes Surg*. 2017;27(9): 2479-2487.
16. Kular KS, Manchanda N, Cheema GK. Seven years of mini-gastric bypass in type II diabetes patients with a body mass index < 35 kg/m(2). *Obes Surg*. 2016; 26(7):1457-1462.
17. Mahawar KK, Jennings N, Brown J, Gupta A, Balupuri S, Small PK. "Mini" gastric bypass: systematic review of a controversial procedure. *Obes Surg*. 2013;23(11): 1890-1898.
18. Wang W, Wei PL, Lee YC, Huang MT, Chiu CC, Lee WJ. Short-term results of laparoscopic mini-gastric bypass. *Obes Surg*. 2005;15(5):648-654.
19. Piazza L, Ferrara F, Leanza S, et al. Laparoscopic mini-gastric bypass: short-term single-institute experience. *Updates Surg*. 2011;63(4):239-242.
20. Chevallier JM, Arman GA, Guenzi M, et al. One thousand single anastomosis (omega loop) gastric bypasses to treat morbid obesity in a 7-year period: outcomes show few complications and good efficacy. *Obes Surg*. 2015;25(6):951-958.
21. Noun R, Riachi E, Zeidan S, Abboud B, Chalhoub V, Yazigi A. Mini-gastric bypass by mini-laparotomy: a cost effective alternative in the laparoscopic era. *Obes Surg*. 2007;17(11):1482-1486.
22. Georgiadou D, Sergentanis TN, Nixon A, Diamantis T, Tsigris C, Psaltopoulou T. Efficacy and safety of laparoscopic mini gastric bypass. A systematic review. *Surg Obes Relat Dis*. 2014;10(5):984-991.
23. Bruzzi M, Rau C, Voron T, Guenzi M, Berger A, Chevallier JM. Single anastomosis or mini-gastric bypass: long-term results and quality of life after a 5-year follow-up. *Surg Obes Relat Dis*. 2015;11(2):321-326.
24. Musella M, Susa A, Greco F, et al. The laparoscopic mini-gastric bypass: the Italian experience: outcomes from 974 consecutive cases in a multicenter review. *Surg Endosc*. 2014;28(1):156-163.
25. Mahawar KK, Kumar P, Carr WR, et al. Current status of mini-gastric bypass. *J Minim Access Surg*. 2016;12(4):305-310.
26. Musella M, Susa A, Manno E, et al. Complications following the mini/one anastomosis gastric bypass (MGB/OAGB): a multi-institutional survey on 2678 patients with a mid-term (5 years) follow-up. *Obes Surg*. 2017;27(11):2956-2967.
27. Saarinen T, Räsänen Salo J, et al. Bile reflux scintigraphy after mini-gastric bypass. *Obes Surg*. 2017;27(8): 2083-2089.
28. Runkel M, Pauthner M, Runkel N. The first case report of a carcinoma of the gastric cardia (AEG II) after OAGB-MGB. *Obes Surg*. 2020;30(2):753-754.
29. Ruiz-Tovar J, Carbajo MA, Jimenez JM, Luque-de-Leon E, Ortiz-de-Solorzano J, Castro MJ. Are there ideal small bowel limb lengths for one-anastomosis gastric bypass (OAGB) to obtain optimal weight loss and remission of comorbidities with minimal nutritional deficiencies? *World J Surg*. 2019;44(3):855-862. doi:10.1007/s00268-019-05243-0.
30. Jedamzik J, Eilenberg M, Felsenreich DM, Krebs M, Ranzenberger-Haider T, Langer FB, Prager G. Impact of limb length on nutritional status in one-anastomosis gastric bypass: 3-year results. *Surg Obes Relat Dis*. 2019;16(4):476-484.
31. Ahuja A, Tantia O, Goyal G, et al. MGB-OAGB: effect of biliopancreatic limb length on nutritional deficiency, weight loss, and comorbidity resolution. *Obes Surg*. 2018;28:3439-3445. https://doi.org/10.1007/s11695-018-3405-7.
32. Benamro F, Bhandari M, Gusani R, Khurana M, Rajvaidya A, Fobi M. Lengthening of the common channel improves hypoalbuminemia and intractable diarrhea after OAGB/MGB. *Surg Obes Relat Dis*. 2020;16(6):P817. https://doi.org/10.1016/j.soard.2020.01.002.
33. Khalaj A, Kalantar Motamedi MA, Mousapour P, Valizadeh M, Barzin M. Protein-calorie malnutrition requiring revisional surgery after one-anastomosis-mini-gastric bypass (OAGB-MGB): case series from the Tehran Obesity Treatment Study (TOTS). *Obes Surg*. 2019;29(6):1714-1720. doi:10.1007/s11695-019-03741-7.
34. Jammu GS, Sharma R. A 7-year clinical audit of 1107 cases comparing sleeve gastrectomy, Roux-En-Y gastric bypass, and mini-gastric bypass, to determine an effective and safe bariatric and metabolic procedure. *Obes Surg*. 2016;26(5):926-932.
35. Lee WJ, Ser KH, Lee YC, Tsou JJ, Chen SC, Chen JC. Laparoscopic Roux-en-Y vs. mini-gastric bypass for the treatment of morbid obesity: a 10-year experience. *Obes Surg*. 2012;22(12):1827-1834.

24

Single Anastomosis Duodenoileostomy and Sleeve Gastrectomy

Angel Reyes, MD

A 38-year-old female with a body mass index (BMI) of 52 kg/m^2 and obesity-related comorbidities including type 2 diabetes mellitus, hypertension, hyperlipidemia, and polycystic ovary syndrome is in your office because she wants to pursue metabolic (bariatric) surgery. She is taking simvastatin (Zocor) and metformin, and recently started insulin. She has completed a nutritional evaluation and behavioral health assessment, and is medically fit to undergo surgery. She is interested to know more about the single anastomosis duodenoileostomy and sleeve gastrectomy (SADI-S) procedure because she read on the Internet that it was safer.

1. **Which of the following statements is true about the SADI-S procedure?**
   - A. It carries a risk of bile reflux >5%.
   - B. It has a lower type 2 diabetes remission rate than Roux-en-Y gastric bypass (RYGB).
   - C. It is an option as a revisional procedure after a failed sleeve gastrectomy (SG).
   - D. There is a higher risk of vitamin B_1 deficiencies due to potential malabsorption of fat.

2. **The hormonal changes that explain this patient's decreased hunger sensation and her improved glycemic metabolism after metabolic surgery include which of the following?**
   - A. Increased orexin and increased neuropeptide Y (NPY)
   - B. Decreased ghrelin and increased glucagon-like peptide 1 (GLP-1)
   - C. Decreased ghrelin and decreased leptin
   - D. Increased orexin and increased GLP-1

3. **Regarding the technical aspect of SADI-S, which of the following is true?**
   - A. Vertical SG, 150-cm common channel, 150-cm alimentary limb
   - B. Horizontal partial gastrectomy, 250-cm alimentary limb, 50-cm common channel
   - C. Vertical SG, pylorus sparing, 300-cm common channel
   - D. Small gastric pouch, 150-cm alimentary limb, 60-cm biliopancreatic limb

4. **Which of the following is the most common complication of SADI-S?**
   - A. Duodenal stump leak
   - B. Internal hernia
   - C. Diarrhea
   - D. Retrograde filling of the afferent limb

5. **Compared to a RYGB, the SADI-S procedure has which of the following?**
   - A. A higher risk of marginal ulcers
   - B. Greater absorption of dietary fat
   - C. Less midterm weight loss
   - D. Less postprandial serum glucose variability

6. **In addition to diet modification and antidiarrheal medication, what else should be considered as an etiology of her bowel movement frequency?**

A. Dumping syndrome
B. Short biliopancreatic limb
C. Short common channel
D. Celiac disease

ANSWERS

1. **C.** SADI-S is a modification of the biliopancreatic diversion with duodenal switch (BPD-DS). SADI-S is also called Stomach Intestinal Pylorus Sparing (SIPS) surgery. The difference between these two procedures is the absence of a second anastomosis with SADI-S. The reported incidence of bile reflux after SADI-S is 0.1%. Several explanations for this low rate of bile reflux are the preservation of the pylorus valve and the dilution of bile with intestinal and pancreatic secretions as it travels through the small intestine.[1,2,4,9,10,11,20]

   The diabetes type 2 remission rate (defined as HgbA1c <6% without antidiabetic medications) for 1 to 4 years for SADI-S has been reported to be 72.4%, 70.3%, 64.4%, and 70.5%, respectively. A retrospective matched cohort study by Cottam et al compared the rate of type 2 diabetes remission of SADI-S versus RYGB. The SADI-S remission rate was significantly higher than for RYGB patients at every HgbA1c level measured.[9]

   The SG procedure has become the most common bariatric procedure performed in the United States, and worldwide as well as of 2014. The SG has been offered as a first step in patients with a BMI > 50 or high-risk patients. *For patients with insufficient weight loss after an SG (failed sleeve), conversion to a SADI-S is a good option, as it adds an intestinal bypass component to a mostly restrictive procedure.* For patients that develop gastroesophageal reflux after an SG, a conversion to RYGB is preferred. The small gastric pouch of the gastric bypass reduces intragastric pressure and the quantity of acid-secreting cells. The Roux-en-Y anatomy of the small bowel diverts all biliopancreatic secretions from the gastroesophageal junction.

   Micronutrient deficiencies are common after metabolic/bariatric surgery procedures. The etiology of these deficiencies is related to decreased acidity, which can occur after every procedure that alters the volume of the stomach (except gastric banding). The other mechanisms that place bariatric surgery patients at risk of nutritional deficiencies are rerouting of the food transit, avoiding the duodenum and proximal small bowel where most of the absorption occurs, and decreasing the time in contact with the small bowel as it occurs with predominantly malabsorptive procedures, such as the duodenal switch and SADI-S. SADI-S and BPD-DS have an increased risk of malabsorption of the fat-soluble vitamins A, D, E, and K. There is also a risk of deficiencies of water-soluble vitamins such as thiamine (B1), B12, biotin, and vitamin C. Thiamine deficiency can be exacerbated by vomiting, poor dietary intake, and noncompliance to oral supplements, but not by decreased fat absorption. The most common complication after SADI-S procedure is diarrhea.

   The patient underwent an SADI-S procedure. She is in your office today for her scheduled 12-month follow-up. Her current BMI is 28. She is no longer taking metformin or insulin. She has not felt hungry since she underwent surgery.

2. **B.** The metabolic/bariatric procedures result in anatomic changes to the gastrointestinal tract that affect the hunger and satiety signals to the hypothalamus. These changes will translate into long-term weight loss, and also the remission of diabetes, even before significant weight loss has occurred. One of the earliest mechanisms that contribute to weight loss as well as glycemic improvement is caloric restriction. This is due to the reduction of the size of the stomach to a small pouch in the case of RYGB, or a long gastric tube in the case of SG, SADI-S, and BPD-DS. The procedures that also have an intestinal bypass component (i.e., SADI-S, RYGB, BPD-DS) will reduce caloric intake by bypassing a portion of the small bowel involved in the absorption of macronutrients and reducing the transit of food through the small intestine. The caloric restriction component is effective only for the first weeks to months after surgery. In addition, these metabolic/bariatric procedures will produce a change in the hormones involved with hunger/satiety and glucose metabolism almost immediately after surgery. This metabolic effect of the surgery will have a lasting effect and correlates with the findings of improvement of diabetes type 2 before any significant weight loss takes place. To understand this concept, we need to discuss the hunger/satiety mechanisms of the central nervous system and hypothalamus, the incretin mechanisms of the gastrointestinal tract, and the relationship between the two.

In the central nervous system, there are several clusters of neurons localized in different areas of the hypothalamus. The pro-opiomelanocortin/cocaine-amphetamine regulated peptides (POMC-CART) and the neuropeptide Y–agouti-related peptide–gamma-aminobutyric acid (NPY-AgRP-GABA) control satiety and hunger, respectively, and both are located in the arcuate nucleus (ARC) of the hypothalamus. The POMC-CART and NPY-AgRP-GABA neurons are referred to as *first-order neurons.* The POMC-CART neurons produce alpha-melanocyte-stimulating hormone (α-MSH) when stimulated by leptin and insulin. α-MSH will then stimulate melanocortin-4 (MC4) receptors located in the paraventricular nucleus (PVN), activating the neurons in this center and exerting a positive effect on fullness. α-MSH also stimulates melanocortin-3 (MC3) receptors located in the NPY-AgRP center, inhibiting the release of both NPY and AgRP and causing fullness. The NPY-AgRP-GABA neurons are inhibited by leptin, insulin, and PYY, and stimulated by ghrelin and orexin. So ghrelin and orexin promote hunger, while leptin, insulin, and PYY create feelings of fullness. The POMC-CART and NPY-AgRP centers regulate each other; when one of them is stimulated, it inhibits the effects of the other.

The PVN has direct projections to the nucleus tractus solitarius (NTS). The PVN projections to the NTS have the net effect of inhibiting food intake. The PVN also receives input from the midbrain and the gastrointestinal tract via NTS afferent signals. The next is the lateral hypothalamic area (LHA), where orexin-producing neurons are located. Orexin neurons correspond to the so-called feeding center. Orexin production is stimulated by ghrelin, fasting, and hypoglycemia, and inhibited by leptin and hyperglycemia. Orexin neurons project to the ARC NPY neurons, stimulating secretion of NPY. The NPY neurons also project to the PVN, and orexin-containing nerve fibers are in close association with the NPY projections to PVN. NPY receptor activation of PVN neurons causes a strong inhibition of the fullness signal. The PVN and LHA neurons are referred as *second-order neurons.*

These centers in the hypothalamus also have receptors to peripheral molecules such as leptin, insulin, ghrelin, and PYY. These peripheral signals are the ones that are directly affected after bariatric/metabolic surgery, and they will mediate the changes in hunger and satiety seen postoperatively.

Ghrelin is an orexigenic hormone secreted mostly from the X/A cells of the stomach fundus. It is the only known peripheral orexigenic hormone. The secretion of ghrelin is cyclical, with levels rising during fasting and decreasing after a meal. SADI-S reduces the levels of ghrelin when the stomach fundus is resected after creation of the sleeve. When ghrelin levels decrease, so does the stimulation of orexin and NPY-AgRP-GABA neurons, thus reducing hunger and feeding signals to the hypothalamus. At the same time, the inhibition on POMC-CART and the PVN satiety signals from NPY-AgRP is removed. The combined effect is a predominant satiety, a fullness state.

The effects of leptin and insulin are affected during obesity due to overnutrition causing insulin resistance in the brain, and a proinflammatory state of obesity causing local inflammation in the hypothalamus. Leptin levels are increased in obesity, but its effect on the central nervous system is blunted due to leptin resistance. In the central nervous system, the effect of insulin depends on an intact leptin-signaling system. Leptin levels will decrease with decreased adiposity.

Peptide-tyrosine-tyrosine (PYY) belongs to the peptide polypeptide family and is secreted by the L cells in the ileum in response to a meal. PYY has affinity for the neuropeptide Y2 receptor (Y2R) located in the NPY-AgRP, effectively inhibiting these neurons and reducing the sensation of hunger. The PYY level increases after bariatric/metabolic procedures, especially those that alter the gastrointestinal anatomy such as SADI-S. The nutrient-rich chyme travels to the ileum and stimulates these L cells, causing a marked increase in PYY levels—higher than you would expect after a meal in a normal subject. Other effects of PYY are a decrease in gastric emptying via the ileal break mechanism.

The glucose metabolism after metabolic surgery is affected by a different set of molecules known as *incretins.* Incretins increase the secretion of insulin in response to oral glucose, and they include GLP-1, glucagon-like peptide-2 (GLP-2), and glucose-dependent insulinotropic peptide (GIP). They are also secreted by the L cells in the terminal ileum except for GIP, which is secreted by the K cells in the duodenum. GLP-1 effects include improved insulin secretion in response to a meal and other effects similar to PYY, like decreased gastric emptying via ileal braking. The metabolic procedures that involve bypassing a segment of the proximal small bowel

(RNYGB, BPD-DS, SADI-S) produce an increase of these incretins immediately after surgery. The increase in GLP-1 has been proven to occur after SG as well, even though this procedure does not bypass a segment of the small bowel. There is increased gastric emptying after SG, as well as a rapid transit of nutrient-rich chyme to the distal ileum, stimulating the L cells and hence increasing GLP-1 levels after a meal.

Adiponectin is an adipokine secreted by the healthy adipose tissue. Its levels are decreased in obesity, type 2 diabetes, and insulin resistance. In obese individuals, the levels of adiponectin are inversely related to those of leptin. Metabolic surgery and nonsurgical weight loss produce an increase of adiponectin, despite a reduction of fat mass, and a decrease of leptin (Figure 24-1).[19,21]

3. **C.** SADI-S is the most recent metabolic surgical procedure endorsed by the ASMBS as an option to treat obesity. The procedure was proposed in 2007 by Sanchez-Pernaute and Antonio Torres as a modification of the duodenal switch. The original version of the procedure by Sanchez et al is constructed with a vertical sleeve over a 56-Fr bougie, and they initially used a 200-cm common channel but increased the length to 250 cm, which saw the nutritional deficiency rate decrease from 8% to 1%. The procedure was modified by Cottam and has an SG created over a 40-Fr bougie, which preserves the pylorus, and a loop of small bowel (common channel) is anastomosed at 300 cm from the ileocecal valve to the duodenum (Figure 24-2).

Long-term weight loss outcomes after SADI are comparable to DS. Long-term data is from Spain. Comorbid resolution is also comparable. The 300-cm limb provides excellent weight loss in the super obese minus the side effects of macronutrient deficiency and frequent loose stools or diarrhea.

The gastric bypass procedure is considered the gold standard of bariatric procedures. The procedure entails a lesser curve-based gastric pouch with a volume of approximately 30 ml, a biliopancreatic limb of 60 cm, and an alimentary limb of 150 cm. There are two anastomoses, a proximal gastrojejunal anastomose and a jejuno-jejunal anastomose connecting the biliopancreatic and alimentary limbs (Figure 24-3).

The biliopancreatic diversion procedure was originally described by Nicola Scopinaro in 1979.

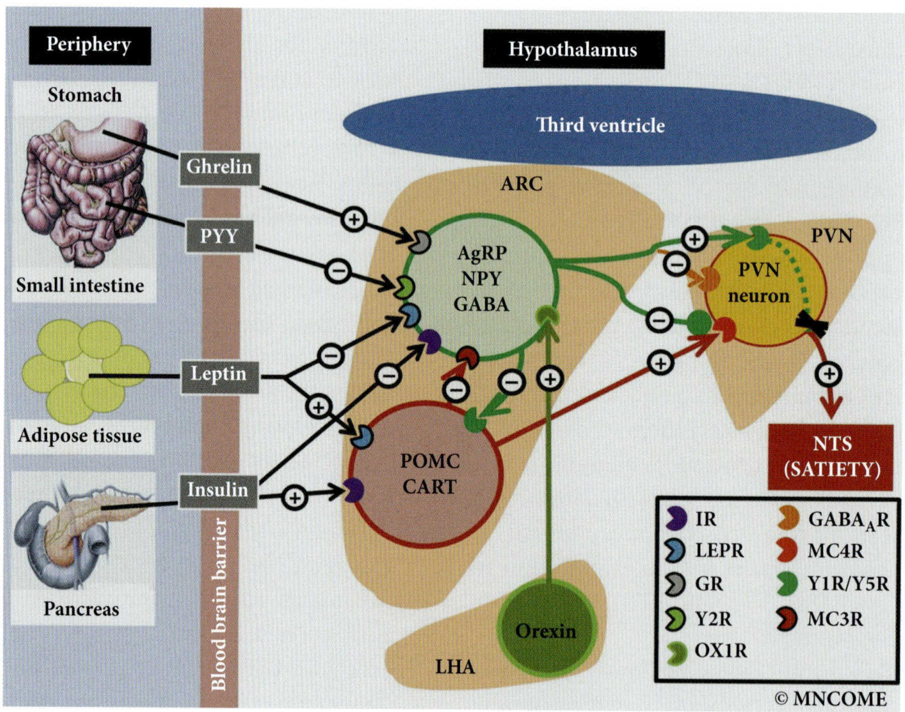

Figure 24-1 Interaction between peripheral hormones and the hypothalamic centers of satiety and hunger. (Reproduced with permission from Gonzalez-Campoy JM, Hurley DL, Garvey WT. *Bariatric Endocrinology: Evaluation and Management of Adiposity, Adiposopathy and Related Diseases*. Switzerland: Springer International Publishing; 2019.)

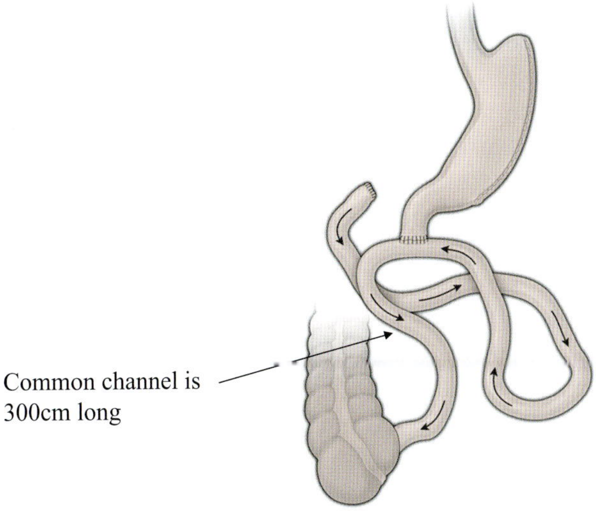

Figure 24-2 SADI-S. (Reproduced with permission from Doherty GM: *CURRENT Diagnosis & Treatment Surgery, 15th ed.* New York, NY: McGraw Hill; 2020.)

It involves a distal gastrectomy with an alimentary limb of 250 cm and a common channel of 50 cm. The procedure had a larger gastric pouch, as opposed to the gastric bypass procedure. However, it was associated with postgastrectomy syndromes such as marginal ulcer, dumping syndrome, and diarrhea.

The BPD-DS was first performed by Hess and Hess in 1988. The duodenal switch differs from the Scopinaro BPD, in that the pylorus is preserved and the gastrectomy is done in a sleeve fashion. By preserving the pylorus, there is less risk of marginal ulcers and dumping syndrome. The alimentary limb is usually 150 cm long, and the common channel is about 150 cm long as well (Figure 24-4).[2,4,9,12,20]

4. **D.** SADI-S is a modification of the traditional duodenal switch that involves only one anastomosis rather than the traditional Roux-en-Y reconstruction. This modification simplifies the operation and eliminates the risk of a second anastomosis. The reported risk of anastomotic leak, marginal ulcer, anastomotic stricture, and bile reflux is 0.6%, 0.1%, 0.3%, and 0.1%,

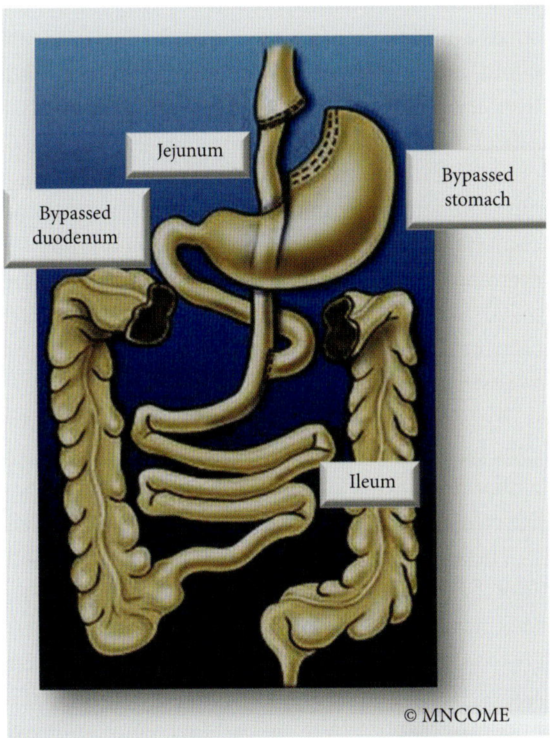

Figure 24-3 RYGB. (Reproduced with permission from Gonzalez-Campoy JM, Hurley DL, Garvey WT. *Bariatric Endocrinology: Evaluation and Management of Adiposity, Adiposopathy and Related Diseases.* Switzerland: Springer International Publishing; 2019.)

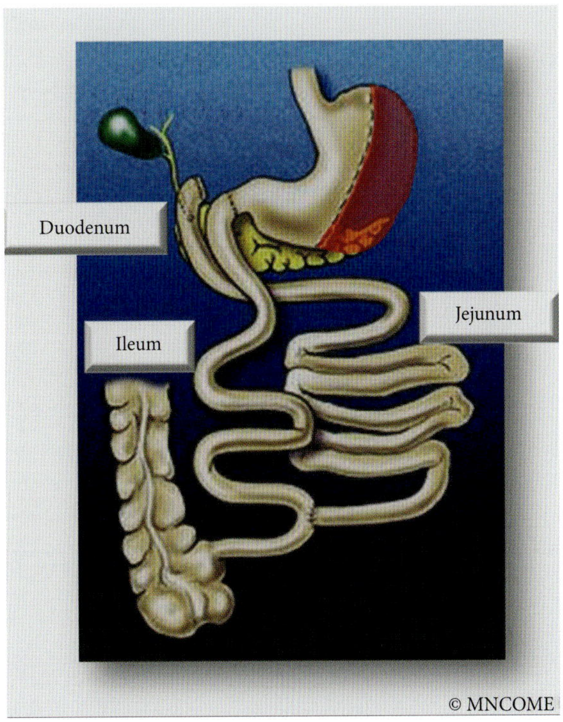

Figure 24-4 BPD-DS. (Reproduced with permission from Gonzalez-Campoy JM, Hurley DL, Garvey WT. *Bariatric Endocrinology: Evaluation and Management of Adiposity, Adiposopathy and Related Diseases.* Switzerland: Springer International Publishing; 2019.)

respectively. Even though there is no mesenteric window created because there is only one anastomosis and no Roux-en-Y reconstruction, there is a risk of internal hernia. An internal hernia can occur at the potential space created when the loop of small bowel is brought anterior to the transverse colon to create the single anastomosis. Although rare, this complication has been reported by Cottam et al recently. One way to decrease the risk of this complication is by suturing the afferent limb to the omentum, fixating the limb in order to prevent it from twisting around the anastomosis like a volvulus.

Duodenal stump leak is also a potential complication of SADI-S. A technique used by Cottam and Roslin preserves the blood supply to the duodenal stump. In this technique, the gastroepiploic perforators are divided at a point 3 cm distal to the pylorus. At this point, the dissection of the duodenum stops at the gastroduodenal artery, preserving the branches of the pancreaticoduodenal arch and the supraduodenal artery (Figure 24-5).

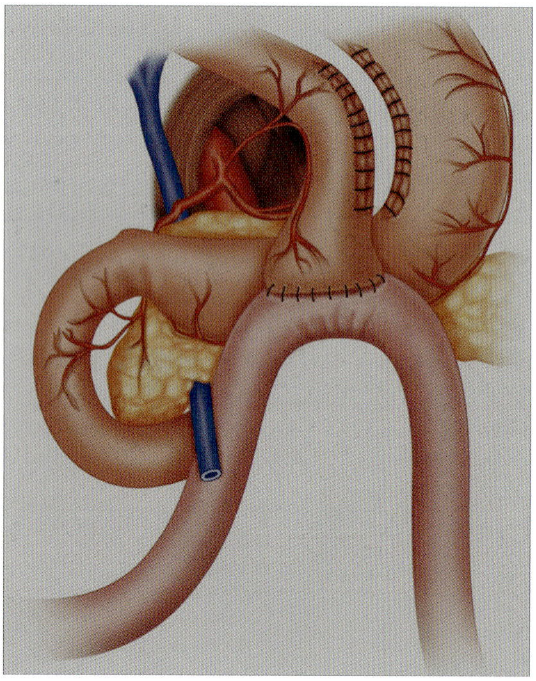

Figure 24-5 Blood supply to the duodenum. (Reproduced with permission from Nguyen NT, Brethauer SA, Morton JM, et al: *The ASMBS Textbook of Bariatric Surgery, 2nd ed.* Switzerland: Springer International Publishing; 2020.)

Intussusception is not a complication of SADI-S. Malabsorptive procedures such as SADI-S and the duodenal switch bypass about two-thirds of the small bowel to create a common channel measuring 150 to 300 cm. The benefits of this configuration are greater weight loss and a higher remission rate of type 2 diabetes compared to the gastric bypass procedure. The downside is a higher risk of macronutrient and micronutrient deficiencies, such as hypoproteinemia. The rate of occurrence of hypoproteinemia is 1.3% to 2%.

Retrograde filling of the afferent limb is a rare complication of the loop anastomosis of the SADI-S procedure. This complication can cause symptoms resembling a partial small bowel obstruction, but it can be prevented by suturing the afferent limb (i.e. the biliopancreatic limb) to the antrum of the stomach. The most common complication related to SADI-S procedure is chronic diarrhea, seen in 2% of patients. In most patients, it can be treated with dietary changes, and medications such as Lomotil.[5,6,9,15,17,20]

5. **D.** Malabsorptive procedures such as SADI-S and the duodenal switch bypass about two-thirds of the small bowel to create a common channel measuring about 150 to 300 cm. The benefits of this configuration are greater weight loss and a higher remission rate of diabetes type 2 compared to the gastric bypass procedure. The downside is a higher risk of macronutrient and micronutrient deficiencies with poor compliance with vitamin supplementation, and diet choices. There is more fat malabsorption after SADI-S compared to gastric bypass. The midterm (36 months) weight loss after SADI-S is comparable to gastric bypass (86% versus 79.9%).

   By preserving the pylorus, there is less risk of marginal ulcers and dumping syndrome. The reported rate of marginal ulcers after SADI-S is 0.1%, and the average rate of marginal ulcers after RYGB is 4% to 5%.

   There is less postprandial glucose variability after SADI-S compared to gastric bypass surgery. This has been measured directly using continuous glucose monitoring, with a higher average percentage of time in both hyperglycemic and hypoglycemic ranges observed in patients who underwent RYGB.[3,9,12,14]

   The patient returns at 18 months after surgery and reports having 6 to 8 loose bowel movements a day. She is following a low carb diet and takes a multivitamin twice a day. Her laboratory workup was unremarkable except for protein 5.0 (6–8 g/dL), and albumin 2.0 (3.5–5 g/dL).

A full workup is done, including checking for *Clostridium difficile* toxins, which was negative. She was also evaluated by a nutritionist to ensure that a proper diet was followed. On physical exam, there is mild peripheral edema.

6. C. This patient's diarrhea is likely secondary to a common channel measuring less than 200 cm. Loose stools after SADI-S or duodenal switch (DS) is not uncommon and is frequently related to dietary indiscretions. The first-line therapy is dietary restriction, avoiding carbohydrates such as bread, pasta, and refined sugars. There is a 65% fat malabsorption after SADI-S with a 300-cm common channel. Patients need to be aware of this to avoid excessive flatulence and steatorrhea. Stool testing should be done to rule out infectious etiologies, and then an antidiarrheal should be used to decrease the frequency of bowel movements. Macronutrient, micronutrient, and electrolyte deficiencies can be significant in a patient with daily diarrhea. This patient has clinical hypoproteinemia with peripheral edema, and also blood chemistry indices showing hypoalbuminemia and abnormal protein levels. She should be considered for a revision of the SADI-S procedure to lengthen the common channel by an additional 200 to 300 cm.

A short biliopancreatic limb has no relevance, and in fact it will make the common channel longer because there is a loop anastomosis. Dumping syndrome is unlikely, given that the pyloric valve is preserved. Lactose intolerance can cause diarrhea, but on this patient, who has already modified her diet, it is unlikely. Celiac disease is an immunologic condition resulting from the small bowel mucosa interacting with gluten. It may present with diarrhea, steatorrhea, and nutritional deficiencies, as well as other clinical signs such as skin rashes and joint pain. Serologic tests can be used to diagnose celiac disease.[7,8,12,16,17]

REFERENCES

1. Neichoy BT, Schiederjan B, Cottam DR, et al. Stomach intestinal pylorus-sparing surgery for morbid obesity. *JSLS*. 2018;22(1):1-6.
2. Roslin M, Tugertimur B, Zarabi S, Cottam D. Is there a better design for bariatric procedure? The case for a single anastomosis duodenal switch. *Obes Surg*. 2018;28(12): 4077-4086.
3. Sánchez-Pernaute A, Rubio SA, Cabrerizo L, Ramos-Levi A, Pérez-Aguirre E, Torres A. Single -anastomosis duodenoileal bypass as a second step after sleeve gastrectomy. *Surg Obes Relat Dis*. 2015;11:351-355.
4. Gebelli JP, Garcia Ruiz de Gordejuela A, Cardoso Ramos A, et al. SADI-S with right gastric artery ligation: technical systematization and early results. *Arq Bras Cir Dig*. 2016;29(Supl.1):85-90.
5. Surve A, Zaveri H, Cottam D. A safer and simpler technique of duodenal dissection and transection of the duodenal bulb for duodenal switch. *Surg Obes Relat Dis*. 2016;12(4):923-924.
6. Vilallonga R, Balibrea JM, Curell A, et al. Technical options for malabsorption issues after single anastomosis duodenoileal bypass with sleeve gastrectomy. *Obes Surg*. 2017;27(12):3344-3348.
7. Surve A, Zaveri H, Cottam D. A step-by-step surgical technique video with two reported cases of common channel lengthening in patients with previous stomach intestinal pylorus sparing surgery to treat chronic diarrhea. *Surg Obes Relat Dis*. 2017;13:706-709.
8. Cottam A, Cottam D, Zaveri H, et al. An analysis of mid-term complications, weight loss, and type 2 diabetes resolution of stomach intestinal pylorus-sparing surgery (SIPS) versus Roux-en-Y gastric bypass (RYGB) with three-year follow up. *Obes Surg*. 2018;28(9):2894-2902.
9. Zaveri H, Surve A, Cottam D, et al. Mid-term 4-year outcomes with single anastomosis duodenal-ileal bypass with sleeve gastrectomy surgery at a single US center. *Obes Surg*. 2018;28(10):3062-3072.
10. Sánchez-Pernaute A, Rubio SA, Cabrerizo L, Ramos-Levi A, Pérez-Aguirre E, Torres A. Single-anastomosis duodenoileal bypass with sleeve gastrectomy (SADI-S) for obese diabetic patients. *Surg Obes Relat Dis*. 2015;11(5): 1092-1098.
11. Surve A, Cottam D, Sánchez-Pernaute A, et al. The incidence of complications associated with loop duodeno-ileostomy after single-anastomosis duodenal switch procedures among 1328 patients: a multicenter experience. *Surg Obes Relat Dis*. 2018;14(5):594-602.
12. Grueneberger JM, Karcz-Socha I, Marjanovic G, et al. Pylorus preserving loop duodeno-enterostomy with sleeve gastrectomy-preliminary results. *BMC Surg*. 2014;20. https://doi.org/10.1186/1471-2482-14-20.
13. Ramos-Levi AM, Sánchez-Pernaute A, Marcuello C, et al. Glucose variability after bariatric surgery: is prediction of diabetes remission possible? *Obes Surg*. 2017;27(12): 3341-3343.
14. Surve A, Cottam D, Horsley B. Internal hernia following primary laparoscopic SADI-S: the first reported case. *Obes Surg*. 2020;30(5):2066-2068.
15. Horsley B, Cottam D, Cottam A, et al. Bowel reconstruction to treat chronic diarrhea and hypoproteinemia following single anastomosis duodenal-ileal bypass with sleeve gastrectomy: a single-site experience. *Obes Surg*. 2019;29(8):2387-2391.

16. Martini F, Paolino L, Marzano E, et al. Single-anastomosis pylorus-preserving bariatric procedures: review of the literature. *Obes Surg*. 2016;26(10):2503-2515.
17. Romero F, Nicolau J, Flores L, et al. Comparable early changes in gastrointestinal hormones after sleeve gastrectomy and Roux-en-Y gastric bypass surgery for morbidly obese type 2 diabetic subjects. *Surg Endosc*. 2012;26(8):2231-2239.
18. Nguyen NT, Brethauer SA, Morton JM, Ponce J, Rosenthal RJ, Eds. *The ASMBS Textbook of Bariatric Surgery*. 2nd ed. Springer International Publishing, Switzerland; 2020.
19. Gonzalez-Campoy JM, Hurley DL, Garvey WT. *Bariatric Endocrinology: Evaluation and Management of Adiposity, Adiposopathy and Related Diseases*. 2019. Springer International Publishing, Switzerland; 2019.

25.1

Adjustable Gastric Band

Kinga A. Powers, MD, PhD, and Kevin K. Seeras, DO

A 52-year-old female with a body mass index (BMI) of 43 kg/m^2, with a medical history of noninsulin-dependent DM, hypertension, severe gastroesophageal reflux disease (GERD), hyperlipidemia, and osteoarthritis, presents to the emergency room (ER) with acute onset of nausea, retching, dysphagia, and inability to tolerate liquids for 4 hours. The patient had a laparoscopic adjustable gastric banding (LAGB) procedure performed 15 years earlier, and she has not seen her surgeon for 10 years. Further investigation reveals that she had a transabdominal hysterectomy 3 years ago. She does not recall the last time she had fluid inserted or removed from her band, but she states she has gained weight steadily for the last 5 years. The lowest BMI she can recall was 38 kg/m^2, and she states that she was never able to discontinue any of her medications for her comorbidities. On exam, her abdomen is soft, minimally tender in the upper abdomen, and nondistended, with no evidence of peritoneal signs. Her vital signs are heart rate 82, blood pressure 152/89, temperature 98.8°, and respiration rate 16.

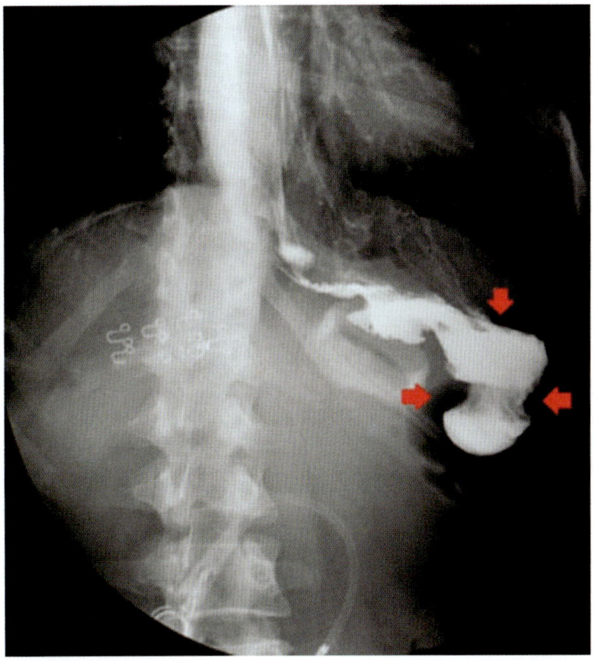

Figure 25-1 Upper GI study-the red arrows indicated contrast in the stomach and do not represent a leak.

1. Regarding this scenario, which of the following steps should be immediately taken?

A. Plain abdominal X-ray, followed by upper gastrointestinal swallow (UGI) study
B. Emergent esophagogastroduodenoscopy (EGD)
C. Immediate operative exploration
D. Nasogastric tube insertion
E. Removal of fluid from the port of the gastric band and follow-up with a bariatric surgeon

2. In the ER, you obtain an UGI study, the results of which are demonstrated in Figure 25-1. You attempt to remove fluid but find that there is none within the band. Which of the following statements regarding this diagnosis is most correct?

A. The pathology is more common with the perigastric technique of band placement.
B. The adoption of the gastric imbrication technique has reduced the incidence of some of these complications.

C. This image shows concentric pouch enlargement.
D. The incidence is less (1–5%) with proper technique. We can make it more wrong at 30%.
E. Figure 25-1 most likely represents a posterior fundus prolapse, with a characteristic horizontal band position.

3. **Emptying he band partially relieves the patient's symptoms, but she cannot tolerate solid food. The patient is taken to the operating room, and the band is removed laparoscopically. Intra-operatively, you determine that there is minimal edema or peri-band tissue inflammation. Which of the following is the best option at this time?**
   A. Conversion to a laparoscopic sleeve gastrectomy (SG)
   B. Conversion to a roux-en-y gastric bypass (RYGB)
   C. Replacement with a new LAGB
   D. Fenestrate any scarring on the stomach from the band because this can still cause restriction
   E. Multidisciplinary evaluation for a possible revision in the future

4. **Regarding elective bariatric revision surgery for LAGB, which of the following statements is most accurate?**
   A. Conversion to a SG is contraindicated in patients with GERD.
   B. Single-stage conversion to RYGB requires a longer length of hospital stay.
   C. When comparing a conversion to RYGB against primary RYGB, the revisional surgery patients experience less weight loss at 2 years.
   D. Single-stage conversion to RYGB as opposed to biliopancreatic diversion with duodenal switch (BPD-DS) has a similar complication rate.
   E. Conversion to a SG has a similar percentage of excess weight loss (% EWL) as conversion to RYGB.

ANSWERS

1. **A.** Acute gastric prolapse secondary to band slippage is a common late complication following adjustable gastric banding (LAGB). Patients will present with symptoms of proximal obstruction such as epigastric pain, nausea, vomiting, reflux, dysphagia, and intolerance of oral intake. Symptoms may also be chronic in nature (e.g., chronic partial prolapse) and may be similar to those with concentric gastric pouch dilation (due mostly to an overtight band).[1]

Immediate management of acute gastric prolapse should include prompt diagnosis and treatment to avoid secondary complications such as ischemia and necrosis of a herniated stomach. Diagnosis of gastric band slippage is confirmed radiographically, most commonly with plain abdominal X-ray and UGI. Abdominal X-ray will demonstrate abnormal positioning of the band (horizontal or pointing toward the left hip) versus normal (pointing to the left shoulder from the 8 o'clock to the 2 o'clock position, as shown in Figure 25-2). The UGI will demonstrate contrast filling of the enlarged/prolapsed fundus and failure of contrast to pass into the distal stomach.[2] If a prolapse is seen, the next step in treatment of this acute condition is immediate removal of any port fluid. This may be done under fluoroscopic guidance.[3] If the patient is subsequently able to swallow comfortably, she can be discharged to follow up with a bariatric surgeon for removal and revision.

Although computed tomography (CT) imaging and EGD may detect band slippage with stomach prolapse, they are not the typical initial studies performed, and this may delay diagnosis/treatment. If there is concern about strangulation of a prolapsed stomach (presenting with fevers, tachycardia, leukocytosis,

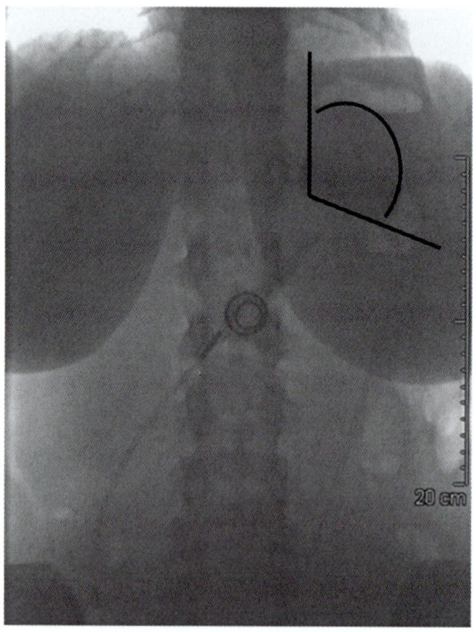

Phi angle 100°

Figure 25-2 Normal band position, pointing to the left shoulder from the 8 o'clock to the 2 o'clock position. (Reproduced with permission from Zinner MJ, Ashley SW, Hines OJ. *Maingot's Abdominal Operations, 13th ed.* New York, NY: McGraw Hill; 2019.)

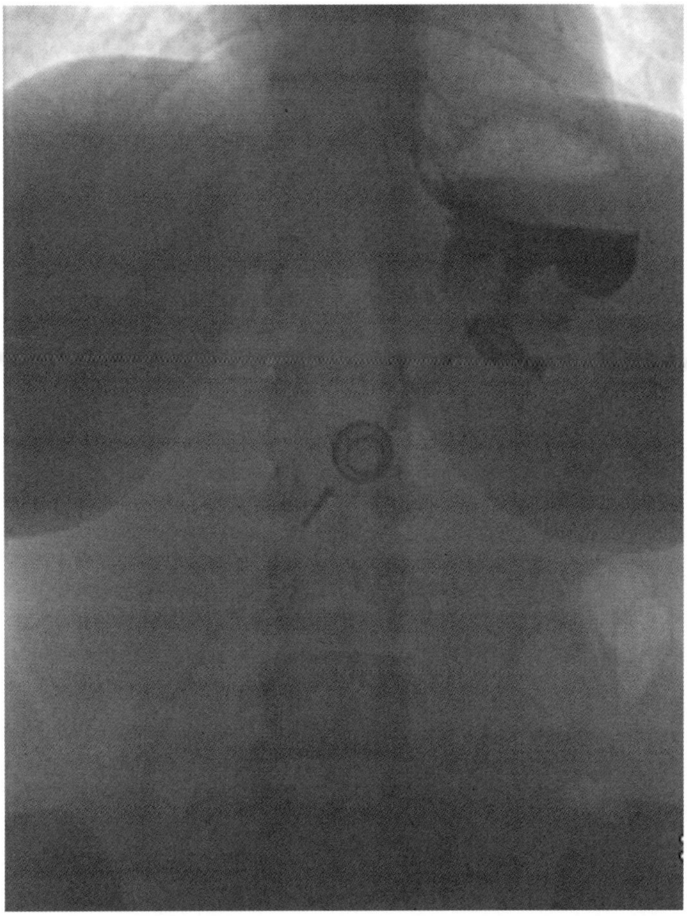

Figure 25-3 Anterior slip. (Reproduced with permission from Zinner MJ, Ashley SW, Hines OJ. *Maingot's Abdominal Operations, 13th ed.* New York, NY: McGraw Hill; 2019.)

severe upper abdominal pain), these modalities would be helpful in making that diagnosis. Evidence of strangulation requires immediate removal of the band and may require resection of the ischemic stomach.

The patient is presenting with acute symptoms of a proximal obstruction. Although small bowel obstruction secondary to adhesions is a possibility, acute gastric prolapse must first be ruled out, as it is an acute pathology that is treated differently.

2. **B.** This scenario concerns an anterior slippage of the band, and its incidence is reduced by adding a gastric plication when it is initially placed. LAGB was once one of the most common weight loss procedures due to its ease of placement, reversibility, low cost, and minimal recovery time.[4] It is considered the safest bariatric procedure, with a 1-year mortality rate of .08%, a 30-day morbidity rate of 3%, and a long-term complication rate of 12%, although the total revision rate is about 40% due to failed weight loss.[5–8] The initial technique of band placement employed the perigastric technique, which involved the dissection of all retrogastric attachments. This led to unacceptably high rates of posterior gastric prolapse and led to the adoption of the pars flaccida technique, in which the retrogastric attachments are kept in place, leaving the posterior portion of the band embedded in the retroperitoneal tissues and resulting in a decrease in posterior gastric prolapse. The addition of gastrogastric plication has been shown to decrease the rate of anterior band slippage. Prolapse is the most common band-related complication, requiring reoperation with an incidence of 1% to 5%, but prior to the abovementioned modifications in techniques, it had an incidence of 25%.[9,10] If the band needs to be removed emergently, it would be important to undo

this plication as well and fenestrate any scarring on the stomach from the band because this can still cause restriction and maintain the prolapse.

Band slippage can be classified as Types I to V (Figure 25-4) (Table 25-1) and have different etiologies.

Concentric pouch dilation can have a similar presentation to chronic gastric prolapse secondary to band slippage. Diagnosis is also done via upper GI swallow imaging, and management differs in the delayed setting. Initial management is similar, in that removing the band fluid is the first course of action; however, subsequent management will differ and may not require any operative intervention. If symptoms resolve as well as pouch dilation on repeat imaging, no operative intervention will be required, and continued use of the band with monitored refilling can proceed. If pouch dilation or symptoms persist, surgical intervention is warranted, which may include band removal/repositioning and/or conversion to another weight loss procedure.[11]

3. **E.** This patient's acute problem, poor intake by mouth, needs to be resolved, and although she will likely gain weight when the band is removed, a revision bariatric procedure should not be done without a multidisciplinary evaluation for surgery, and not in an acute setting. When considering an acute patient such as in this scenario, a thorough preoperative evaluation will not be completed, as urgent surgery is required. The primary goal of intervention in a gastric prolapse will be reduction of the stomach contents to prevent ischemia and relieve the obstruction, which is done primarily via band removal.

Revisional bariatric surgery for a laparoscopic adjustable gastric band (LAGB) includes many options. Indications for a revision include failure of weight loss, weight regain, comorbidity recurrence, and complications related to the band/port. The best course of action in a revisional case of LAGB utilizes several factors, which include the indication for revision, the condition of the patient, and the condition

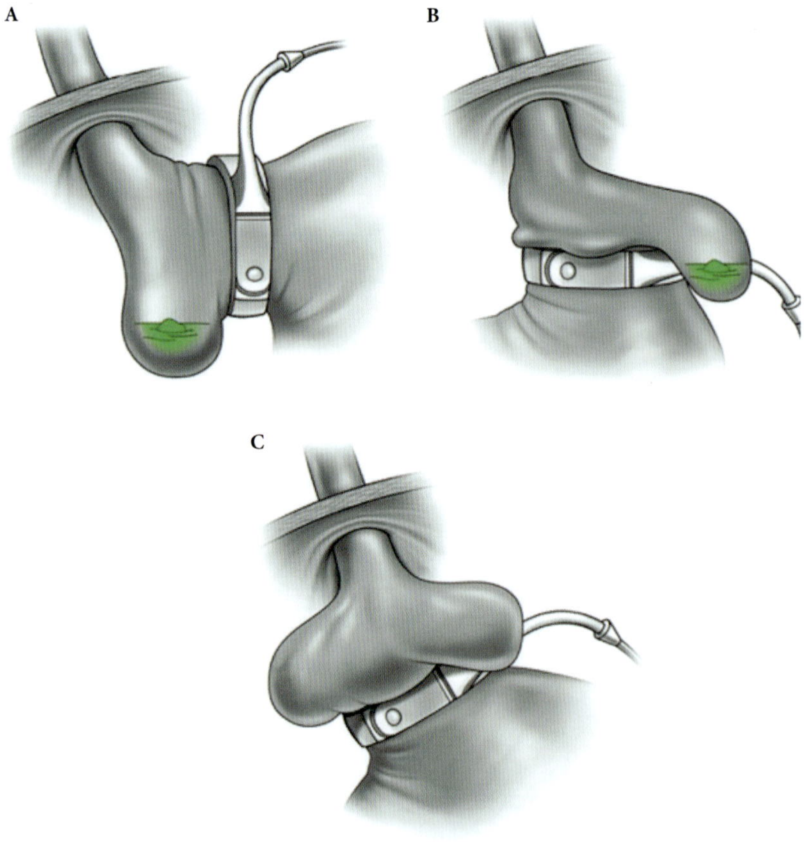

Figure 25-4 (**A**)Posterior band slippage with gastric prolapse, (**B**) Anterior band slippage with gastric prolapse, (**C**) Concentric pouch dilation. (Reproduced with permission from Nguyen NT, Brethauer SA, Morton JM, et al. *The ASMBS Textbook of Bariatric Surgery, 2nd ed.* Switzerland: Springer International Publishing; 2020.)

Table 25-1 TYPES OF BAND SLIPPAGES

Type	Etiology	AXR/UGI Imaging Description
I–Anterior slip (Figures 25-3, 25-4A)	Insufficient anterior fixation → downward migration of the band	Horizontal band position (rotated clockwise)
II–Posterior slip (Figure 25-4B)	Perigastric approach → cephalad migration of the posterior stomach through the band	Vertical band position (rotated counterclockwise)
III–Concentric pouch enlargement (Figure 25-4C, 25-5)	Tight band with or without overeating → progressive pouch dilation	Enlargement of the proximal gastric pouch without a change in the angle of the band
IV–Immediate postop slip	Technical error → low placement of the band	
V–Type I or II, with associated gastric necrosis	Acute pouch dilation → ischemia and necrosis	

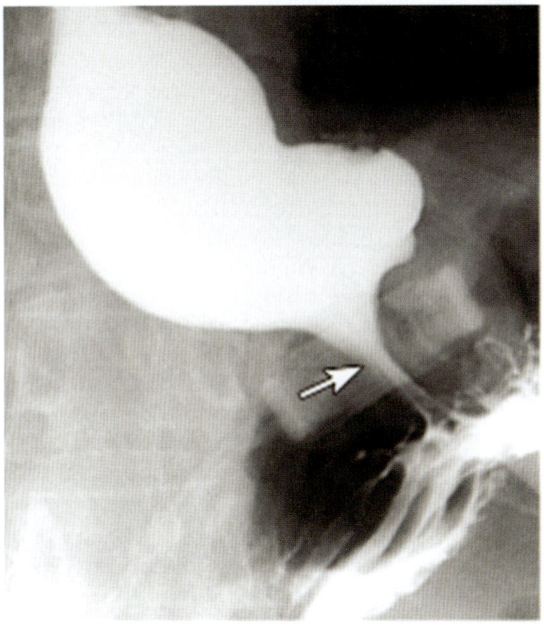

Figure 25-5 Concentric pouch enlargement. (Reproduced with permission from Levine MS, Carucci LR. Imaging of bariatric surgery: normal anatomy and postoperative complications. *Radiology*. 2014;270(2):327-341.)

of the tissues intra-operatively. However, success with revision is more variable than a de novo operation, and it is still highly dependent on patient circumstances. As such, a revision should not be conducted in the acute setting.

When considering a revision, repositioning and replacement of a band in this patient would not be appropriate in this case, as the patient has experienced failure of weight loss/weight regain with the original band and further treatment with this procedure would be futile. This technique may be considered in a patient who had an initial response to treatment but has had weight regain secondary to a band complication.[12]

As this patient has seen failure of her LAGB in terms of weight loss and comorbidity resolution, a conversion to a different weight loss procedure is indicated. Were this not an acute situation, this conversion could be completed in a one- or two-stage fashion. A recent systematic review demonstrated no differences in morbidity/mortality when comparing one or two staged techniques; however, there may have been a selection bias when considering a two-stage approach for LAGB-related complications as the indication for revision.[13]

4. **C.** In the outpatient setting, the most common indication for LAGB revisional surgery is failure of weight loss, weight regain, or both. Options for these patients include conversion to a different procedure, such as RYGB, laparoscopic sleeve gastrectomy (SG), BPD-DS, one anastomosis gastric bypass (OAGB), and Stomach Intestinal Pylorus Sparing Procedure (SIPS). The most common of these is RYGB, followed by SG. While revision with rebanding has been done in the past, the results are poor and lead to continued inadequate weight loss and need for further operations.[14]

Regarding conversion to RYGB versus primary RYGB, the former showed significantly higher intraoperative and postoperative complications, as well as lower weight loss and the need for interventions at 24 months.[15] The single-stage approach was evaluated and compared to the two-stage approach and found to be no different in terms of perioperative morbidity/mortality, but single-stage operations had a shorter length of hospital stay.[16]

Regarding conversion to SG as opposed to primary SG, there were no significantly higher complication rates between the two groups. The %EWL was lower in the conversion group at 6–12 months, but similar at 24 months.[17] The single-stage operation has similar complication rates as two-stage conversion. There was a significant increase in BMI after the first stage while waiting for the conversion surgery in the two-stage approach, which led to the recommendation of a single-stage operation when able.[13] While SG can be complicated by GERD, its preoperative presence in this patient may be caused by the band and prolapse. In fact, it may be improved simply by removing the band. As such, conversion to a SG is not contraindicated.

Regarding conversion to SG from RYGB, overall complication and reoperation rates are higher for RYGB, but with equivalent leak rates. There is a slight %EWL advantage for conversion to RYGB, and the benefits are seen most often in RYGB patients who have a higher initial BMI.[18]

Regarding conversion to BPD-DS, overall complication rates are high, with a 14% leak rate. It demonstrates the best %EWL rate, 66.2%, which is comparable to its primary operation counterpart.[19]

REFERENCES

1. Egan RJ, Monkhouse SJW, Meredith HE, Bates SE, Morgan JDT, Norton SA. The reporting of gastric band slip and related complications; a review of the literature. *Obes Surg*. 2011;21(8):1280-1288.
2. Beitner M, Kurian MS. Laparoscopic adjustable gastric banding. *Abdom Imag*. 2012;37(5):687-689. doi:10.1007/s00261-012-9864-8.
3. Manganiello M, Sarker S, Tempel M, Shayani V. Management of slipped adjustable gastric bands. *Surg Obes Relat Dis*. 2008;4(4):534-538. doi:10.1016/j.soard.2007.11.003.
4. Nguyen NT, Vu S, Kim E, Bodunova N, Phelan MJ. Trends in utilization of bariatric surgery, 2009–2012. *Surg Endosc*. 2016;30(7):2723-2727. doi:10.1007/s00464-015-4535-9.
5. Hutter MM, Schirmer BD, Jones DB, Ko CY, Cohen ME, Merkow RP, Nguyen NT. On behalf of the ACS-BSCN advisory committee. First report from the American College of Surgeons–bariatric surgery center network: laparoscopic sleeve gastrectomy has morbidity and effectiveness positioned between the band and the bypass. *Ann Surg*. 2012;254(3):410-422.
6. Smith MD, Patterson E, Wahed AS, et al. Thirty-day mortality after bariatric surgery: independently adjudicated causes of death in the longitudinal assessment of bariatric surgery. *Obes Surg*. 2011;21(11):1687-1692.
7. Nguyen NT, Hohmann S, Nguyen XM, Elliott C, Masoomi H. Outcome of laparoscopic adjustable gastric banding and prevalence of band revision and explantation at academic centers: 2007–2009. *Surg Obes Relat Dis*. 2012;8(6):724-727.
8. Carelli AM, Youn HA, Kurian MS, Ren CJ, Fielding GA. Safety of the laparoscopic adjustable gastric band: 7-year data from a U.S. center of excellence. *Surg Endosc*. 2010;24(8):1819-1823.
9. Snow JM, Severson PA. Complications of adjustable gastric banding. *Surg Clin North Am*. 2011;91(6):1249-1264. doi:10.1016/j.suc.2011.08.008.
10. Himpens J, Cadiére G-B, Bazi M, Vouche M, Cadiére B, Dapri G. Long-term outcomes of laparoscopic adjustable gastric banding. *Arch Surg*. 2011;146(7):802-807.
11. Arias IE, Radulescu M, Stiegeler R, et al. Diagnosis and treatment of megaesophagus after adjustable gastric banding for morbid obesity. *Surg Obes Relat Dis*. 2009;5(2):156-159.
12. Abu-Gazala S, Keidar A. Conversion of failed gastric banding into four different bariatric procedures. *Surg Obes Relat Dis*. 2012;8(4):400-407.
13. Dang JT, Switzer NJ, Wu J, et al. Gastric band removal in revisional bariatric surgery, one-step versus two-step: a systematic review and meta-analysis. *Obes Surg*. 2016;26(4):866-873. doi:10.1007/s11695-016-2082-7.
14. Müller MK, Attigah N, Wildi S, et al. High secondary failure rate of rebanding after failed gastric banding. *Surg Endosc*. 2008;22(2):448-453. doi:10.1007/s00464-007-9450-2.
15. Worni M, Østbye T, Shah A, et al. High risks for adverse outcomes after gastric bypass surgery following failed gastric banding. *Ann Surg*. 2013;257:279-286.
16. Debergh I, Defoort B, De Visschere M, et al. A one-step conversion from gastric banding to laparoscopic Roux-en-Y gastric bypass is as safe as a two-step conversion: a comparative analysis of 885 patients. *Acta Chir Belg*. 2016;116(5):271-277.
17. Silecchia G, Rizzello M, Angelis FD, et al. Laparoscopic sleeve gastrectomy as a revisional procedure for failed laparoscopic gastric banding with a "2-step approach": a multicenter study. *Surg Obes Relat Dis*. 2014;10:626-631.
18. Brethauer SA, Kothari S, Sudan R, et al. Systematic review on reoperative bariatric surgery American Society for Metabolic and Bariatric Surgery Revision Task Force. *Surg Obes Relat Dis*. 2014;10:952-972.
19. Topart P, Becouarn G, Ritz P. Biliopancreatic diversion with duodenal switch or gastric bypass for failed gastric banding: retrospective study from two institutions with preliminary results. *Surg Obes Relat Dis*. 2007;3(5):521-525.

25.2
Sleeve

Kinga A. Powers, MD, PhD, and Kevin K. Seeras, DO

A 42-year-old male presents to your office for evaluation of weight regain. He had a laparoscopic sleeve gastrectomy (SG) performed 3 years ago at another facility with an initial BMI of 52 kg/m^2, as well as hypertension. Postoperatively, he experienced weight loss with a maintained BMI of 34 kg/m^2 for approximately 2 years, along with remission of his hypertension. Over the last year, he has been experiencing weight regain and now has a BMI of 46 kg/m^2 and again requires medication for his hypertension. He insists that he has kept up with the recommended diet and exercises regularly. He has no other surgical history. You are unable to obtain his operative reports. He is otherwise in good health, as reported by his primary care physician, and is inquiring about further weight loss procedures. Initially, you counsel the patient on diet and lifestyle modifications and trial conservative management; however, the patient continues to experience weight regain.

1. **Which of the following is a technical reason during the initial operation that may contribute to failure of weight loss after a SG?**
   A. A bougie size of 42 Fr
   B. Concomitant hiatal hernia repair
   C. Complete fundus resection
   D. A 4-cm antrum
   E. Omental pexy to the greater curvature

2. **The patient has an initial workup including an upper gastrointestinal swallow study (UGI), an esophagogastroduodenoscopy (EGD), and three-dimensional CT reconstruction with volume estimation. The patient is scheduled for a revisional surgery. Which of the following operations is the most appropriate for the scenario presented?**
   A. Resleeve in the patient with retained gastric fundus and proximal dilation on imaging.
   B. Conversion to a Roux-en-Y gastric bypass (RYGB) in a patient with no symptoms of gastroesophageal reflux disease (GERD) and a retained fundus.
   C. Resleeve in the patient with a twist in the sleeve causing a stricture
   D. Conversion to a biliopancreatic diversion with duodenal switch (BPD-DS) in a patient with severe GERD.
   E. Addition of a laparoscopic adjustable gastric band (LAGB) to SG in a patient with no abnormal gastric sleeve dilation.

3. **You elect to perform a conversion to an RYGB. Which of the following statements regarding revisional surgery of a sleeve gastrectomy is most correct?**
   A. Conversion to BPD-DS will yield greater %EWL with similar perioperative and postoperative complications.
   B. A resleeve technique will yield a %EWL of over 50% at 12 months.
   C. Conversion to RYGB is more effective for weight recidivism than it is for refractory GERD symptoms following SG.
   D. The overall complication rate of SG to RYGB conversion is similar to that of a primary RYGB.
   E. Conversion to BPD-DS will yield greater %EWL with less post-operative nutritional deficiencies.

4. Which of the following technical aspects of conversion of SG to RYGB is a best attempt to decrease the incidence of anastomotic leak?

A. Abdominal drain placement
B. Resection of the remnant stomach to reduce parietal cell mass
C. Use of a staple height of 2.5 mm when encountering thickened tissue
D. Preservation of the left gastric pedicle
E. Use of staple line reinforcement

ANSWERS

1. A. SG is now the most common weight loss operation performed in the United States today.[1] The American Society for Metabolic and Bariatric Surgery (ASMBS) had supported SG as a stand-alone procedure in 2007; thus, long-term data are being published. One study has shown that revisions are performed in 19.9% of SG in the long term.[2] Indications for revisional surgery in SG can be complications of the original surgery (leak, stenosis, stricture, refractory GERD), weight loss failure/weight recidivism, or a planned second-stage operation.

Major reasons for weight regain/inadequate weight loss following SG include anatomical (technical and acquired) and patient selection, patient education, and inadequate lifestyle modification. Patients with an initial BMI >50 kg/m^2 have a greater likelihood of inadequate weight loss response when SG is the definitive procedure.[3] Patients who are noncompliant with diet modifications, specifically eating of sweets and other high-calorie foods, are likely to experience failure of weight loss with all bariatric procedures. In SG patients, GERD, dysphagia, and vomiting can be early side effects of the operation, leading to maladaptive eating habits to alleviate the symptoms. Gastric pouch sizes dilate over the first year and can lead to poor eating habits as well. Studies have demonstrated improved outcomes when these behaviors are monitored and corrected with close follow-up within comprehensive weight loss programs.[4]

Technical considerations of SG during the index operation, leading to poor weight loss results, include inadequate sleeve volume, bougie size >40 Fr, retained fundus, and large amount of retained antrum.[5,6] Concomitant hiatal hernia repair or omental pexy has no impact on postsurgical weight loss. Beginning the staple line 4 cm proximal to the pylorus is a common practice and has not been associated with failure of weight loss or weight regain.

2. A. A preoperative workup of a patient presenting with failure of weight loss or weight recidivism after a SG begins with a thorough history and physical exam. Lifestyle and diet modifications should first be attempted, as noncompliance would affect subsequent operations as well. Delineation of the anatomic reasons for weight loss failure should be evaluated with contrast UGI and EGD, with or without CT (with volume estimates of the pouch). Options for revisional surgery are either resleeve or conversion to a different operation, such as: RYGB, one anastomosis gastric bypass (OAGB), BPD-DS, and single anastomosis duodeno-ileostomy with sleeve gastrectomy SADI-S.

Resleeve can be considered in a patient with either weight recidivism or <50% EWL at 1-year postoperation, with either a dilated gastric body or a retained/persistent fundus on preoperative investigation.[7] Another consideration for resleeve is in a patient with weight recidivism and a gastric volume >250 cc as determined by CT volumetry.[8] Proximal gastric/fundus dilation can be secondary to a midbody stricture, not a retained fundus. In this case, a resleeve is *not* advised, as there is an increased risk of a staple line blowout from increased pressure. Resleeve and DS are not recommended in the setting of refractory/severe GERD.

Conversion operations have many options, with the most common being RYGB, especially for patients with GERD.

The addition of an LAGB to a failed sleeve gastrectomy has been described by Greenstein and Jacob as producing good weight loss results. However, in that case, there was radiographic evidence of proximal pouch dilation.[9] Here, there was adequate sleeve restriction, making this choice incorrect.

3. B. Outcomes of the resleeve technique for weight loss failure or weight recidivism have been reported in small sample studies. Results from three studies have demonstrated 57%, 58%, and 74.1% EWL at 12, 12, and 20 months postoperation.[7,10,11]

Outcomes of SG to RYGB conversion showed 60% and 48% EWL at 12 and 24 months, respectively, in a systematic review.[12] Overall complication rates have been reported as high as 31% and they are much more significant compared to the primary

RYGB.[13] Conversion to RYGB is extremely effective for refractory GERD following SG, with remission rates between 75% and 100% and considered more effective in GERD treatment versus weight loss failure.[13–15]

Outcomes of SG to BPD-DS were evaluated in studies compared to RYGB conversion. RYGB and DS had 23% and 59% EWL, respectively, at 34 months postoperation, DS demonstrated higher perioperative and short-term postoperative complications.[16] Another single-institution retrospective study demonstrated superior %EWL for BPD-DS versus RYGB and increased nutritional deficiencies for the BPD-DS group.[17]

4. D. Anastomotic leaks have an increased incidence in revisional bariatric surgery. When converting SG to RYGB, the pouch is created by stapling through the prior SG staple line, and this thicker tissue will most likely require upsizing of the staple height. Regardless of the staple maker, staple height ranges from 2.5 mm to 4.5 mm, with the taller staple heights used for thicker tissue. The left gastric vessels must be preserved, and if compromised, will necessitate an esophago-jejunostomy creation, which confers a much higher leak rate compared to a gastro-jejunostomy (GJ) anastomosis. Abdominal drain placement is at the surgeon's discretion, but that will not prevent leaks. Remnant gastrectomy will not prevent leaks and compromises enteral access, should it be needed. Additional methods to prevent leaks that are used include the judicious use of intraoperative endoscopy, leak tests, and anastomotic reinforcement/buttress; however, those technical aspects will need to be studied in larger studies to prove their effectiveness in leak prevention.

REFERENCES

1. Lee YC, Lee WJ, Lee TS, et al. Prediction of successful weight reduction after bariatric surgery by data mining technologies. *Obes Surg.* 2007;17(9):1235-1241.
2. Clapp B, Wynn M, Martyn C, Foster C, O'Dell M, Tyroch A. Long term (7 or more years) outcomes of the sleeve gastrectomy: a metaanalysis. *Surg Obes Relat Dis.* 2018;14(6):741-747.
3. Csendes A, Burgos AM, Martinez G, Figueroa M, Castillo J, Díaz JC. Loss and regain of weight after laparoscopic sleeve gastrectomy according to preoperative BMI: late results of a prospective study (78–138 months) with 93% of follow-up. *Obes Surg.* 2018;28:3424-3430.
4. Moroshko I, Brennan L, O'Brien P. Predictors of dropout in weight loss interventions: a systematic review of the literature. *Obes Rev.* 2011;12(11):912-934.
5. Weiner RA, Theodoridou S, Weiner S. Failure of laparoscopic sleeve gastrectomy—further procedure? *Obes Facts.* 2011;4(Suppl 1):42-46.
6. Wang Y, Yi XY, Gong LL, Li QF, Zhang J, Wang LH. The effectiveness and safety of laparoscopic sleeve gastrectomy with different sizes of calibration: a systematic review and meta-analysis. *Int J Surg.* 2018;49:32-38.
7. Iannelli A, Schneck AS, Noel P, Ben Amor I, Krawczykowski D, Gugenheim J. Re-sleeve gastrectomy for failed laparoscopic sleeve gastrectomy: a feasibility study. *Obes Surg.* 2011;21(7):832-835.
8. Nedelcu M, Noel P, Iannelli A, Gagner M. Revised sleeve gastrectomy (re-sleeve). *Surg Obes Relat Dis.* 2015;11(6):1282-1288. doi:10.1016/j.soard.2015.02.009.
9. Greenstein AJ, Jacob BP. Placement of a laparoscopic adjustable gastric band after failed sleeve gastrectomy. *Surg Obes Relat Dis.* 2008;4(4):556-558. doi:10.1016/j.soard.2008.05.002.
10. Noel P, Nedelcu M, Nocca D, et al. Revised sleeve gastrectomy: another option for weight loss failure after sleeve gastrectomy. *Surg Endosc.* 2014;28(4):1096-1102. doi:10.1007/s00464-013-3277-9.
11. AlSabah S, Alsharqawi N, Almulla A, et al. Approach to poor weight loss after laparoscopic sleeve gastrectomy: re-sleeve vs. gastric bypass. *Obes Surg.* 2016;26(10):2302-2307. doi:10.1007/s11695-016-2119-y.
12. Cheung D, Switzer NJ, Gill RS, Shi X, Karmali S. Revisional bariatric surgery following failed primary laparoscopic sleeve gastrectomy: a systematic review. *Obes Surg.* 2014;24(10):1757-1763. doi:10.1007/s11695-014-1332-9.
13. Casillas RA, Um SS, Zelada Getty JL, Sachs S, Kim BB. Revision of primary sleeve gastrectomy to Roux-en-Y gastric bypass: indications and outcomes from a high-volume center. *Surg Obes Relat Dis.* 2016;12(10):1817-1825. doi:10.1016/j.soard.2016.09.038.
14. Parmar CD, Mahawar KK, Boyle M, Schroeder N, Balupuri S, Small PK. Conversion of sleeve gastrectomy to Roux-en-Y gastric bypass is effective for gastroesophageal reflux disease but not for further weight loss. *Obes Surg.* 2017;27(7):1651-1658.
15. Quezada N, Hernández J, Pérez G, Gabrielli M, Raddatz A, Crovari F. Laparoscopic sleeve gastrectomy conversion to Roux-en-Y gastric bypass: experience in 50 patients after 1 to 3 years of follow-up. *Surg Obes Relat Dis.* 2016;12(8):1611-1615.
16. Homan J, Betzel B, Aarts EO, van Laarhoven KJ, Janssen IM, Berends FJ. Secondary surgery after sleeve gastrectomy: Roux-en-Y gastric bypass or biliopancreatic diversion with duodenal switch. *Surg Obes Relat Dis.* 2015;11(4):771-777. doi:10.1016/j.soard.2014.09.029.
17. Carmeli I, Golomb I, Sadot E, Kashtan H, Keidar A. Laparoscopic conversion of sleeve gastrectomy to a biliopancreatic diversion with duodenal switch or a Roux-en-Y gastric bypass due to weight loss failure: our algorithm. *Surg Obes Relat Dis.* 2015;11(1):79-85.

25.3

RYGB Revision

Kinga A. Powers, MD, PhD, and Kevin K. Seeras, DO

A 48-year-old female who is 36 months postop from a roux-en-y-gastric bypass (RYGB) presents to your clinic with complaints of weight regain over the last 6 months. Her preoperative BMI was 42 kg/m^2, and her medical comorbidities included hypertension and diabetes mellitus. At 24 months postoperatively, her BMI was 30 kg/m^2, with resolution of her hypertension and diabetes. Currently, though, the patient has a BMI of 40 kg/m^2, with redevelopment of her hypertension and diabetes requiring medications. She has no complaints and feels fine otherwise. She states that she no longer feels full quickly as she did in the 2 years postoperatively, and she has been having larger meals; however, she does not keep a food diary. She states that she has not changed her exercise regimen. She denies any tobacco, non-steroidal anti-inflammatory drug (NSAID), or alcohol use. She has no other surgical history. Abdominal exam is considered normal, and her vital signs area all within normal limits.

1. **The patient in this scenario has seen a failure of her RYGB in the form of weight recidivism and comorbidity redevelopment. What should be the first step in management?**
   A. EGD
   B. An upper gastrointestinal swallow (UGI) contrast study
   C. A conversion to Biliopancreatic diversion with duodenal switch (BPD-DS)
   D. Enrollment in programs to encourage lifestyle modification
   E. Trial of weight loss medications

2. **The patient undergoes nutritional and psychosocial assessments and has followed a strict diet and exercise program for 3 months, with no improvement in her weight loss. The patient undergoes a preoperative workup for revisional surgery that includes EGD and a UGI contrast study. EGD reveals a gastric pouch measuring 8 cm long and 6 cm wide, with a gastro-jejunal (GJ) anastomosis measuring 3 cm in diameter. EGD and UGI studies fail to demonstrate a gastrogastric fistula, and no ulceration is noted. Which of the following true?**
   A. This patient has a dilated GJ anastomosis, allowing more food consumption.
   B. This patient requires further imaging to rule out a gastrogastric fistula.
   C. This patient's larger pouch size is the most common reason for her weight regain.
   D. The large gastric pouch in this patient is related to increased secretion of the hormone ghrelin, which is partially responsible for larger meal consumption and weight regain.
   E. There is rarely an anatomic reason for weight regain.

3. **She has been evaluated by a psychiatrist, a registered dietitian, and a bariatrician. The team has determined that the best chance of long-term success is with a revision. When considering RYGB revisions, which of the following procedures results in the most significant long-term %EWL?**

A. Conversion to BPD-DS
B. Conversion to single anastomosis duodenal switch or single anastomosis duodenal ileal bypass(SADI-S)
C. Conversion to distal bypass
D. Revision of the GJ anastomosis using gastric plication or argon plasma coagulation
E. Stapled reduction of the Roux/anastomosis/pouch complex

ANSWERS

1. **D.** RYGB has mostly successful long-term outcomes; however, up to one-third of patients have inadequate weight loss (<50% EWL) or unacceptable weight regain (with or without comorbidity relapse).[1,2] Indications for revisional surgery in RYGB patients are failure of weight loss/weight regain and complications of the surgery. Primary failure is described as <50% EWL post-RYGB at 1 year. Weight regain with redevelopment of comorbidities constitutes failure of RYGB and is also an indication for revisional surgery.[3] The patient will most likely have to regain enough weight to meet the initial National Institutes of Health (NIH) criteria for bariatric surgery to be considered a candidate for this procedure.

   Initial management of a patient with failed weight loss or weight regain in RYGB patients is similar to that of other failed weight loss procedures. Patients must be evaluated for compliance to the recommended lifestyle and diet modification. Further investigation should search for anatomic reasons for weight regain. This includes review of prior operative report and postop course, EGD, and contrast UGI study. An enlarged gastric pouch, a gastrogastric fistula, and a large gastrojejunostomy have all been implicated as structural causes for weight regain. Anatomic factors may influence surgical decision-making; thus, an immediate schedule of conversion to a SS-DS is inappropriate.

   Pharmacologic treatment of a failed RYGB does not have substantial evidence to prove its efficacy; however, it can be a useful adjunct for patients who are starting to regain weight after bariatric surgery and may be used before patients meet the criteria for surgery.

2. **A.** Three abnormal anatomic features related to the gastric pouch have been implicated in weight recidivism following RYGB; pouch dilation, GJ anastomosis dilation, and gastrogastric fistula. These abnormalities are involved in the reduction of the restrictive component of the RYGB. Abnormal anatomic findings exist in 71.2% of patients experiencing weight regain; 58.9% have a dilated GJ, 28.8% have an enlarged pouch, and 12.3% have both.[4]

   Regarding gastrogastric fistula, incidence ranges from 1% to 2.6% and can be secondary to failure to divide the stapled stomach (incidence of 50%), staple line leaks, perforated ulcers, and foreign bodies.[5] Gastro-gastric pathology can lead to weight regain. The most sensitive test for detecting gastro-gastric fistulas is a UGI contrast study. Techniques to manage gastro-gastric fistula include resection of the portion of excluded stomach involved, as well as the fistula tract. In cases with anastomotic pathology, a formal GJ resection and reanastomosis may be required.[6–8]

   Regarding stomal dilation, dilated GJ anastomoses are stomas >2 cm.[9] GJ stomal dilation is directly related to weight recidivism. There is a clear correlation described in the literature, in which a small GJ stoma (<1 cm) is associated with superior %EWL.[10,11]

   Regarding pouch dilation, that is defined as >6 cm in length and >5 cm wide.[9] Larger pouch sizes correlate with inadequate weight loss and weight regain, but not as strongly as GJ anastomosis dilation does.[12] A larger pouch size at 6 and 12 months postoperatively directly correlates with an inferior %EWL, as it plays a restrictive role in weight loss in the form of early satiety when appropriately sized. This patient's weight loss went well for 2.5 years before she experienced weight regain. The role of ghrelin in this situation is unknown.

3. **A.** In terms of weight regain following RYGB, there are many therapeutic options available. In general, there are endoscopic and surgical procedures.

   Endoluminal therapies are low risk and indicated by the presence of enlarged GJ anastomosis or a gastric pouch (goals: GJ anastomosis 1.2–1.5 cm and a pouch that is 3 cm long and 3 cm wide). The GJ anastomosis may be narrowed using endoluminal plications, sclerosing agent injections, and argon plasma coagulation. The dilated pouch may be narrowed with endoluminal plication techniques only. Plication platforms (ROSE, StomaphyX, Overstitch) have had good short-term success, but questionable long-term results.[13–17] When considering management of the GJ stoma dilation, combined use of argon plasma coagulation followed by Overstitch full-thickness, purestring suture has had excellent short-term results and moderate results at 12 months.[18–23] Sclerotherapy results are also promising.

Surgical options include but are not limited to GJ revision, laparoscopic adjustable gastric band (LAGB) of the gastric pouch, limb-lengthening procedures, stapled pouch/anastomosis reduction, and conversion to BPD-DS. A review has demonstrated a complication rate of 20% to 33%, with a leak rate >10% for these revisions.[24]

Salvage gastric banding is typically indicated in patients with dilated GJ stomas and gastric pouches (although they can be used in all patients). Further, 1- and 2-year %EWL ranged from 17.6% to 41.3% and 42.5% to 48.7%, respectively. The greatest benefit was seen in patients with dilation and BMI <42.[25–27] Reoperation rates range from 14% to 29%, and there is an increase in perioperative complications when compared to primary LAGB. In addition, it is associated with the lysis of adhesions.[28]

Stapled reduction of the pouch and anastomosis and the blind end of the Roux limb is indicated in patients who have dilated pouch and/or anastomoses. It involves a linear stapler sequentially fired along the Roux limb, GJ, and gastric pouch over a bougie (32–40 Fr), which reduces the gastric pouch and narrows the anastomosis. Incidentally, the blind jejunal (candy cane) limb is resected as well (Figure 25-6).

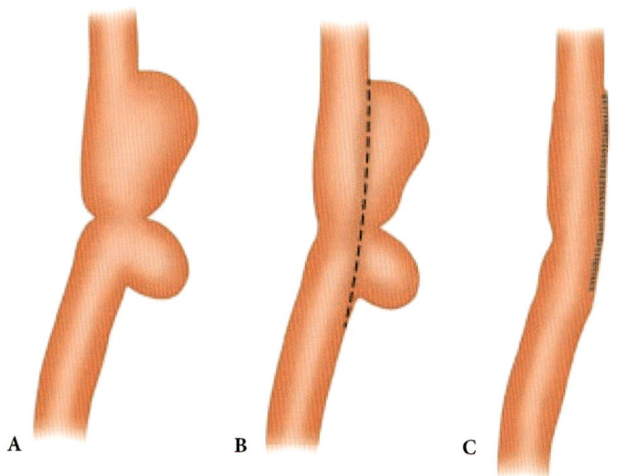

Figure 25-6 Stapled reduction of the pouch and anastomosis and the blind end of the Roux limb. (A) RYGB with enlarged pouch and enlarged proximal Roux limb (candy cane). (B) Projected staple line for reduction of both the pouch and Roux limb. (C) Reduce RYGB pouch and Roux limb.

Complete resection and revision of GJ anastomosis is associated with improved %EWL as opposed to stapled reduction, but it has increased perioperative and postoperative risk.

Conversion to distal bypass is indicated in patients with weight loss failure following RYGB without concomitant pouch/stomal dilation. In addition, it may be beneficial in patients with dense adhesions around the pouch. Two techniques include Sugerman and Brolin, both of which reduce the common channel length (CCL). The Sugerman technique involves transection of the Roux limb proximal to the jejuno-jejunal anastomosis and reanastomosis of the jejuno-jejunal farther down the common channel, in essence lengthening the biliopancreatic (BP) limb. The Brolin technique involves transection of the BP limb proximal to the jejuno-jejunal anastomosis and also reanastomosis of the jejuno-jejunal farther down the common channel (Figure 25-7). These techniques resulted in excellent weight loss and resolution of comorbidities, but with dismal long-term complications of macronutrient/micronutrient deficiency (a 30%–100% rate of hypoalbuminemia), intractable diarrhea, total parenteral nutrition (TPN), liver failure, and a high rate of reoperation.[29–33]

Conversion to BPD-DS is indicated for failure of RYGB in a patient with a very high BMI. The steps of the procedure are as follows (Figure 25-8):

1. Division of the Roux limb and gastric pouch (resection of GJ anastomosis)
2. Creation of a gastrogastrostomy between the pouch and the medial end of remnant stomach, which can be done with a linear/circular stapler, or in a hand-sewn fashion (a circular stapler with 25-mm anvil has the highest stricture rate)
3. A wide SG over a 60-Fr bougie
4. Duodenal transection 3 cm distal to the pylorus
5. Trans-section of the BP limb proximal to the jejuno-jejunal anastomosis
6. Anastomosis of the Roux limb to the transected BP limb
7. Construction of the duodenoileostomy
8. Construction of the ileoileostomy

The outcomes of a series of 12 patients undergoing the operation demonstrated 79.4% EWL. and 4 patients required management of gastrogastrostomy strictures (three-quarters were resolved with endoscopic management).[34] These results are similar to those of primary BPD-DS in terms of weight loss and comorbidity

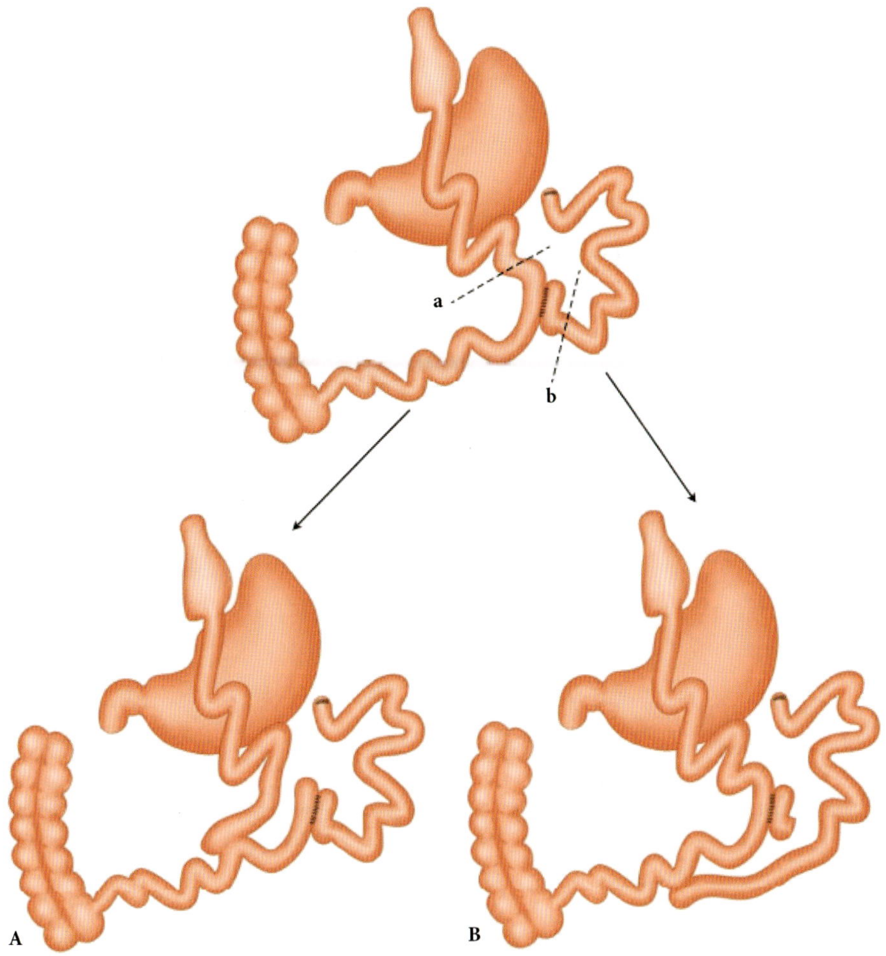

Figure 25-7 Distal bypass techniques for weight regain. (A) Elongating the biliopancreatic limb (Sugerman technique); (B) Elongating the Roux limb (Brolin technique).

resolution, but further investigation is required to determine long-term complication rates. Converting this to a SADI-S has very little research literature or data support.

REFERENCES

1. Higa K, Ho T, Tercero F, Yunus T, Boone K. Laparoscopic Roux-en-Y gastric bypass: 10-year follow-up. *Surg Obes Relat Dis*. 2011;7:516-525.
2. Cooper T, Simmons E, Webb K, Burns J, Kushner R. Trends in weight regain following Roux-en-Y gastric bypass (RYGB) bariatric surgery. *Obes Surg*. 2015;25: 1474-1481.
3. Hubbard VS, Hall WH. National Institutes of Health Consensus Development Conference Draft statement: gastrointestinal surgery for severe obesity. *Obes Surg*. 1991;1:257-265.
4. Yimcharoen P, Heneghan HM, Singh M, et al. Endoscopic findings and outcomes of revisional procedures for patients with weight recidivism after gastric bypass. *Surg Endosc*. 2011;25(10):3345-3352. doi:10.1007/s00464-011-1723-0.
5. Yao DC, Stellato TA, Schuster MM, Graf KN, Hallowell PT. Gastrogastric fistula following Roux-en-Y bypass is attributed to both surgical technique and experience. *Am J Surg*. 2010;199(3):385-386.
6. Pauli EM, Beshir H, Mathew A. Gastrogastric fistulae following gastric bypass surgery-clinical recognition and treatment. *Curr Gastroenterol Rep*. 2014;16(9):405.
7. Salimath J, Rosenthal RJ, Szomstein S. Laparoscopic remnant gastrectomy as a novel approach for treatment of gastrogastric fistula. *Surg Endosc*. 2009;23:2591-2595.
8. Tucker ON, Szomstein S, Rosenthal RJ. Surgical management of gastro-gastric fistula after divided laparoscopic Roux-en-Y gastric bypass for morbid obesity. *J Gastrointest Surg*. 2007;11:1673-1679.
9. Brethauer SA, Nfonsam V, Sherman V, Udomsawaengsup S, Schauer PR, Chand B. Endoscopy and upper gastrointestinal contrast studies are complementary in evaluation of weight regain after bariatric surgery. *Surg Obes Relat Dis*. 2006;2(6):643-650. doi:10.1016/j.soard.2006.07.012.
10. Horgan S, Jacobsen G, Weiss GD, et al. Incisionless revision of post-Roux-en-Y bypass stomal and pouch

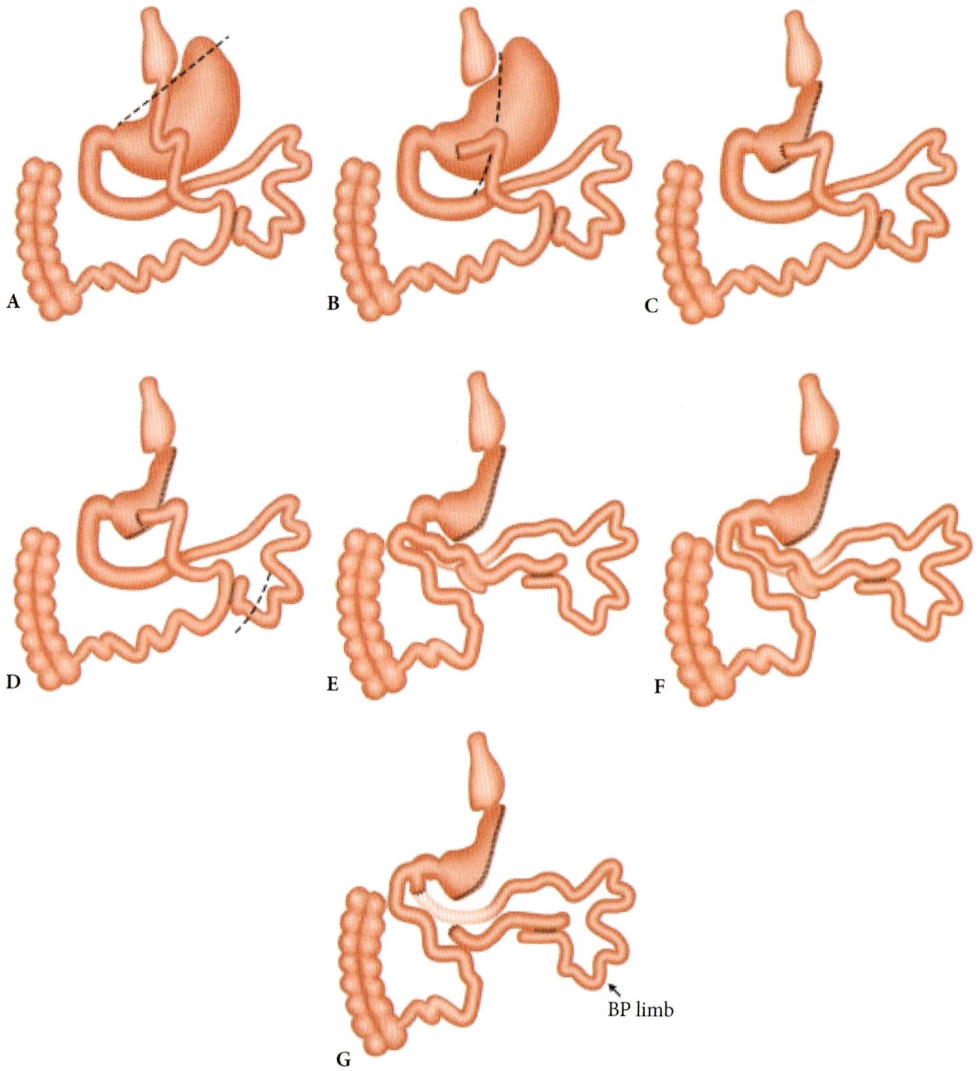

Figure 25-8 Converting a RYGB to a BPD. (A)Resection of GJ anastomosis; (B) Resection of greater curvature of the distal stomach; (C) Gastro-gastrostomy to create a Sleeve; (D) Resection of previous JJ anastomosis; (E) division of duodenum and anastomosis of previous Roux limb to previous BP limb; (F) onstruction of duodenal-ileal anastomosis; (G) construction of ileo-ileal anastomosis.

dilation: multicenter registry results. *Surg Obes Relat Dis.* 2010;6(3):290-295.

11. Thompson CC, Jacobsen GR, Schroder GL, Horgan S. Stoma size critical to 12-month outcomes in endoscopic suturing for gastric bypass repair. *Surg Obes Relat Dis.* 2012;8(3):282-287.
12. Roberts K, Duffy A, Kaufman J, Burrell M, Dziura J, Bell R. Size matters: gastric pouch size correlates with weight loss after laparoscopic Roux-en-Y gastric bypass. *Surg Endosc.* 2007;21(8):1397-402.
13. Raman SR, Holover S, Garber S. Endolumenal revision obesity surgery results in weight loss and closure of gastric-gastric fistula. *Surg Obes Relat Dis.* 2011;7(3):304-308.
14. Gallo AS, DuCoin CG, Berducci MA, et al. Endoscopic revision of gastric bypass: holy grail or epic fail? *Surg Endosc.* 2016;30(9):3922-3927. B. Hodgens et al. 389
15. Mikami D, Needleman B, Narula V, Durant J, Melvin WS. Natural orifice surgery: initial US experience utilizing the StomaphyX device to reduce gastric pouches after Roux-en-Y gastric bypass. *Surg Endosc.* 2010;24(1): 223-228.
16. Ong'uti SK, Ortega G, Onwugbufor MT, Ivey GD, Fullum TM, Tran DD. Effective weight loss management with endoscopic gastric plication using StomaphyX device: is it achievable? *Surg Obes Relat Dis.* 2013;9(1):113-117.
17. Yimcharoen P, Heneghan HM, Singh M, et al. Endoscopic findings and outcomes of revisional procedures for patients with weight recidivism after gastric bypass. *Surg Endosc.* 2011;25(10):3345-3352.
18. Thompson CC, Chand B, Chen YK, et al. Endoscopic suturing for transoral outlet reduction increases weight loss after Roux-en-Y gastric bypass surgery. *Gastroenterology.* 2013;145(1):129-137e3.
19. Jirapinyo P, Dayyeh BK, Thompson CC. Gastrojejunal anastomotic reduction for weight regain in Roux-en-Y gastric bypass patients: physiological, behavioral, and

anatomical effects of endoscopic suturing and sclerotherapy. *Surg Obes Relat Dis*. 2016;12(10):1810-1816.
20. Jirapinyo P, Kroner PT, Thompson CC. Purse-string transoral outlet reduction (TORe) is effective at inducing weight loss and improvement in metabolic comorbidities after Roux-en-Y gastric bypass. *Endoscopy*. 2018;50(4):371-377.
21. Kumar N, Thompson CC. Comparison of a superficial suturing device with a full-thickness suturing device for transoral outlet reduction (with videos). *Gastrointest Endosc*. 2014;79(6):984-989.
22. Kumar N. Weight loss endoscopy: development, applications, and current status. *World J Gastroenterol*. 2016;22(31):7069-7079.
23. Brunaldi VO, Jirapinyo P, de Moura DTH, et al. Endoscopic treatment of weight regain following Roux-en-Y gastric bypass: a systematic review and meta-analysis. *Obes Surg*. 2018;28(1):266-276.
24. Hallowell PT, Stellato TA, Yao DA, Robinson A, Schuster MM, Graf KN. Should bariatric revisional surgery be avoided secondary to increased morbidity and mortality? *Am J Surg*. 2009;197(3):391-396.
25. Bessler M, Daud A, DiGiorgi M, Inabnet W, Schrope B, Olivero-Rivera L, Davis D. Adjustable gastric banding as revisional bariatric procedure after failed gastric bypass—intermediate results. *Surg Obes Relat Dis*. 2010;6:31-35.
26. Irani K, Youn A, Ren-Fielding C, Fielding G, Kurian M. Midterm results for gastric banding as salvage procedure for patients with weight loss failure after Roux-en-Y gastric bypass. *Surg Obes Relat Dis*. 2011;7:219-224.
27. Uittenbogaart M, Leclercq WK, Luijten AA, van Dielen FMh. Laparoscopic adjustable gastric banding after failed Roux-En-Y gastric bypass. *Obes Surg*. 2016;45: 539-552.
28. Aminian A, Corcelles R, Daigle C, Chand B, Brethauer S, Schauer P. Critical appraisal of salvage banding for weight loss failure after gastric bypass. *Surg Obes Relat Dis*. 2015;11:607-611.
29. Sugerman H, Kellum J, DeMaria E. Conversion of proximal to distal gastric bypass for failed gastric bypass for superobesity. *J Gastrointest Surg*. 1997;1:517-525.
30. Brolin R, Cody R. Adding malabsorption for weight loss failure after gastric bypass. *Surg Endosc*. 2007;21: 1924-1926.
31. Rawlins L, Teel D, Hedgcorth K, Maguire J. Revision of Roux-en-Y gastric bypass to distal bypass for failed weight loss. *Surg Obes Relat Dis*. 2011;7:45-49.
32. Fobi MA, Lee H, Igwe D Jr, et al. Revision of failed gastric bypass to distal Roux-en-Y gastric bypass: a review of 65 cases. *Obes Surg*. 2001;11:190-195.
33. Ghiassi S, Higa K, Chang S, Ma P, Lloyd A, Boone K, DeMaria E. Conversion of standard Roux-en-Y gastric bypass to distal bypass for weight loss failure and metabolic syndrome: 3-year follow-up and evolution of technique to reduce nutritional complications. *Surg Obes Relat Dis*. 2018;14:554-561.
34. Parikh M, Pomp A, Gagner M. Laparoscopic conversion of failed gastric bypass to duodenal switch: technical considerations and preliminary outcomes. *Surg Obes Relat Dis*. 2007;3:611-618.

25.4

Ulcer

Kinga A. Powers, MD, PhD, and Kevin K. Seeras, DO

A 46-year-old female underwent a laparoscopic Roux-en-Y gastric bypass (RYGB) at your institution 6 months ago. She has demonstrated the expected amount of weight loss, and her hypertension is now controlled without medications. Her immediate post-operative course was without complications. She developed symptoms 2 months after surgery, related to an autoimmune disorder, for which her rheumatologist prescribed her non-steroidal anti-inflammatory drugs (NSAIDs). She developed a marginal ulcer at her gastro-jejunal (GJ) anastomosis, which was treated with a proton pump inhibitor (PPI) and Carafate, and on subsequent EGD, she appeared to have healed at 3 months postoperation. She now presents for her 6-month post-operative visit with a 1-month history of dysphagia, early satiety, and intolerance of large pieces of solid food. When questioned further, she admits to stopping her PPI and has experienced nocturnal epigastric pain off and on. She denies tobacco, alcohol, or chronic steroid use, but she admits to occasionally taking Motrin. The patient's vital signs are within normal limits, and her abdominal exam reveals a soft, nondistended, and nontender abdomen.

1. **What is the best next step to take in the workup and management of this patient?**
    A. Contrast upper gastrointestinal swallow (UGI) study
    B. CT scan
    C. Esophagogastroscopy with roux limb enteroscopy
    D. PPI, sucralfate, and misoprostol prescription
    E. Diagnostic laparoscopy

2. **You perform an upper endoscopy, which shows an active ulcer on the jejunal side of the GJ anastomosis in addition to stenosis of the GJ measuring about 6 mm in diameter. An UGI study is obtained showing a 7-cm-long x 6-cm-wide gastric pouch with no gastrogastric fistula. You place the patient back on PPI and sucralfate therapy and plan a repeat endoscopy in 8 weeks. Which of the following is the most common cause of recurrent marginal ulceration in this patient?**
    A. Continued foreign body reaction, inflammation, and ulceration from a suture or staple.
    B. Prostaglandin release and the resultant decrease in jejunal mucosal barriers
    C. Hyperacidity affecting the jejunal mucosa
    D. Increased secretion of gastrin and stomach acid
    E. Gastrogastric fistulae

3. **Upon repeat endoscopy, the ulceration has completely healed. The diameter of the GJ anastomosis remains at 6 mm, and the patient is still experiencing dysphagia, early satiety, and intolerance of larger solid foods. What is the best next step to take?**
    A. Placement of gastrostomy tube in the remnant stomach for feeding
    B. Operative revision of the gastrojejunal anastomosis
    C. Continued PPI therapy and a repeat endoscopy in another 8 weeks
    D. Endoscopic dilation with a balloon or bougie
    E. Operative gastric pouch reduction

4. **You have performed six endoscopic dilations without relief of symptoms or sustained patency of GJ anastomosis. The decision is made to proceed with a surgical intervention. The patient is optimized medically, and there are no micronutrient deficiencies. A preoperative serum albumin level was drawn and resulted in a reading of 3.2. Which of the following operations are most appropriate?**
   A. Gastric pouch reduction and gastrojejunostomy re-creation
   B. Total gastrectomy and esophagojejunostomy creation
   C. Resection of the gastrojejunostomy with reanastomosis of the pouch and Roux limb
   D. Resection of the gastrojejunostomy with reanastomosis of the pouch and Roux limb, and remnant stomach feeding tube placement
   E. Resection of the gastrojejunostomy with reanastomosis of the pouch and Roux limb and parietal cell vagotomy

5. **Which of the following must be performed during this operation for optimal results?**
   A. Lysis of all adhesions within the abdomen and pelvis
   B. Surgical drain placement adjacent to anastomosis
   C. Roux limb length of at least 75 cm
   D. Limited dissection of the gastric pouch and remnant
   E. Preservation of the right gastric pedicle

ANSWERS

1. **C.** Marginal ulcer formation at the gastrojejunal anastomosis after RYGB is one of the most common chronic complications of the procedure, with an incidence ranging from 0.6% to 25%, with an average of 4% to 5%.[1-3] Patients with marginal ulcers may be asymptomatic or express symptoms of burning epigastric pain, nausea, vomiting, dysphagia, bleeding, and perforation. The workup for a patient with suspected marginal ulceration should initially be with an upper endoscopy revealing the ulceration (gastric/stomal versus jejunal), as well as any concomitant stenosis, foreign body, or fistula. As such, patients may also get immediate relief with a concomitant dilation or foreign body (suture, staple) removal. Further delineation with contrast UGI will define anatomy and identify a large gastric pouch or a gastrogastric fistula (a CT scan may be helpful, but UGI is most sensitive for a gastro-gastric fistula).[4]

   Although PPI, misoprotal, and sucralfate are viable treatment options, treatment of a marginal ulcer without endoscopic evidence of pathology is not acceptable.

   Immediate operative exploration with laparoscopy would not be appropriate in this scenario, as the symptoms are suggestive of stomal ulceration and stenosis, which can be best diagnosed with endoscopy. Laparoscopy may be appropriate if there is a high index of suspicion for internal hernia with bowel obstruction, which is not the case in this patient.

2. **C.** Ulcers at the GJ anastomosis are either on the gastric or the jejunal side. Gastric stomal ulcers are related to ischemia. Jejunal ulcers are secondary to gastric acid exposure without a bicarbonate buffer. Several factors are linked to marginal ulcer formation, including the following:

   - A large gastric pouch results in a larger parietal cell mass, leading to increased stomach acid formation and resultant marginal ulceration. Studies reveal that a pouch greater than 50 ml predisposes patients to marginal ulcer formation, and limiting the pouch to just include the cardia reduces the rate of marginal ulcer to 0.6% at 3 years postoperation.[9] Another cohort demonstrated that every additional centimeter of length to the gastric pouch increases the relative risk of marginal ulcer formation by 14%.[10]
   - NSAID use results in COX inhibition resulting in decreased prostaglandin production which reduces mucosal protection and leads tomarginal ulcer formation (one-third of all marginal ulcers are a result of NSAID use).[1] This is the most common cause of marginal ulcers.
   - Tobacco use leads to local ischemia, which impairs healing. It is implicated in more than one-third of marginal ulcer cases and is linked to recurrent disease and higher rates of perforation.[5]
   - Hypertension, diabetes, anticoagulation use, and chronic steroid use have all been implicated in marginal ulcer development.[6]
   - Alcohol consumption historically has been implicated in marginal ulcer development, but there is currently no research to support this.

- The use of permanent sutures when constructing the anastomosis results in chronic foreign body inflammatory reaction and marginal ulceration. Disolving suture has been shown to decrease marginal ulcer rates.[7,8]
- *Heliobacter pylori* infection's effect on the development on marginal ulcers after a RYGB is not entirely clear and needs further studies. It colonizes the gastric antrum, not the fundus, in order to exert its effects. Some authors propose routine testing and eradiation in the preoperative preparation for RYGB.
- Gastrogastric fistulae allow increased acid exposure of the jejunum from the gastric acid produced in the remnant stomach. Patients may present with recurrent ulceration in addition to weight regain. In a series of 1,292 patients, the incidence of marginal ulcer development was 53.5% in patients with a gastro-gastric fistula as opposed to 4.2% in patients without gastro-gastric fistula.[4] Causes of a gastrogastric fistula include incomplete gastric transection at index operation (noncutting stapler), foreign bodies, ischemia, and contained leakage.

3. **D.** GJ stomal stenosis/stricture (defined as a diameter of <10 mm or the inability to pass an adult endoscope) is relatively common following RYGB, with reported rates between 3% and 32%.[11,12] Etiology of GJ strictures are multifactorial and include tension on the anastomosis resulting in partial ischemia, scar formation, recurrent marginal ulcers, anastomotic leaks, NSAID/tobacco/alcohol use, and various surgical techniques. When considering the creation of a GJ anastomosis, hand-sewn techniques have the lowest stricture rates compared to circular and linear stapler techniques (<4% for hand-sewn, <7% for linear, and up to 31% for circular). Circular stapled techniques may reduce stenotic complication rates by 50% when a 25-mm stapler is used, as opposed to a 21-mm stapler; however, it is also associated with higher rates of weight loss failure.[13–15]

   Initial management of symptomatic GJ stenosis is with endoscopic dilation. This can be done with balloon dilation or Savary bougie dilators. Repeat endoscopy should be performed every 2 weeks until the endoscope passes freely through the stoma and the symptoms have resolved (the goal diameter of stoma is 12 mm). Endoscopic removal of any foreign body (suture or staple) is recommended to prevent recurrence of stenosis.

   Regarding balloon dilation, reported overall success rate ranges from 61% to 95%, and when performed early (within 90 days), the success rate ranges from 95% to 98%. This concluded that early strictures are more amenable to dilation than late strictures, which more often require revisional surgery.[16] Similar good results are reported for bougie dilation, with a 100% overall success rate.[17] The overall complication rate of balloon dilation is between 2% and 5%, with the two most significant complications being perforation and bleeding.[18]

4. **D.** Revisional surgery for recalcitrant marginal ulcers and/or stenosis that has failed medical/endoscopic management classically involves resection of the gastrojejunostomy to healthy/perfused tissue with redone gastrojejunostomy.

   Resection of the excluded stomach does not confer a significant benefit to prevention of marginal ulcers and is not routinely done.[19] Indications for this is in the setting of remnant stomach bleeding or gastrogastric fistula.

   The addition of a truncal vagotomy is recommended by some centers for chronic marginal ulcers requiring revision of the GJ, but supporting data are limited.[20]

   Total gastrectomy should be performed only when there is vascular compromise of the remaining lesser curvature vasculature, leading to an unviable gastric pouch. This will require the creation of an esophagojejunostomy, which is more technically challenging, with high anastomotic complication rates.[21]

   Placement of a feeding tube in the remnant stomach will provide early postoperative nutritional support in these malnourished patients.

   Gastric pouch reduction is a treatment for weight regain in RYGB patients. It would not address the anastomotic stricture.

5. **C.** Optimal results in the scenario presented in these questions must focus on removal of the pathology, prevention of recurrence, and limitation of postoperative complications. Key technical aspects to a successful operation in a recalcitrant marginal ulcer case with concomitant stenosis are as follows:

   - Ensure the integrity of the left gastric pedicle (if compromised, esophagojejunal anastomosis will be needed). There is no right gastric pedicle. This structure gets its name because it comes off the left gastric artery.
   - Create a clear/open plane between the excluded stomach and a pouch to definitively exclude a gastrogastric fistula. This would require a full dissection of the gastric pouch.

- Perform a resection of the gastrojejunostomy to healthy, well-perfused tissue utilizing a linear stapler (may need increased staple heights to accommodate thicker gastric tissue).
- Lengthen the Roux limb to at least 75 cm if necessary (any bile reflux will contribute to recurrent ulceration and stricture).
- Recreate a tension-free GJ anastomosis (utilize the hand-sewn technique if previous stapled techniques led to a foreign body reaction).
- Place a remnant stomach gastrostomy tube in patients at risk for malnutrition.

Complete lysis of adhesions is not required in the absence of adhesive bowel obstruction.

Surgical drain placement near anastomosis is surgeon dependent.

REFERENCES

1. Coblijn UK, Goucham AB, Lagarde SM, Kuiken SD, Wagensveld BA. Development of ulcer disease after Roux-en-Y gastric bypass, incidence, risk factors, and patient presentation: a systematic review. *Obes Surg*. 2014;24:299-309.
2. Ying VWC, Kim SHH, Khan KJ, et al. Prophylactic PPI help reduce marginal ulcers after gastric bypass surgery: a systematic review and meta-analysis of cohort studies. *Surg Endosc*. 2015;29:1018-1023.
3. Carrodeguas L, Szomstein S, Soto F, et al. Management of gastro-gastric fistulas after divided Roux-en-Y gastric bypass surgery for morbid obesity: analysis of 1,292 consecutive patients and review of literature. *Surg Obes Relat Dis*. 2005;1(5):467-474.
4. Carrodeguas L, Szomstein S, Soto F, et al. Management of gastrogastric fistulas after divided Roux-en-Y gastric bypass surgery for morbid obesity: analysis of 1,292 consecutive patients and review of literature. *Surg Obes Relat Dis*. 2005;1(5):467-474. doi:10.1016/j.soard.2005.07.003
5. Carr WRJ, Mahawar KK, Balupuri S, Small PK. An evidence-based algorithm for the management of marginal ulcers following Roux-en-Y gastric bypass. *Obes Surg*. 2014;24:1520-1527.
6. Coblijn UK, Lagarde SM, Castro SMM, Kuiken SD, Wagensvekl BA. Symptomatic marginal ulcer disease after Roux-en-Y gastric bypass: incidence, risk factors and management. *Obes Surg*. 2015;25:805-811.
7. Rasmussen JJ, Fuller W, Ali MR. Marginal ulceration after laparoscopic gastric bypass: an analysis of predisposing factors in 260 patients. *Surg Endosc*. 2007;21:1090-1094.
8. Vasquez JC, Wayne Overby D, Farrell TM. Fewer gastrojejunostomy strictures and marginal ulcers with absorbable suture. *Surg Endosc*. 2009;23(9):2011-2015. doi:10.1007/s00464-008-0220-6.
9. Palermo M, Acquafresca PA, Rogula T, Duza GE, Serra E. Late surgical complications after gastric by-pass: a literature review. *Arq Bras Cir Dig*. 2015;28(2):139-143.
10. Edholm D, Ottosson J, Sundbom M. Importance of pouch size in laparoscopic Roux-en-Y bypass: a cohort study of 14,168. *Surg Endosc*. 2016;30:2011-2015.
11. Csendes A, Burgos AM, Burdiles P. Incidence of anastomotic strictures after gastric bypass: a prospective consecutive routine endoscopic study 1 month and 17 months after surgery in 441 patients with morbid obesity. *Obes Surg*. 2009;19:269-273.
12. Ahmad J, Martin J, Ikramuddin S, Schauer P, Slivka A. Endoscopic balloon dilation of gastroenteric anastomotic stricture after laparoscopic gastric bypass. *Endoscopy*. 2003;35:725-728.
13. Kravetz AJ, Reddy S, Murtaza G, Yenumula P. A comparative study of hand-sewn versus stapled gastrojejunal anastomosis in laparoscopic Roux-en-Y gastric bypass. *Surg Endosc*. 2011;25:1287-1292.
14. Gonzalez R, Lin E, Venkatesh KR, Bowers SP, Smith CD. Gastrojejunostomy during laparoscopic gastric bypass: analysis of 3 techniques. *Arch Surg*. 2003;138:181-184.
15. Kravetz AJ, Reddy S, Murtaza G, Yenumula P. A comparative study of handsewn versus stapled gastrojejunal anastomosis in laparoscopic Roux-en-Y gastric bypass. *Surg Endosc*. 2011;25(4):1287-1292. doi:10.1007/s00464-010-1362-x
16. Yimcharoen P, Heneghan H, Chand B, et al. Successful management of gastrojejunal strictures after gastric bypass: is timing important?. *Surg Obes Relat Dis*. 2012;8(2):151-157. doi:10.1016/j.soard.2011.01.043 Fernández-Esparrach G, Bordas J, Llach J, et al. Endoscopic dilation with Savary-Gilliard bougies of stomal strictures after laparosocopic gastric bypass in morbidly obese patients. *Obes Surg*. 2008;18:155-161.
17. Ukleja A, Afonso BB, Pimentel R, Szomstein S, Rosenthal R. Outcome of endoscopic balloon dilation of strictures after laparoscopic gastric bypass. *Surg Endosc*. 2008;22:1746-1750.
18. Csendes A, Burgos AM, Altuve J, Bonacic S. Incidence of marginal ulcer 1 month and 1 to 2 years after gastric bypass: a prospective consecutive endoscopic evaluation of 442 patients with morbid obesity. *Obes Surg*. 2009;19(2):135-138. doi:10.1007/s11695-008-9588-6.
19. Hunter J, Stahl RD, Kakade M, Breitman I, Grams J, Clements RH. Effectiveness of thoracoscopic truncal vagotomy in the treatment of marginal ulcers after laparoscopic Roux-en-Y gastric bypass. *Am Surg*. 2012;78(6):663-668.
20. Esquivel CM, Ampudia C, Fridman A, Moon R, Szomstein S, Rosenthal RJ. Technique and outcomes of laparoscopic-combined linear stapler and hand-sutured side-to-side esophagojejunostomy with Roux-en-Y reconstruction as a treatment modality in patients undergoing proximal gastrectomy for benign and malignant disease of the gastroesophageal junction. *Surg Laparos Endos Percutan Tech*. 2014;24(1):89-93.
21. Esquivel CM, Ampudia C, Fridman A, Moon R, Szomstein S, Rosenthal RJ. Technique and outcomes of laparoscopic-combined linear stapler and hand-sutured side-to-side esophagojejunostomy with Roux-en-Y reconstruction as a treatment modality in patients undergoing proximal gastrectomy for benign and malignant disease of the gastroesophageal junction. *Surg Laparos Endos Percutan Tech*. 2014;24(1):89-93.

SECTION 5

Outcomes Short-Term

26

Sleeve Gastrectomy Versus Roux-en-Y Gastric Bypass Versus Biliopancreatic Diversion with Duodenal Switch

W. James Melvin, MD, and Dana Telem MD, MPH

You are meeting a 45-year-old woman with a body mass index (BMI) of 50 kg/m^2, type 2 diabetes, obstructive sleep apnea (OSA), and hypertension who has been referred to the clinic for evaluation of bariatric surgery. She has had several friends get weight loss surgery before but has also heard about Roux-en-Y gastric bypass (RYGB), sleeve gastrectomy (SG), and biliopancreatic diversion with duodenal switch (BPD-DS). She is interested in hearing about the comparative risks and benefits of each operation. They know that you are a surgeon who is comfortable with and has adequate experience in all three operations, and you perform them primarily in a laparoscopic fashion.

1. **Regarding the expected weight loss, which of the following is correct?**
    - A. Long-term (i.e., five years) expected weight loss is definitively greater and clinically relevant with RYGB in comparison to SG.
    - B. BPD-DS predicts more excess weight loss (EWL) compared to RYGB.
    - C. After initial weight loss, weight recidivism is equivalent among all three procedures.
    - D. Expected weight loss at 1 year is equivalent between BPD-DS and SG.

2. **She is especially interested in how her potential operation would affect her type 2 diabetes, as many of her family members have had diabetes-related complications. Which of the following is correct?**
    - A. BPD-DS is less effective at resolving type 2 diabetes than RYGB.
    - B. RYGB is less effective at resolving type 2 diabetes than RYGB.
    - C. BPD-DS is more effective at resolving type 2 diabetes than SG.
    - D. SG is more effective than BPD-DS at resolving type 2 diabetes.

3. **Regarding the risk of short-term complications, which of the following is correct?**
    - A. The risk of 30-day mortality is similar with SG, RYGB, and BPD-DS.
    - B. The risk of gastrointestinal leak is higher in RYGB than in SG.
    - C. The risk of venous thromboembolism (VTE) is higher in RYGB than in SG.
    - D. Patients who have undergone bariatric surgery have had equivalent rates of wound complications (such as dehiscence, infection, and hematoma) with SG, RYGB, and BPD-DS.

4. **Regarding the risk of long-term complications, which of the following is correct?**
    - A. Internal hernia is not a known risk of BPD-DS.
    - B. Malnutrition and nutrient deficiency are more of a concern with BPD-DS than with RYGB or SG.

C. SG patients have similar rates of postoperative gastrointestinal reflux than patients with RYGB.
D. The rate of reoperation needed for revision of the original procedure is higher with RYGB compared to SG.

5. The patient is wondering how permanent her potential operation of choice would be and some reasons why revisional surgery might be needed. Which of the following reoperations would be the most appropriate?

A. SG again due to insufficient weight loss following SG
B. BPD-DS for medically refractory gastrointestinal reflux following SG
C. Proximal jejunojejunostomy for protein calorie malnutrition following BPD-DS
D. RYGB for protein calorie nutrition following BPD-DS

ANSWERS

1. **B.** BPD-DS has been shown to deliver the greatest amount of lasting (five-year) weight loss, measured as the percentage of EWL at multiple time points compared to SG and RYGB. BPD-DS typically result in a lasting EWL of between 70% and 80%, compared to 60% to 70% for RYGB and 50% to 55% from SG. This has been shown in large data sets such as the Metabolic and Bariatric Surgery Accreditation and Quality Improvement Program (MBSAQIP)[1] and Michigan Bariatric Surgery Collaborative (MBSC),[2] small, prospective randomized trials,[3] and large metanalyses highlighted by Buchwald et al in 2009.[4] Large multicenter data sets show that clinicians who routinely use BPD-DS typically offer this operation to patients with a higher preoperative BMI on average where such a difference will be more clinically relevant, as described by Prachand et al in 2010,[5] typically in cases of supermorbid obesity where BMI >50.[1,4,6]

   Historically, it has been thought that RYGB offered more weight loss than SG, at respective 5-year EWL of 60% to 70% as opposed to 50% to 55%,[7] and this has been supported by 5-year second end-point data from the STAMPEDE randomized control trial[8] and retrospective multicenter data sets from large databases like the MBSC or MBSAQIP. However, other recent randomized trials out of Europe (such as SM-BOSS and SLEEVEPASS) have shown no statistical difference in EWL between SG and RYGB at multiple time points, including after 5 years.[9,10] These studies, although randomized, offer smaller patient cohorts compared to large database studies and could be underpowered to detect EWL differences between SG and RYGB, because if true differences exist between the two operations, it is likely small. As SG has become the most common bariatric surgery performed in recent years, upcoming long-term data will help crystallize comparisons to RYGB. Furthermore, the SG technique has changed over the past several years and may influence outcomes at the present time.

   Classically, bariatric surgery is characterized by initial weight loss to a nadir over the first year to year and a half, followed by a plateau phase, and then many patients experience some degree of reclamation of excess body weight[11] over subsequent years before reaching a new set point. This is well described in both RYGB,[11] and especially in SG,[12] and in a subset of these patients, an additional malabsorptive operation can be offered due to the degree of weight regain. However, this is not typically seen with patients who get BPD-DS as their index operation. Behavioral factors must be at the forefront of the differential when evaluating patients for postoperative weight recidivism.

2. **C.** One of the key long-term benefits offered by bariatric surgery is thought to be the improvement and prevention of weight-related comorbid conditions such as diabetes, hypertension, hyperlipidemia, OSA, and osteoarthritis. Due to its significance with morbidity and mortality, the effect on diabetes resolution is especially scrutinized. The STAMPEDE randomized control trial established that bariatric surgery (either SG or RYGB) combined with medical therapy was superior to medical therapy alone at reducing patients' hemoglobin A1c.[8] Furthermore, a seminal meta-analysis by Buchwald et al in 2009[4] reported that 78% of patients achieved complete resolution of type 2 diabetes following bariatric surgery, and 86% of patients demonstrated improvement in glycemic control.

   In terms of differences in achieving control of type 2 diabetes between the three major modern bariatric surgeries, it is important to note that all three operations are effective at this goal. However, BPD-DS shows that the vast majority of patients are able to achieve lasting remission (normoglycemia without medication) of type 2 diabetes, as demonstrated in meta-analyses like that of Buchwald et al, with 95.9% of patients at 2 years, as well as in long-term data for smaller studies, such as Bolckmans et al, which showed a total remission in 87.5% of patients at 10+ years following BPD-DS.[13] This is superior to RYGB and SG, especially when long-term weight recidivism is taken into account.

The quantifiable difference in glycemic control between SG and RYGB is more nuanced. In the STAMPEDE trial, there was no statistical difference in hemoglobin A1c measured at 5 years between the RYGB and SG groups; however, patients with RYGB were taking fewer medications for treatment of type 2 diabetes.[8] A recent retrospective study performed using pharmacy claim information assessed that patients with RYGB had a 12% increased probability of achieving remission of type 2 diabetes and 42% decreased probability of subsequently relapsing compared to SG patients.[14] However, it should again be noted that both procedures are effective and 88% of the 2,746 patients experienced remission, with 22.5% of cases relapsing after mean follow-up of about 2.5 years. Another study by Lewis et al published in 2019 evaluated pharmaceutical claims at 2 years postsurgery and found that SG was 20% less likely to induce remission of type 2 diabetes compared to RYGB.[15] For this question, it would be important to counsel this patient on the impact of this increased ability to deliver remission of type 2 diabetes with RYGB compared to SG, given that her satisfaction with the operation may be more closely tied to glycemic control than the average patient due to her family history of diabetic complications.

3. **A.** Multiple modern studies of various levels of evidence have shown that 30-day mortality rates (<0.5%) between laparoscopic bariatric operations are not statistically different. As the less common and more technically challenging operation, BPD-DS is sometimes thought to be riskier than its competitors. However, with experienced teams, single-center 30-day mortality outcomes for BPD-DS are similar to RYGB/SG,[3,5,16] and large database retrospective reviews showed that at least in terms of mortality, it is similar to RYGB/SG.[1] The rate of minor complications and serious complications for BPD-DS is typically shown to be higher, with some variability. For instance, the rate of gastrointestinal leak was shown to be several times higher than SG and RYGB in the MBSAQIP and MSBC multicenter data, but it was not seen in all reported single-center studies as previously mentioned. Some of the data lack cohort matching or failure to fully account for higher historic percentage of open surgery performed with BPD-DS[6] due to laparoscopic complexity. This is compounded by BPD-DS patients having higher preoperative BMI and an increased number of preoperative comorbidities.[1]

Historically, SG was associated with higher gastrointestinal leak rates than RYGB; however, this difference has disappeared in recent years. Overall, leak rates in bariatric surgery have decreased over the past two decades. Modern leak rates between SG and RYGB are comparable at 0.7%, well illustrated by Hutter et al in a 28,000-patient longitudinal study published in 2011.[17] A further important study analyzing American College of Surgeons (ACS) National Surgical Quality Improvement Program (NSQIP) data for laparoscopic SG and RYGB procedures performed between 2010 and 2011 showed similar rates of intra-abdominal abscess/sepsis (as surrogate for leaks); at 0.6% for both operations.[18] This study did show decreased rates of serious morbidity with SG compared to RYGB, however, including wound infection, sepsis, and 30-day readmission and reoperation. Taking these data together also suggests that leaks from SG are less likely to cause intra-abdominal catastrophe and more likely to be self-limited compared to leaks in RYGB. It is also noteworthy that BPD-DS is well established to have increased rates of anastomotic leaking (1%–4%) compared to SG or RYGB,[1,6,13] although some experienced centers have demonstrated prospective single-center data that shows equivalent rates of gastrointestinal leaking[5,16] to both SG and RYGB.

VTE not only is an important quality metric in postoperative populations, but it also has a significant effect on morbidity and mortality. It has been shown in multiple multicenter retrospective data that there is no difference in VTE rates between laparoscopic SG and RYGB;[19] however, ACS NSQIP data from 2010 to 2011 showed increased rate of VTE in SG compared to RYGB, at a rate of 0.47% to 0.21%.[18]

Wound complications have decreased in incidence since the widespread adoption of laparoscopic techniques for bariatric surgery. BPD-DS has been shown in multicenter databases to be associated with increased rates of wound complications compared to SG and RYGB. Finks et al looked at

MBSC data in 2011 and found that the risk of minor and serious wound complications with BPD-DS is 4.9% and 4.6%, respectively, comparable to open gastric bypass.[6] Criticism of this study would appropriately argue that about 75% of the BPD-DS procedures in MBSC were open, and there were more comorbidities in the BPD-DS group. However, Martinovski et al (2017) analyzed MBSAQIP data, selecting for laparoscopic or robotic BPD-DS, and also found statistically increased risk of wound complications compared to RYGB, at 2.5% vs. 1.55%.[1] However, this population also had increased comorbidities compared to RYGB. To further expand on the differential risk of wound complications, modern ACS NSQIP data suggests lower risk of wound infection with laparoscopic SG compared to RYGB, at 0.06% vs 0.2%.[18]

4. **B.** Regardless of operative complexity and average operative time, the main long-term drawback of BPD-DS is the risk of long-term malabsorption, protein calorie malnutrition, and micronutrient deficiency[13] compared to RYGB and DS. In fact, reoperation/revision for malabsorption-related complications is needed on occasion, ranging from as low as 0.6% at mean follow-up of 7.3 years (as described by Marceau et al)[20] to 4.7% as reported by Hamoui et al,[21] or 10% as reported by Risstat et al[22] All bariatric surgery patients are at risk for malnutrition and micronutrient deficiencies, but small changes to common channel length (CCL) and variability between patients lead to BPD-DS being a less forgiving operation than RYGB and DS in this regard. A CCL of 75 to 150 cm is associated with less need for revision compared to 50 cm.[21] In a prospective randomized trial, 7% of BPD-DS patients with CCL of 100 cm were noted to have anemia and hypoalbuminemia at only 1 year postoperatively.[3] Active involvement of specialized dieticians and extensive preoperative and postoperative patient education and coaching are critical to avoid and mitigate malabsorption-related complications with bariatric surgery, especially BPD-DS.

Following alongside malabsorption, the risk of diarrhea is higher in BPD-DS compared to RYGB and SG. Risstat et al showed that 63% of BPD-DS patients at 5 years postoperatively reported altered bowel function causing social limitations, and an average daily amount of bowel movements of 3.0; compared to 25% of RYGB patients developing altered bowel function causing social limitations and an average of 1.8 daily bowel movements.[22] Likewise, in a recent large cohort study, Elias et al reported the rate of diarrhea 5 years postoperatively to be 11.3% in BPD-DS, 2.7% in RYGB, and 5.8% in SG,[23] suggesting no significant increase in diarrhea with RYGB over preoperative baseline. The increase in postoperative diarrhea seen in SG patients is attributed by the authors to increase in concomitant increase in acid-related symptoms in SG, but possibly also due to changes in gastric function, diet, and gut microbiota from the procedure.[23] Overall, diarrheal symptoms should be taken in context within overall patient quality of life because only a small minority of BPD-DS patients report dissatisfaction with their surgery (2%–5%),[20,24] despite having high rates of postoperative diarrhea. Further large, robust data are also warranted to better understand these outcomes in patients—and is often overlooked as illustrated by lack of reporting these symptoms in the SM-BOSS and SLEEVEPASS trials.

Internal hernia is a known risk of BPD-DS;[25] however, due to small operative volume at specialized centers, there are no robust data on its prevalence in comparison to the risk of internal hernia with RYGB, where it a well-known long-term complication. Incidence of internal hernia following RYGB is 2.5%, with reported ranges from 0.5% to 11%, and closure of mesenteric defects with nonabsorbable suture reduces incidence.[26] This is clearly shown by the SLEEVEPASS trial, in which 17 out of 120 (14%) RYGB patients underwent reoperation for suspected internal hernia by year 5, as this group did not close mesenteric defects routinely during the study.[10] SG is not known to have internal hernias.

The intersection of gastrointestinal reflux (GERD) and bariatric surgery is an area of active research. It is established that SG is more likely to fail to improve or worsen reflux symptoms than RYGB.[7,9,10,12] In the SLEEVEPASS randomized trial, 7 out of 120 (5.8%) SG patients underwent conversion to RYGB by year 5 due to refractory reflux, and 11 more required daily proton pump inhibitors. All the SLEEVEPASS patients had preoperative endoscopy to exclude patients with large hiatal hernia, but they received no formal reflux evaluation.[10] In the SM-BOSS trial, 31% of patients had worsening GERD symptoms, and 25% improved following SG; in as opposed to RYGB, where 60% saw remission and only 6% worsened.[9] North American data are consistent with these European randomized trials in that they also show that in patients with preoperative GERD, RYGB offers clear benefits to these patients for their symptoms,[27] and GERD increases the risk of revisional surgery needed for SG (0.6% from 0.3%). Of further concern are limited data showing increased incidence of Barrett's esophagus (15%) in patients with de novo GERD who are post-SG.[28]

Preoperative Barrett's was considered a relative contraindication to SG; however, it may be appropriate in selected patients. Some surgeons will perform omentopexy[29] to the sleeve, in part to reduce postoperative GERD, but this has not been definitively shown to offer benefits.[30] When counseling patients on the risk of GERD with SG, it is important to discuss the slightly decreased risks of short-term morbidity with the procedure in contrast to the increased risk of worsening GERD and the opportunity cost of potentially eliminating their GERD symptoms if they elect to undergo RYGB. An individualized approach with adequate preoperative evaluation in these patients is key. Less robust data on BPD-DS suggests higher rate of postoperative GERD compared to RYGB as well;[22] it is unclear what relationship there is between SG and BPD-DS regarding GERD risk.

Overall risk of reoperation has been investigated between SG, RYGB, and BPD-DS. Howard et al showed in a large retrospective Medicare beneficiary cohort study between SG and RYGB that at 5 years, SG has a lower risk of reoperation (defined by any abdominal operation such as hernia or biliary) compared to RYGB with a hazard ratio of 0.66 (0.59–0.73).[31] However, need for bariatric-specific revision was higher in SG compared to RYGB in this same cohort, with a hazard ratio of 3.41 (2.44–4.74).[31] Similarly, another large observational study by Courcoulas et al of a comparatively younger patient cohort (PCOR database) showed SG with a lower risk of reintervention (all procedures excluding endoscopy) after five years compared to RYGB with a hazard ratio of 0.72 (0.65–0.79) and no significant difference seen in bariatric-specific revisionary surgery between SG and RYGB.[32] There is more limited multicenter data about long-term reoperative risk for BPD-DS, especially specific to laparoscopic BPD-DS; and what single-center data exists is greatly influenced by specific operative technique such as CCL, gastric pouch size, and variability in follow-up nutritional regimens. However, what data does exist suggest a high rate of reoperation necessary in BPD-DS patients over the long-term. Risstad et al randomized patients to laparoscopic RYGB versus laparoscopic BPD-DS and followed outcomes for 5 years; they found that 44% of patients with BPD-DS required additional operation compared to 9% of RYGB patients.[22] Similarly, in other large single-center series at 5 years of follow-up, significant portions (37%, 75%)[24,33] of BPD-DS patients required reoperative intervention. Regarding bariatric-specific revision, this only seems to play a part in the total reoperative risk for BPD-DS. In a 2015 metanalysis of BPD-DS; the bariatric-specific revision rate ranged from 2% to 5% in most series,[34] and was 10% in Risstad et al,[22] typically related to malnutrition or excessive diarrhea/steatorrhea.

5. C. When considering elective reoperation following bariatric surgery, a careful and thorough assessment is critical before heading to the operating room. One must investigate for possible technical errors with the index operation, rule out long-term anatomic complications, optimize medical management, and address modifiable patient behaviors. Infrequently, the aforementioned workup will lead to clear evidence that revisionary bariatric surgery is necessary to address ongoing quality-of-life issues for the patient or achieve the patient's original goals for bariatric surgery.

As previously discussed, BPD-DS creates the risk for protein malnutrition, refractory diarrhea, and micronutrient deficiencies. Incidence of revisional surgery for this in BPD-DS ranges from 0.7% to ~5% for CCL >50 cm in multiple single-center studies with long follow-up.[34] There are multiple options for revision and reversal; however, laparoscopic creation of side-to-side anastomosis between the proximal alimentary and biliopancreatic limbs is described as a straightforward way to achieve this,[34] and the patient will still be left with SG anatomy.

In the setting of inadequate weight loss after SG, in a patient who has a functional gastric sleeve without evidence of dilation, if the person undergoes a second operation, it should be a procedure that adds malabsorption to their restrictive anatomy. If weight loss or resolution of type 2 diabetes is the primary goal, laparoscopic DS/BPD should be performed.[35] If the patient has significant risk factors for duodenal switch (DS) or has significant GERD, conversion to RYGB should be considered.[35] Recently, repeat sleeve gastrectomy (reSG) has been performed with increasing frequency, typically in patients with inadequate weight loss associated with primary sleeve dilation (posterior fundal gastric pouch as a result of inadequate initial operation) or secondary dilation (homogenous dilated gastric tube >250 mL on volumetric computed tomography).[36] Limited single-center data reports that the reSG procedure is relatively safe, and offers promising results at rescuing weight loss with 5-year follow-up,[36,37] especially for patients with primary dilation, with one series reporting 72% of these patients maintaining at least 50% EWL after 5 years.[37] More robust and larger data analyses of this revisionary procedure are warranted. However, if comfortable with the procedure, it is reasonable to offer reSG to the appropriate patient with a diagnosed dilation of their existing SG compared to revision with a RYGB or BPD-DS.

REFERENCES

1. Martinovski M, Navratil A, Zeni T, et al. Minimally invasive Roux-en-Y gastric bypass versus biliopancreatic diversion with duodenal switch: results from the Metabolic and Bariatric Surgery Accreditation and Quality Improvement Program (MBSAQIP). *SOARD*. 2017;13(10):S18.
2. Martinovski M, Kemmeter P, Birkmeyer N, Carlin A, Finks J. A matched cohort comparison of laparoscopic biliopancreatic diversion with duodenal switch and Roux-en-Y gastric bypass. *SOARD*. 2015;11(6):S22.
3. Sovik TT, Taha O, Aasheim ET, et al. Randomized clinical trial of laparoscopic gastric bypass versus laparoscopic duodenal switch for superobesity. *BJS*. 2010;97(2):160-166.
4. Buchwald H, Estok R, Fahrbach K, et al. Weight and type 2 diabetes after bariatric surgery: systemic review and meta-analysis. *Am J Med*. 2009;122(3):248-256e5.
5. Prachand VN, Ward M, Alverdy JC. Duodenal switch provides superior resolution of metabolic comorbidities independent of weight loss in the super-obese (BMI ≥ 50 kg/m^2) compared with gastric bypass. *J Gastrointest Surg*. 2010;14:211-220.
6. Finks JF, Kole KL, Yenumula PR, et al. Predicting risk for serious complications with bariatric surgery. *Ann Surg*. 2011;254(4):633-640.
7. Bohdjalian A, Langer FB, Shakeri-Leidenmühler S, et al. Sleeve gastrectomy as sole and definitive bariatric procedure: 5-year results for weight loss and ghrelin. *Obes Surg*. 2010;20:535-540.
8. Schauer PR, Bhatt DL, Kirwan JP, et al. Bariatric surgery versus intensive medical therapy for diabetes— 5-year outcomes. *N Eng J Med*. 2017;376(7):641-651.
9. Peterli R, Wölnerhanssen BK, Peters T, et al. Effect of laparoscopic sleeve gastrectomy vs laparoscopic Roux-en-Y gastric bypass on weight loss in patients with morbid obesity: the SM-BOSS randomized clinical trial. *JAMA*. 2018;319(3):255-265.
10. Salminen P, Helmiö M, Ovaska J, et al. Effect of laparoscopic sleeve gastrectomy vs laparoscopic Roux-en-Y gastric bypass on weight loss at 5 years among patients with morbid obesity: the SLEEVEPASS randomized clinical trial. *JAMA*. 2018;319(3):241-254.
11. King WC, Hinerman AS, Belle SH, Wahed AS, Courcoulas AP. Comparison of the performance of common measures of weight regain after bariatric surgery for association with clinical outcomes. *JAMA*. 2018;320(15): 1560-1569.
12. Himpens J, Dobbeleir J, Peeters G. Long-term results of laparoscopic sleeve gastrectomy for obesity. *Ann Surg*. 2010;252(2):319-324.
13. Bolckmans R, Himpens J. Long-term (>10 Yrs) outcome of the laparoscopic biliopancreatic diversion with duodenal switch. *Ann Surg*. 2016;264(6): 1029-1037.
14. Gonzalez AG, Canner JK, Alsulaim HA, Steele K. Remission and relapse of type 2 diabetes mellitus after bariatric surgery: vertical sleeve gastrectomy vs Roux-en-Y gastric bypass. *JACS*. 2017;225(4):S18.
15. Lewis KH, Arterburn D, Zhang F, et al. Comparative effectiveness of vertical sleeve gastrectomy versus Roux en Y gastric bypass for diabetes treatment. *Ann Surg*. 2021;273(5):940-948.
16. Polega, J, Barreto T, Kemmeter K, Koehler T, Davis A, Kemmeter P. A matched cohort study of laparoscopic bilipancreatic diversion with duodenal switch and sleeve gastrectomy performed by one surgeon. *SOARD*. 2017;13:411-414.
17. Hutter MM, Schirmer BD, et al. First report from the American College of Surgeons Bariatric Surgery Center Network: Laparoscopic sleeve gastrectomy has morbidity and effectiveness between the band and the bypass. *Ann Surg*. 2011;254:410-422.
18. Young MT, Gebhart A, Phelan MJ, Nguyen NT. Use and outcomes of laparoscopic sleeve gastrectomy vs laparoscopic gastric bypass: analysis of the American College of Surgeons NSQIP. *JACS*. 2015;220(5):880-885.
19. Goitein D, Raziel A, Szold A, et al. Assessment of perioperative complications following primary bariatric surgery according to the Clavien–Dindo classification: comparison of sleeve gastrectomy and Roux-Y gastric bypass. *Surg Endosc*. 2016;30:273-278.
20. Marceau P, Biron S, Hould FS. Duodenal switch: long-term results. *Obes Surg*. 2007;17:1421-1430.
21. Hamoui N, Chock B, Anthone GJ, Crookes PF. Revision of the duodenal switch: indications, technique, and outcomes. *JACS*. 2007;204(4):603-608.
22. Risstad H, Sovik TT, Engstrom M, Aasheim ET, et al. Five-year outcomes after laparoscopic gastric bypass and laparoscopic duodenal switch in patients with body mass index of 50 to 60. *JAMA Surg*. 2015;150(4): 352-361.
23. Elias K, Hedberg J, Sundbom M. Prevalence and impact of acid-related symptoms and diarrhea in patients undergoing Roux-en-Y gastric bypass, sleeve gastrectomy, and biliopancreatic diversion with duodenal switch. *SOARD*. 2020;16:520-528.

24. Sethi M, Chau M, Youn A, Jiang Y, Fielding G, Ren-Fielding C. Long-term outcomes after biliopancreatic diversion with and without duodenal switch: 2-, 5-, and 10-year data. *SOARD*. 2016;12:1697-1705.
25. Khwaja HA, Stewart DJ, Magee CJ, Javed SM, Kerrigan DD. Petersen hernia complicating laparoscopic duodenal switch. *SOARD*. 2012;8:236-238.
26. Chowbey P, Baijal M, Kantharia NS, et al. Mesenteric defect closure decreases the incidence of internal hernias following laparoscopic Roux-en-Y gastric bypass: a retrospective cohort study. *Obes Surg*. 2016;26:2029-2034.
27. DuPree CE, Blair K, Steele SR, Martin MJ. Laparoscopic sleeve gastrectomy in patients with preexisting gastroesophageal reflux disease: a national analysis. *JAMA Surg*. 2014;149(4):328-334.
28. Felsenreich DM, Kefurt R, Schermann M, et al. Reflux, sleeve dilation, and Barrett's esophagus after laparoscopic sleeve gastrectomy: long-term follow-up. *Obes Surg*. 2017;27:3092-3101.
29. Filho AM, Silva LB, Godoy ES, et al. Omentopexy in sleeve gastrectomy reduces early gastroesophageal reflux symptoms. *Surg Laparosc Endosc Percutan Tech*. 2019;29(3): 155-161.
30. Afaneh C, Costa R, Pomp A, et al. A prospective randomized controlled trial assessing the efficacy of omentopexy during laparoscopic sleeve gastrectomy in reducing postoperative gastrointestinal symptoms. *Surg Endosc*. 2015;29:41-47.
31. Howard R, Chao GF, Yang J, et al. Comparative safety of sleeve gastrectomy and gastric bypass up to 5 years after surgery in patients with severe obesity. *JAMA Surg*. October 6, 2021. doi:10.1001/jamasurg.2021.4981
32. Courcoulas A, Coley RY, Clark JM, et al. Interventions and operations 5 years after bariatric surgery in a cohort from the US National Patient-Centered Clinical Research Network Bariatric Study. *JAMA Surg*. 2020;155(3):194-204
33. Strain GW, Torghabeh MH, Gagner M, et al. The impact of biliopancreatic diversion with duodenal switch over 9 years. *Obes Surg*. 2017;27:787-794.
34. Topart PA, Becouarn G. Revision and reversal after biliopancreatic diversion for excessive side effects of ineffective weight loss: a review of the current literature on indications and procedures. *SOARD*. 2015;11:965-972.
35. Carmeli I, Golomb I, Sadot E, Kashtan H, Keidar A. Laparoscopic conversion of sleeve gastrectomy to a biliopancreatic diversion with duodenal switch or a Roux-en-Y gastric bypass due to weight loss failure: our algorithm. *SOARD*. 2015;11:79-87.
36. Nedelcu M, Noel P, Iannelli A, Gagner M. Revised sleeve gastrectomy (re-sleeve). *SOARD*. 2015;11:1282-1288.
37. Noel P, Nedelcu A, Eddbali I, et al. Five-year results after resleeve gastrectomy. *SOARD*. 2020;16:1186-1191.

27

Conventional Versus MGB/OAGB

Shawn Tsuda, MD, MBA, FACS, and Angel J. Rivera Aponta, MD

1. **When deciding between conventional Roux-en-Y gastric bypass (RYGB) versus mini-gastric bypass/one-anastomosis gastric bypass (MGB/OAGB), the surgeon should be aware of which of the following? See Figure 27-1.**
   A. MGB/OAGB results in poorer patient satisfaction in the long term.
   B. MGB/OAGB has less efficacy in weight loss in comparison with RYGB.
   C. The incidence of marginal ulcer is higher in RYGB than MGB/OAGB.
   D. MGB/OAGB has more malabsorptive effects compared to RYGB.

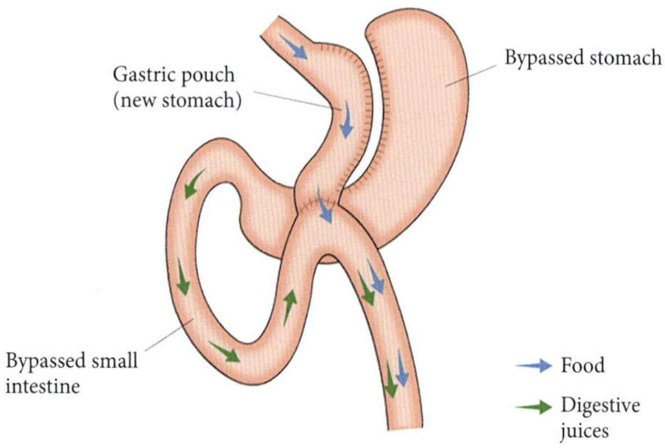

Figure 27-1 MGB/OAGB

2. **A 50-year-old male presents to the emergency department with worsening epigastric pain, nausea, and vomiting 15 days after an MGB/OAGB. He is hemodynamically stable. Computed tomography (CT) of the abdomen and pelvis shows a dilated loop of bowel proximal to the gastrojejunostomy. What is the most appropriate management?**
   A. Enteroenterostomy
   B. Observation, nasogastric tube, and antiemetics
   C. Esophagogastroduodenoscopy
   D. Intravenous fluids and antibiotics

3. **A 60-year-old man had an MGB/OAGB for morbid obesity 1 year ago. For the last 4 months, he has been complaining of burning epigastric pain and emesis of dark fluid. The pain has been unrelieved by acid suppression and is aggravated by both oral intake and recumbent position. Upper endoscopy shows mildly erythematous mucosa with no evidence of stricture or ulcer. Biopsy shows internalization of gastric glands with inflammation. He has failed medical management with prokinetic agents, antispasmodic therapy, cholestyramine, and dietary modification. What is the most likely diagnosis?**
   A. Zollinger–Ellison syndrome
   B. Delayed gastric emptying
   C. Efferent loop syndrome
   D. Alkaline reflux gastritis

ANSWERS

1. **D.** MGB-OAGB has stronger malabsorptive effects compared to RYGB.[1] In a study by Lee et al., about 40% of revisions after MGB/OAGB were due to malnutrition.[2] MGB/OAGB has comparable efficacy in weight loss in comparison with RYGB.[3] In addition,

MGB/OAGB has results in weight loss, comorbidity treatment, and patient satisfaction in both the short and long term that are comparable to RYGB.[4–8] The incidence of marginal ulcer with MGB/OAGB is 1% to 6% in multiple studies, which is similar to RYGB.[9,10] Finally, the overall incidence of leak is reported as 0.1% to 1.9% by Mahawar et al. in their systematic review.[11] This incidence is comparable with the leak rates in RYGB (0.1%–5.6%).[12]

2. **A.** Afferent loop syndrome is a mechanical issue wherein the afferent loop becomes partially or completely obstructed. MGB/OAGB is associated with a risk of afferent loop syndrome, due to its similarity to the anatomy of Billroth II operations.[13] Surgical correction is indicated for this mechanical problem. A long afferent limb is usually the underlying problem, so treatment involved the elimination of this loop. Remedies include conversion to Roux-en-Y or an enteroenterostomy below the stoma.

   Antibiotics can be used to treat bacterial overgrowth that can occur in afferent limbs that do not have good peristalsis. Patients will typically present with chronic abdominal pain and the diagnosis can be made via an esophagogastroduodenoscopy or suspected and treated empirically.

3. **D.** Bile reflux can be complication of Billroth II and OAGB as a consequence of retrograde bile passage at the anastomotic site. Bile reflux gastritis results from exposure of the gastric mucosa to bile, pancreatic secretions, and duodenal contents. Musella et al. reported an overall 4% rate for bile reflux in OAGB and found a statistical correlation between postoperative reflux with pouches shorter than 9 cm.[14] Bile gastritis is a diagnosis of exclusion because of the low specificity of the endoscopic findings and histologic findings (internalization of gastric glands with inflammation). Zollinger–Ellison syndrome and other postgastrectomy syndromes should be ruled out prior to operative repair aimed at correction of this condition.

   Conversion to Roux-en-Y gastrojejunostomy with Roux limb of at least 40 cm is associated with symptomatic relief in most patients. Distal Braun enteroenterostomy has been shown to improve symptoms of bile reflux gastritis in about 50% of patients.

REFERENCES

1. Lee WJ, Ser KH, Lee YC, Tsou JJ, Chen SC, Chen JC. Laparoscopic Roux-en-Y vs. mini-gastric bypass for the treatment of morbid obesity: a 10-year experience. *Obes Surg*. 2012;22(12):1827-1834.
2. Lee WJ, Lee YC, Ser KH, et al. Revisional surgery for laparoscopic minigastric bypass. *Surg Obes Relat Dis*. 2011; 7:486-491.
3. Disse E, Pasquer A, Espalieu P, et al. Greater weight loss with the omega loop bypass compared to the Roux-en-Y gastric bypass: a comparative study. *Obes Surg*. 2014;24: 841-846.
4. Kular KS, Manchanda N, Rutledge R. A 6-year experience with 1,054 mini-gastric bypasses- first study from Indian subcontinent. *Obes Surg*. 2014;24:1430-1435.
5. Musella M, Susa A, Greco F, et al. The laparoscopic minigastric bypass: the Italian experience: outcomes from 974 consecutive cases in a multicenter review. *Surg Endosc*. 2014;28:156-163.
6. Padwal R, Klarenbach S, Wiebe N, et al. Bariatric surgery: A systematic review and network meta-analysis of randomized trials. *Obes Rev*. 2011;12:602-621.
7. Milone M, Di Minno MN, Leongito M, et al. Bariatric surgery and diabetes remission: sleeve gastrectomy or mini-gastric bypass? *World J Gastroenterol*. 2013;19: 6590-6597.
8. Moszkowicz D, Rau C, Guenzi M, et al. Laparoscopic omega-loop gastric bypass for the conversion of failed sleeve gastrectomy: early experience. *J Visc Surg*. 2013;150: 373-378.
9. Rutledge R. The mini-gastric bypass: experience with the first 1,274 cases. *Obes Surg*. 2001;11(3):276-280.
10. Rutledge R, Walsh TR. Continued excellent results with the mini-gastric bypass: six-year study in 2,410 patients. *Obes Surg*. 2005;15(9):1304-1308.
11. Mahawar KK, Jennings N, Brown J, et al. "Mini" gastric bypass: systematic review of a controversial procedure. *Obes Surg*. 2013;23:1890-1898.
12. Jacobsen HJ, Nergard BJ, Leifsson BG, et al. Management of suspected anastomotic leak after bariatric laparoscopic Roux-en-Y gastric bypass. *Br J Surg*. 2014;101:417-423.
13. Kassir R, Blanc P, Lointier P, Breton C, Debs T, Tiffet O. Laparoscopic revision of an omega loop gastric bypass to treat afferent loop syndrome. *Obes Surg*. 2015;25(10): 1976⊠1978. doi:10.1007/s11695-015-1805-5.
14. Musella M, Susa A, Manno E, et al. Complications following the mini/one anastomosis gastric bypass (MGB/ OAGB): a multi-institutional survey on 2678 patients with a mid-term (5 years) follow-up. *Obes Surg*. 2017;27: 2956-2967.

28

Single-Anastomosis Duodeno-Ileal Bypass (SADI)

Caitlin Halbert, DO, MS

QUESTION STEM 1

A 54-year-old female with a body mass index (BMI) of 44 kg/m^2 and medical history notable for type 2 diabetes mellitus, hypertension, and hyperlipidemia presents for evaluation for bariatric surgery. The patient is interested in pursuing a malabsorptive procedure for both weight loss and comorbidity resolution.

1. **Which of the following accurately describes the technical difference between biliopancreatic diversion with duodenal switch (BPD/DS) and single-anastomosis duodeno-ileal bypass with sleeve gastrectomy (SADI-S)?**
   A. SADI-S involves a more restrictive approach by performing a sleeve gastrectomy over a 32 French bougie.
   B. SADI-S serves as a simplification of the BPD/DS that uses a sleeve gastrectomy over a 54 French bougie, followed by SADI-S with a 200-cm to 300-cm common channel.
   C. BPD/DS is a pylorus-preserving procedure whereas SADI-S requires division of the stomach proximal to the pylorus.
   D. SADI-S requires mesenteric opening, increasing susceptibility for internal hernia, compared to BPD/DS, which does not.
   E. SADI-S and BPD/DS require the same amount of operative time to complete.

2. **In regards to the short-term complications following different bariatric surgical techniques, which of the following is correct?**
   A. SADI-S has similar marginal ulceration rates when compared to Roux-en-Y gastric bypass (RYGB).
   B. The leak rate of SADI-S is significantly higher than that of BPD/DS.
   C. Overall incidence of short-term complications is lower in SADI-S than RYGB.
   D. SADI-S has a lower incidence of malnutritional when compared to BPD/DS.
   E. RYGB has a lower incidence of dumping syndrome compared to the SADI-S.

3. **In regards to excess weight loss (EWL) 2 years after surgery, which of the following is correct?**
   A. EWL with RYGB is superior to BPD/DS.
   B. EWL with SADI-S is better than BPD/DS.
   C. There is no difference in EWL between BPD/DS and RYGB.
   D. SADI-S and BPD/DS both have superior excess weight loss compared to SG and RYGB.
   E. BPD/DS has the highest EWL of all bariatric procedures

4. **In regards to the resolution of comorbidities associated with morbid obesity after bariatric surgery, which of the following is correct?**
   A. The complete remission of diabetes mellitus 3 years after surgery is equivalent among patients who had RYGB, BPD/DS, and SADI-S.
   B. SADI-S is not as effective as RYGB in resolving diabetes mellitus and hyperlipidemia in morbidly obese patients.

C. Bariatric surgery is not superior to conventional medical therapy in reducing overall mortality in obese patients.
D. Long-term outcomes after bariatric surgery suggest that RYGB is the most successful operation in resolving diabetes mellitus.
E. SADI-S and BPD/DS have been found to have similar diabetes, hyperlipidemia, and hypertension resolution rates, and both are superior to RYGB and SG.

ANSWERS TO QUESTION STEM 1

1. **B.** Despite the clearly superior results in weight loss of the BPD/DS when compared to RYGB and SG, this procedure only accounts for less than 1% of all bariatric procedures due to its technical complexity and complications, notably nutritional deficiencies.[1] With this in mind, the SADI-S was designed as a modification of the BPD/DS, which greatly simplifies the operation while maintaining its restrictive and malabsorptive features.

   Originally described in 2007 by Sanchez-Pernaute, the SADI-S was designed as a simplified version of the BPD/DS that involves obtaining a sleeve gastrectomy over a 54 French bougie, transecting the duodenum at the level of the gastroduodenal artery, leaving a 3 cm to 4 cm proximal duodenal stump, and performing an end-to-side duodeno-ileostomy at a point 200 cm proximal to the ileocecal junction.[2] This anastomosis was described as an antecolic, isoperistaltic stapled anastomosis. The common limb length was later lengthened to 250 cm due to an unacceptably high hypoalbuminemia rate noted in the first series of patients.[3] Subsequent authors have further lengthened this common channel up to 300 cm.[4]

   Both BPD/DS and SADI-S are pylorus-preserving procedures, which brings a theoretical advantage of physiologic gastric emptying, reducing alkaline reflux and dumping syndrome symptoms.[5] SADI-S does not require any opening of the mesentery, with reduction noted in postoperative internal hernia rates when compared to other bariatric surgeries.[6] SADI-S has been shown to require significantly less operative time than BPD/DS,[7] which is attributed to less technical complexity and one less enteric anastomosis. BPD/DS is reconstructed in a Roux-en-Y fashion, whereas SADI-S utilizes an end-to-side duodeno-ileostomy.

2. **C.** In reviewing the incidence of short-term complications associated with SADI-S over a 6-year-period among 1,328 patients, Surve et al. found that the overall leak rate was 0.6%, the marginal ulceration rate was 0.1%, and bile reflux rate was 0.1%.[8] There were no reported cases of internal hernia or volvulus after SADI-S. These short-term complications were noted to be lower than the reported incidence than that associated with RYGB (leak rate 0.1%–5.6%, internal hernia 0.5%–16%, marginal ulceration 0.6%–20%, bile reflux 0.9%). Complication rates were also noted to be higher for the BPD/DS (leak 0.5%–6%, internal hernia 0.4%–18%, marginal ulceration 0.2%–1.9%). The reduced rate of dumping syndrome, alkaline reflux, and marginal ulceration in BPD/DS and SADI-S when compared to RYGB is believed to be due to their postpyloric reconstruction, which is felt to be more physiologic than prepyloric reconstruction.

   Interestingly, despite a longer common limb in SADI-S when compared to BPD/DS, the nutritional data postoperatively is similar, with no statistical difference in the rate of malnutrition.[3]

3. **D.** Although more long-term data is needed to be collected to further evaluate SADI-S in comparison to other more well-established bariatric procedures, the currently available data suggests that it has similar weight loss profile to that of the BPD/DS, with 2-year excess weight loss exceeding 70% to 80%.[9] This is in comparison to the EWL at 2 years of ~70% for RYGB and ~60% for SG. Two-year EWL for VBG has been reported as 70% to 75%, and for laparoscopic adjustable gastric band (LAGB) as 55%, for comparison.[10]

4. **E.** While weight loss remains one of the principal goals of bariatric surgery, the resolution of associated comorbidities may in fact be one of the most significant benefits because this has been shown to reduce overall mortality among obese patients. Overall mortality among bariatric surgery patients has been shown to be reduced compared to matched controls who receive only conventional medical therapy for obesity.[11] Specifically for diabetes mellitus, BPD/DS has been shown to have durable and excellent remission postoperatively, superior to RYGB.[12] Studies examining SADI-S have shown similar results. Torres et al. found complete diabetes remission in noninsulin-dependent diabetics after 3 years to be present in 77%, 90%, and 96% of patients after undergoing RYGB, BPD/DS, and

SADI-S, respectively.[13] Over 20 years of follow-up, BPD/DS has been shown to have a 93% diabetes resolution rate.[14]

QUESTION STEM 2

A 48-year-old man with a BMI of 50 kg/m^2 presents for evaluation for bariatric surgery. He has done some research on various bariatric operations, and has several questions for you about the efficacy and safety of his possible procedural options.

1. **Out of the currently recognized bariatric surgical procedures, which offers the greatest weight loss?**
   A. Roux-en-Y gastric bypass (RYGB)
   B. Sleeve gastrectomy (SG)
   C. Biliopancreatic diversion with duodenal switch (BPD/DS)
   D. Laparoscopic adjustable gastric band (LAGB)
   E. Vertical-banded gastroplasty (VBG)

2. **The patient has read some of the more recent literature about alternatives to BPD/DS, and asks about the long-term safety data on SADI-S. Which of the following is most accurate?**
   A. Long-term follow-up data for SADI-S demonstrates it to be an effective, durable weight loss procedure with good safety profile.
   B. There is not currently enough long-term evidence to provide meaningful comparison of SADI-S to other longstanding procedures.
   C. SADI-S shows unacceptably high recurrence of type 2 diabetes mellitus and hyperlipidemia in long-term follow-up data.
   D. The leak rate following SADI-S surgery is significantly higher than that of RYGB and SG.
   E. The risk of internal hernia after SADI-S is theoretically higher than after other Roux-en-Y procedures.

3. **After answering the patient's questions, you perform further evaluation and learn that he has poorly controlled diabetes mellitus, hypertension, and obstructive sleep apnea. In terms of comorbidity resolution, which of the following is true?**
   A. Early and midterm data show that both weight loss and comorbidity resolution in patients undergoing SADI-S is comparable to BPD/DS.
   B. RYGB remains the best bariatric procedure in terms of resolution of obesity-associated comorbidities.
   C. The long-term (20-year) resolution rate of type 2 diabetes mellitus in patients undergoing BPD/DS is 75%.
   D. Lipid reduction is superior in RYGB.

4. **You recommend that the patient undergoes a restrictive and malabsorptive procedure. He is amenable to this, and is interested in SADI-S; however, he asks what the current national and international guidelines reflect regarding this procedure. Select the most accurate response.**
   A. The International Federation for the Surgery of Obesity and Metabolic Disorders (IFSO) in its 2018 guidelines established SADI-S as a recognized bariatric and metabolic procedure that requires additional study for long-term results.
   B. IFSO summarizes the SADI-S procedure to be superior to BPD/DS in safety profile based on available short- and midterm data.
   C. The American Society of Metabolic and Bariatric Surgery (ASMBS) in 2016 designated the SADI-S procedure as "effective and safe."
   D. No national or international guidelines currently exist regarding SADI-S.
   E. Given its similarity to RYGB, SADI-S has been established as a modified, simpler version of gastric bypass procedures.

ANSWERS TO QUESTION STEM 2

1. **C.** Expected excess weight loss at 2 years after surgery proceeds in the following order, from least to most: LAGB (55%), SG (60%), RYGB (70%), VBG (70%–75%), and BPD/DS (70%–80%).[9,10] The proposed mechanism behind weight loss in restrictive bariatric surgeries involves decreased intake capacity of the stomach as well as changes in gastric emptying. There is also believed to be an effect from the resection of the gastric fundus due to diminished secretion of ghrelin and its subsequent downstream effects on hunger and appetite. Malabsorptive procedures have several suspected contributory mechanisms, including bypass of the duodeno-pancreas region diminishing the incretin effect and decreased exposure of enteric contents to absorptive distal small bowel, resulting in malabsorption.[15] The RYGB procedure is considered to be both a restrictive and malabsorptive procedure, as are the BPD/DS and SADI-S. The LAGB and VBG are considered purely restrictive procedures. The SG

is mainly restrictive but also has hormonal effects as described that assist with metabolic function and weight loss.

2. **B.** While the available literature shows promising weight loss and comorbidity resolution results from the SADI-S procedure, given its inception in 2007, there is a paucity of available long-term data at this time. The available data currently shows it to be a relatively safe procedure, with comparable weight loss results and safety profile to BPD/DS.[16] There have been no reported internal hernias in the literature after SADI-S, and given the lack of mesenteric opening during the procedure, theoretically this would be a very rare complication. The leak rate for SADI-S has been reported to be 0.6%, and the marginal ulcer rate is 0.1%.[8]

3. **A.** Several comparisons of SADI-S to both BPD/DS and RYGB have been performed. In 2017, Torres et al. published an analysis of their data over 10 years of performing the SADI-S procedure.[13] They showed that patients undergoing SADI-S achieved significantly greater weight loss, hypertension resolution, lipid reduction, and diabetes resolution rates than those undergoing RYGB. These findings were comparable to that of BPD/DS. For example, after 3 years of follow-up, patients undergoing RYGB, BPD/DS, and SADI-S had diabetes remission rates of 77%, 89%, and 96%, respectively. Further long-term data is needed for full comparison. Long-term data for BPD/DS shows this procedure to have a 20-year diabetes resolution rate of 93%, currently making it the gold standard.[14] The STAMPEDE trial, which examined RYGB and SG, showed 5-year diabetes resolution to be 29% in RYGB patients and 23% in SG patients.[17]

4. **A.** Both the ASMBS and IFSO have published guidelines regarding SADI-S.[7,16] In 2016, the ASMBS recognized SADI-S as an investigational procedure, with promising early data but insufficient evidence to draw any definitive conclusions regarding "safety, efficacy, and durability" of the procedure. Its guidelines stated that SADI-S should be classified as a modification of the BPD/DS, and remains a procedure that requires institutional review board (IRB) approval at this time. In 2018, IFSO published guidelines that recognized SADI-S as an established bariatric procedure, and went further to say that it appears to have a similar safety profile to BPD/DS; however, IFSO also stated that long-term data from randomized trials was necessary. SADI-S evolved as an alternative to the BPD/DS to reduce the technical complexity and risk of long-term nutritional deficiencies but remains similarly advantageous with regards to weight loss and diabetes resolution. While ultimately at the discretion of the surgeon, patients with higher BMIs and/or diabetes would be ideal candidates for SADI-S.

REFERENCES

1. Kim J. American Society for Metabolic and Bariatric Surgery statement on single-anastomosis duodenal switch. *Surg Obes Relat Dis.* 2016;12(5):944-945. doi:10.1016/j.soard.2016.05.006
2. Sánchez-Pernaute A, Rubio Herrera MA, Pérez-Aguirre E, et al. Proximal duodenal-ileal end-to-side bypass with sleeve gastrectomy: proposed technique. *Obes Surg.* 2007; 17(12):1614-1618.
3. Sánchez-Pernaute A, Herrera MAR, Pérez-Aguirre ME, et al. Single anastomosis duodeno-ileal bypass with sleeve gastrectomy (SADI-S). One to three-year follow-up. *Obes Surg.* 2010;20(12):1720-1726.
4. Cottam A, Cottam D, Portenier D, et al. A matched cohort analysis of stomach intestinal pylorus saving (SIPS) surgery versus biliopancreatic diversion with duodenal switch with two-year follow-up. *Obes Surg.* 2017;27(2):454-461. doi:10.1007/s11695-016-2341-7
5. Martini F, Paolino L, Marzano E, et al. Single-anastomosis pylorus-preserving bariatric procedures: review of the literature. *Obes Surg.* 2016;26(10):2503-2515. doi:10.1007/s11695-016-2310-1
6. Zaveri H, Surve A, Cottam D, et al. Mid-term 4-year outcomes with single anastomosis duodenal-ileal bypass with sleeve gastrectomy surgery at a single US center. *Obes Surg.* 2018;28(10):3062-3072.
7. Topart P, Becouarn G. The single anastomosis duodenal switch modifications: a review of the current literature on outcomes. *Surg Obes Relat Dis.* 2017;13(8):1306-1312. doi:10.1016/j.soard.2017.04.027
8. Surve A, Cottam D, Sanchez-Pernaute A, et al. The incidence of complications associated with loop duodeno-ileostomy after single-anastomosis duodenal switch procedures among 1328 patients: a multicenter experience. *Surg Obes Relat Dis.* 2018;14(5):594-601. doi:10.1016/j.soard.2018.01.020
9. Shoar S, Poliakin L, Rubenstein R, Saber AA. Single anastomosis duodeno-ileal switch (SADIS): a systematic review of efficacy and safety. *Obes Surg.* 2018;28(1):104-113.
10. Schouten R, Wiryasaputra DC, Van Dielen FMH, Van Gemert WG, Greve JWM. Long-term results of bariatric restrictive procedures: a prospective study. *Obes Surg.* 2010;20(12):1617-1626.
11. Arterburn DE, Olsen MK, Smith VA, et al. Association between bariatric surgery and long-term survival. *JAMA.* 2015;313(1):62-70.
12. Buchwald H, Avidor Y, Braunwald E, et al. Bariatric surgery: a systematic review and meta-analysis. *JAMA.* 2004;292(14):1724-1728.

13. Torres A, Rubio MA, Ramos-Leví AM, Sánchez-Pernaute A. Cardiovascular risk factors after single anastomosis duodeno-ileal bypass with sleeve gastrectomy (SADI-S): a new effective therapeutic approach? *Curr Atheroscler Rep*. 2017;19(12).
14. Marceau P, Biron S, Marceau S, et al. Long-term metabolic outcomes 5 to 20 years after biliopancreatic diversion. *Obes Surg*. 2015;25(9):1584-1593.
15. Sánchez-Pernaute A, Rubio MÁ, Cabrerizo L, Ramos-Levi A, Pérez-Aguirre E, Torres A. Single-anastomosis duodenoileal bypass with sleeve gastrectomy (SADI-S) for obese diabetic patients. *Surg Obes Relat Dis*. 2015;11(5): 1092-1098. doi:10.1016/j.soard.2015.01.024
16. Brown WA, Ooi G, Higa K, Himpens J, Torres A. Single anastomosis duodenal-ileal bypass with sleeve gastrectomy/one anastomosis duodenal switch (SADI-S/OADS) IFSO position statement. *Obes Surg*. 2018;28(5):1207-1216.
17. Schauer PR, Bhatt DL, Kirwan JP, et al. Bariatric surgery versus intensive medical therapy for diabetes - 5-year outcomes. *N Engl J Med*. 2017;376(7):641-651.

SECTION 6

Preoperative Preparation

29

Management and Prehabilitation of Bariatric Patients with Cardiac Disease

Judy YR Chen, MD

A 26-year-old woman with a body mass index (BMI) of 57 kg/m^2 and history of childhood obesity since the age of 6, presents with dyspnea on exertion, excessive sweating, and fatigue. This patient also has hypertension, type 2 diabetes mellitus, obstructive sleep apnea (OSA), and hyperlipidemia. Her physical exam shows prominent jugular venous distension, rales at the bases of her lungs bilaterally, a palpable liver edge on abdominal exam as well as pitting edema of both her ankles.

1. **Regarding the impact of obesity on hemodynamics and cardiac function, which is true?**
   A. Increased blood volume
   B. Decreased stroke volume
   C. Eccentric left ventricular hypertrophy
   D. Decreased arterial pressure
   E. Decreased cardiac output

2. **The patient also had a sister with severe obesity, who died of a stroke at age 45. Which of the following patient characteristics increases her chance of having a cardiac complication?**
   A. Hyperlipidemia
   B. BMI >45
   C. Family history of stroke
   D. Female sex
   E. OSA

3. **The patient also has a smoking history consisting of 10 pack-years. She quit 6 months ago when her sister passed away. She drinks 1 to 2 beers a week while watching television and lives alone. She does not perform regular exercise and must take a break due to dyspnea on exertion when walking up a flight of stairs. Of these risk factors, which nonlifestyle most predicts adverse perioperative outcome and can be improved with cardiac prehabilitation?**
   A. Smoking
   B. Psychological support
   C. Alcohol use
   D. Physical inactivity
   E. Inability to walk up two flights of stairs

4. **Which would improve cardiorespiratory fitness in patients with obesity and heart failure?**
   A. Vegan diet
   B. Ketogenic diet
   C. Exercise
   D. Heart transplant
   E. Improved sleep

5. **This patient did not initially undergo bariatric surgery and now presents 15 years later with the same BMI; however, she now also has stage D heart failure due to nonischemic cardiomyopathy. Her left ventricular dysfunction requires a left ventricular assist device (LVAD).**

   Which of the following is correct?

   A. Bariatric surgery should not be performed in patients that requires an LVAD.

B. Bariatric surgery can be used as a bridge to heart transplantation.
C. A heart transplant should be performed prior to undergoing bariatric surgery in these patients.
D. Class I obesity precludes patients from being transplant candidates.
E. Even with successful bariatric surgery, this patient will still need a heart transplant.

ANSWERS

1. **A.** Cardiac morphology and ventricular function changes associated with obesity.[1] A study published by Kenchaiah et al[2] from the Framingham Heart Study shows that heart failure increases in 7% of women and 5% of men for every 1 kg/m^2 increase in BMI. Obesity has a significant impact on hemodynamic properties. Hypertension severity increases due to an increase in circulating blood volume and systemic vascular resistance, typically leading to increased peripheral arterial resistance and afterload with concentric left ventricular hypertrophy.[1-5] Obesity is associated with multiple cardiac comorbidities including hypertension, diabetes, dyslipidemia, and OSA. In an obese patient, cardiovascular risk is more severe with coronary artery disease, heart failure, sudden cardiac death, and arrhythmia given increased total cardiac output and workload.

2. **C.** There are complex factors that presents a challenge in understanding characteristics of patients that have increased perioperative adverse events in bariatric surgery. A scoring system developed from a single site retrospective cohort study proposing the bariatric surgery mortality risks score, identified four independent variables associated with mortality.[6] These four included BMI >50, male sex, hypertension, and venous thrombosis risk.[7] The Longitudinal Assessment of Bariatric Surgery is a prospective, multicenter, observational study of 30-day outcomes in consecutive patients undergoing bariatric procedures. This identified only BMI and history of venous thromboembolisms as independent risk factors for adverse events.[8] Extremes of BMI, inability to walk 200 feet prior to surgery, history of VTE, sleep apnea, and a BMI of 70 was as high as 10% adverse event Longitudinal Assessment of Bariatric Surgery (LABS).[8] Evaluation and individualized risk assessment of a patient's metabolic acuity is essential for achieving best outcomes.[9-11]

3. **D.** Poor physical fitness predicts adverse perioperative outcomes and is consistent across multiple specialties.[12,13] Cardiac and pulmonary rehabilitation demonstrates effectiveness. Screening, assessment, and intervention principles are integral for preoperative understanding of the patient's own metabolic acuity. This allows from using predicted outcomes for optimizing patient selection and informed consent.[12] Cigarette smoking and alcohol drinking are preventable lifestyle risks factors in surgery. Long-term tobacco abstinence reduces the complication risk but the significance of short-term smoking is not as well defined. Preoperative smoking cessation is beneficial and abstinence starting 3 to 8 weeks before surgery will significantly reduce serious postoperative complications due to improved immune function and recovery.[20]

4. **C.** The role of nonpharmacologic interventions for treatment of patients with obesity and heart failure is important.[1] Morbidity and mortality can impact increases in hospital length of stays, readmissions, and a burden on elective surgeries. Lifestyle and behavioral factors can elevate risks, including but not limited to physical inactivity, poor fitness, smoking, hazardous drinking, malnutrition, and adverse psychological factors.[12] Exercise training improves exercise capacity by improving VO_2 and cardiac function, specifically by improving systolic function with left ventricular ejection fraction and cardiac remodeling. Carbone cardiorespiratory fitness (CRF) assessment is through cardiopulmonary exercise testing (CPX); peak oxygen consumption is a primary CRF measure. Exercise capacity is measured through metabolic equivalents (METs).[12,14,15] There is no evidence that the vegan or ketogenic diet or improved sleep improve cardiorespiratory fitness in patients with obesity and heart failure. Obesity is a contraindication for heart transplant.[21]

5. **B.** Bariatric surgery has emerged as an alternative means of improving cardiac status in patients with severe left ventricular dysfunction and heart failure that requires LVADs. There is potential benefit in the high-risk cardiac patient population where bariatric surgery can improve weight loss, cardiac comorbidities, and quality of life.[16] The studies in the literature have been small, but have shown bariatric surgery in patients with cardiomyopathy is feasible and effective. Treatment of obesity with bariatric surgery has

shown significant mean left ventricular ejection fraction and improved functional capacity as measured by NYHA classification.[17–19] In a study by McCloskey, 14 patients with left ventricular ejection fraction <35% underwent bariatric surgery and patients' cardiac function improved significantly to not require heart transplants, while two patients were able to have successful cardiac transplantation after weight loss from bariatric surgery.[19] Contraindications for cardiac transplant include obesity (BMI >35 or weight >140% of ideal body weight).[21]

REFERENCES

1. Carbone S, Levie CJ, Elagizi A, Arena R, Ventura HO. The impact of obesity in heart failure. *Heart Failure Clin.* 2020;16:71-80.
2. Kenchaiah S, Evans JC, Levy D. Obesity and the risks of heart failure. *N Engl J Med.* 2002;347(15):305-313.
3. Lavie CJ. Laddu D, Arena R. Healthy weight and obesity prevention: JACC health promotion series. *J Am Coll Cardiol.* 2018;72(13):1506-1531.
4. Alpert MA, Karthikeyan K, Abdulla O. Obesity and cardiac remodeling in adults: mechanisms and clinical implications. *Prog Cardiovasc Dis.* 2018;61(2):114-123.
5. Artham SM, Lavie CJ, Milani RV, Ventura HO. Obesity and hypertension, heart failure and coronary heart disease- risk factor, paradox and recommendations for weight loss. *Ochsner J.* 2009;9(3):124-132.
6. DeMaria EJ, Portenier D, Wolfe L. Obesity surgery mortality risk score: proposal for a clinically useful score to predict mortality risks in patients undergoing gastric bypass. *Surg Obese Relat Dis.* 2007;3:134-140.
7. DeMaria Ej, Murr M, Byrne TK, et al. Validation of the Obesity Surgery Mortality Risk Score in a multicenter study proves it stratifies mortality risk in patients undergoing gastric bypass for morbid obesity. *Ann Surg.* 2007;246:578-582.
8. Flum DR, Belle SH, King WC, et al. Perioperative safety in the longitudinal assessment of bariatric surgery. *N Engl J Med.* 2009;361:445-454.
9. Ramanan B, Gupta PK, Gupta H, Fang X, Forse RA. Development and validation of a bariatric surgery mortality risk calculator. *J Am Coll Surg.* 2012;214:892-900.
10. Tewksbury C, Geng Z, Foster M, et al. Validation and improvement of a highly predictive bariatric surgery mortality risk calculator to include sleeve gastrectomy using MBSAQIP 2015-2017 data. *Surg Obes Relat Dis.* 2020;16(6):715-731.
11. Gupta PK, Franck C, Miller WJ, Gupta H, Forse RA. Development and validation of a bariatric surgery morbidity risk calculator using the prospective, multicenter NSQIP dataset. *J Am Coll Surg.* 2011;212(3):301-309.
12. Durrand J, Singh SJ, Danjoux G. Prehabilitation. *Clin Med.* 2019;19(6):458-464.
13. Flocke SA, Clark E, Antognoli E. Teachable moments for health behavior change and intermediate patient outcomes. *Patient Educ Couns.* 2014;96:43-49.
14. Moran J, Wilson F. The preoperative use of field tests of exercise tolerance to predict postoperative outcomes in intra-abdominal surgery: a systematic review. *J Clin Anesth.* 2016;35:446-455.
15. Livingston EH, Arteburn D, Schifftner TL, Handerson WG, DePalma RG. National surgical quality improvement program analysis of bariatric operations: modifiable risk factors contribute to bariatric surgical adverse outcomes. *J Am Coll Surg.* 2006;203(5):625-633.
16. Zenilman A, Pechman D, Moran-Atkin E, Choi J. Camacho D. Bariatric surgery in patients with left ventricular assist devices: a safe and effective method of weight loss as a gateway to heart transplantation. *Surg Obes Relat Dis.* 2019;15(10):1780-1784.
17. Punchai S. Hanipah ZN, Sharma G, et al. Laparoscopic sleeve gastrectomy in heart failure patients with left ventricular assist device. *Obesity Surg.* 2019;29:1122-1129.
18. Poirier P, Giles T, Bray GA, et al. Obesity and cardiovascular disease: pathophysiology, evaluation, and effect of weight loss. *Circulation.* 2006;114:898-918.
19. McCloskey C, Ramani G, Mathier M, Mattar S, Courcoulas A, Ramanathan R. Bariatric surgery improves cardiac function in morbidly obese patients with severe cardiomyopathy. *SOARD.* 2007;3(5):503-507.
20. Tonnesen H, Nielsen PR, Lauritzen JB, Moller AM. Smoking and alcohol intervention before surgery: evidence for best practice. *British Journal of Anaesthesia.* 2009;102(3):297-306.
21. Bhagra S, Pettit S, Parameshwar J. Cardiac transplantation: indications, eligibility and current outcomes. *Heart.* 2018;105(3):252-260.

30

Pulmonary Optimization in Bariatric Surgery

Julietta Chang, MD, FACS and Jonathan Carter, MD, FACS, FASMBS

1. A 52-year-old male with a body mass index (BMI) of 44 kg/m^2 presents for evaluation for bariatric surgery. He is a current pack-a-day cigarette smoker and uses a daily inhaled corticosteroid for chronic obstructive pulmonary disease (COPD) and takes one medication for hypertension. His wife reports that he is a loud snorer. Which is correct regarding his preoperative workup?

A. Counseling to stop smoking at least 2 weeks before surgery is needed.
B. A home sleep monitoring study is not required.
C. Referral for an overnight laboratory polysomnography (PSG) is needed.
D. The patient has a low STOP-BANG score and does not need to be screened for obstructive sleep apnea (OSA).

2. The patient underwent a polysomnography and his apnea hypopnea index (AHI) was 34. It is 2 months before his surgical date and he reports that he is abstaining from smoking. Which is accurate?

A. The patient should be fitted for a continuous positive airway pressure device (CPAP).
B. The patient needs no further cessation therapy.
C. The patient is as likely to finish the program as a nonsmoker.
D. The patient is a better candidate for having a laparoscopic sleeve gastrectomy (LSG).

3. On the day of surgery, the patient's cotinine test is negative. He has brought his CPAP with him. He undergoes an uneventful LSG. Which about his postoperative course is correct?

A. The patient does not need any adjustments from his home CPAP settings while in the hospital.
B. The patient should be placed on a continuous pulse oximeter in the immediate postoperative period.
C. Consideration should be made for admission to the intensive care unit.
D. The patient's length of stay (LOS) will likely be longer.

4. It is 6 months after the patient's LSG and he is doing well. He has lost 15% of his total body weight and has been able to reduce the dose of his blood pressure medication. He is wondering if he will be able to stop his COPD medications and his CPAP machine. Which is accurate?

A. The patient will likely continue to need his medications for COPD because it is a product of his many years of smoking, rather than obesity.
B. The patient will still likely require CPAP postoperatively.
C. The patient needs to wait until he loses more weight prior to repeating a PSG.
D. This is a good time to counsel the patient again on smoking cessation.

ANSWERS

1. C. A systematic review of preoperative smoking cessation found that interventions that begin at least 4 to 8 weeks prior to surgery have the most meaningful impact on smoking cessation, and intensive interventions (including multiple interventions and nicotine replacement therapy) yielded greater success with decreased postoperative complications than brief intervention alone.[1]

OSA is common in the obese population with 60% to 70% affected and many underdiagnosed.[2] A meta-analysis of noncardiac surgeries showed that the presence of OSA increased the risk of postoperative complications including desaturations, cardiac events, and unplanned transfers to the ICU.[3] Worse for this patient, the combination of undiagnosed OSA and chronic obstructive pulmonary disease (overlap syndrome) has increased perioperative morbidity.[4] Thus, the bariatric surgeon should screen all preoperative patients for symptoms of sleep apnea.

The gold standard for the diagnosis of OSA is an overnight laboratory PSG that measures the number of desaturation events and their severity.[5] A home sleep study may be used for diagnosis in patients with a high pretest probability for OSA because it tends to underestimate frequency.[6]

The STOP-BANG questionnaire is the best validated screening tool for sleep apnea; sensitivity and specificity of a score ≥3 to detect moderate-to-severe OSA is 93% and 100%, respectively.[7] The STOP-BANG questionnaire uses a mnemonic that assigned 1 point for each condition present: Snoring, Tired (excessive daytime sleepiness), Observed (apneic episodes), Pressure (hypertension), BMI (>35), Age (>50), Neck circumference (>16 inches), Gender (male) for a score of 0-8. Without even being specifically screened with the questionnaire, our patient has a score of at least 5 (snoring, BMI >35, hypertension, age >50, male sex).

2. **A.** A PSG measures AHI, which is calculated by the number of apneic and hypopneic (decreased airflow) events in an hour of sleep. An AHI of 15 or greater is indicative of OSA.[6] This patient has severe sleep apnea (AHI >30) and should be fitted for a CPAP.

   Although the patient reports cessation of tobacco, this may not be accurate, and it is important to continue to offer support and resources to maximize his chances of quitting. The use of a cotinine test that detects byproduct of nicotine in the bloodstream can be used as a confirmatory test of abstinence. In one study, bariatric preoperative patients were required to quit smoking prior to surgery; 13% failed their cotinine test, and of these only one patient admitted to smoking when presented with the positive test results.[8] The cotinine test, however, is limited by the fact that it detects all nicotine byproducts including nicotine replacement therapy up to 7 days after use. Studies show that smokers tend to have higher rates of drop-out from bariatric programs, perhaps in part due to mandatory cessation.[9]

   Smoking is a known risk factor for marginal ulcers after a laparoscopic Roux-en-Y gastric bypass (LRYGB). A recent study showed smoking to confer the greatest risk compared to immunosuppression or nonsteroidal anti-inflammatory drug (NSAID) use in recalcitrant ulcers requiring surgical intervention.[10] Due to the risk of ulceration, it may be safer to offer a sleeve gastrectomy (SG).

3. **B.** CPAP requirements may change postoperatively while in the hospital, and the patient should be on a continuous pulse oximeter to ensure adequate oxygenation because desaturation episodes frequently occur in the first 24 hours after surgery.[11] Surgeons should not be worried about staple line disruption caused by CPAP. Additional monitors such as end-tidal carbon dioxide monitoring may also be required if additional narcotics or sedating medications are anticipated.[5] Routine admission to an intensive care unit for a diagnosis of OSA alone is not necessary.[12]

   One study examined perioperative morbidity and outcomes in patients diagnosed with OSA who started CPAP in the preoperative period, compared with those who scored 3 or more on STOP-BANG but did not undergo PSG, compared with those with a score of <3. Patients on CPAP had similar LOS and complication rates as those with low STOP-BANG scores; however, patients with high STOP-BANG scores who did not undergo PSG had significantly lower SpO_2 postoperatively, longer LOS, and two cases of sudden death compared to the other two groups,[13] underscoring the importance of preoperative diagnosis of OSA and initiation and continuation of CPAP postoperatively.

4. **D.** Although COPD is a chronic disease of the airways, obesity has been shown to be a significant risk factor in acute exacerbations. The mechanism is unclear but may be due to the proinflammatory milieu secondary to the large amount of adipose tissue present in obesity. Sustained weight loss after bariatric surgery has been shown to decrease emergency room visits and hospitalizations for acute COPD exacerbations.[14]

Bariatric surgery has been proven superior to medical therapy including pharmacotherapy for treatment of obesity and, by extension, OSA.[15] Studies show anywhere from 55% to 77% improvement or resolution of OSA after bariatric surgery.[16,17] In one study, the authors found that those with resolution of OSA had greater reduction in weight lost, overall fat, and abdominal subcutaneous fat compared to those without resolution.[16]

The current American Academy of Sleep Medicine clinical guidelines recommends patients undergo retesting for OSA after significant weight loss defined as 10% of body weight or more.[18]

Studies show that there is no long-term effect on smoking cessation with brief preoperative intervention (i.e. the patient will resume smoking postoperatively), while there is some benefit with intensive intervention).[1] Although this patient is not at risk of marginal ulcer disease, smoking any amount increases all-cause mortality,[19] and studies show that repeated counseling is associated with increased likelihood for the patient to quit.[20]

REFERENCES

1. Thomsen T, Villebro N, Møller AM. Interventions for preoperative smoking cessation. *Cochrane Database Syst Rev.* 2014;3(27). doi:10.1002/14651858.CD002294.pub4.
2. Ravesloot MJL, et al. Obstructive sleep apnea is underrecognized and underdiagnosed in patients undergoing bariatric surgery. *Eur Arch Otorhinolaryngol.* 2012; 269:1865-1871. doi:10.1007/s00405-012-1948-0.
3. Kaw R, Chung F, Pasupuleti V, et al. Meta-analysis of the association between obstructive sleep apnoea and postoperative outcome. 2012;109(6):897-906. doi:10.1093/bja/aes308.
4. Raveendran R, et al. Obesity hypoventilation syndrome, sleep apnea, overlap syndrome: perioperative management to prevent complications. *Curr Op Anaesthesiol.* 2017;30(1):146-155.doi:10.1097/ACO.0000000000000421.
5. de Raaff CAL, et al. Perioperative management of obstructive sleep apnea in bariatric surgery: a consensus guideline. *Surg Obesit Relat Dis.* 2017;13:1095-1109. doi:10.1016/j.soard.2017.03.022.
6. Sateia MJ. International classification of sleep disorders-third edition highlights and modifications. *Chest.* 2014;146:1387-1394. doi:10.1378/chest.14-0970.
7. Chung F, Abdullah HR, Liao P. STOP-bang questionnaire a practical approach to screen for obstructive sleep apnea. *Chest.* 2016;149:631-638. doi:10.1378/chest.15-0903.
8. Gormsen J, Hjørne F, Helgstrand F. Cotinine test in evaluating smoking cessation at the day of bariatric surgery. *Scandinavian J Surg.* 2019;109(3). doi:10.1177/1457496919866017.
9. Veldheer S, et al. Completion rates in a preoperative surgical weight loss program by tobacco use status. *Surg Obesity Relat Dis.* 2017;13:842-847. doi:10.1016/j.soard.2017.02.004.
10. Di Palma A, et al. Marginal ulceration following Roux-en-Y gastric bypass: risk factors for ulcer development, recurrence and need for revisional surgery. *Surg Endoscopy.* 2021;35(5):2347-2353. doi:10.1007/s00464-020-07650-0.
11. Ahmad S, et al. Postoperative hypoxemia in morbidly obese patients with and without obstructive sleep apnea undergoing laparoscopic bariatric surgery. *Anesthes Analges.* 2008;107:138-143. doi:10.1213/ane.0b013e318174df8b.
12. Shearer E, et al. Obstructive sleep apnea can be safely managed in a level 2 critical care setting after laparoscopic bariatric surgery. *Surg Obes Relat Dis.* 2013;9:845-849. doi:10.1016/j.soard.2012.09.006.
13. Proczko MA, et al. STOP-Bang and the effect on patient outcome and length of hospital stay when patients are not using continuous positive airway pressure. *J Anesthes.* 2014;28:891-897. doi:10.1007/s00540-014-1848-0.
14. Goto T, et al. Reduced risk of acute exacerbation of copd after bariatric surgery: a self-controlled case series study. *Chest.* 2018;153:611-617. doi:10.1016/j.chest.2017.07.003.
15. Ashrafian H, et al. Bariatric surgery or non-surgical weight loss for obstructive sleep apnoea? a systematic review and comparison of meta-analyses. *Obesity Surg.* 2015;25:1239-1250. doi:10.1007/s11695-014-1533-2.
16. Auclair A, et al. Bariatric surgery-induced resolution of hypertension and obstructive sleep apnea: impact of modulation of body fat, ectopic fat, autonomic nervous activity, inflammatory and adipokine profiles. *Obesity Surg.* 2017;27:3156-3164. doi:0.1007/s11695-017-2737-z.
17. Sillo TO, et al. The impact of bariatric surgery on the resolution of obstructive sleep apnoea. *BMC Research Notes.* 2018;11. doi:10.1186/s13104-018-3484-5.
18. Kapur VK, et al. Clinical practice guideline for diagnostic testing for adult obstructive sleep apnea: an American academy of sleep medicine clinical practice guideline. *J Clin Sleep Med.* 2017;13(3):479-504. doi:10.5664/jcsm.6506.
19. Inoue-Choi M, et al. Association of long-term, low-intensity smoking with all-cause and cause-specific mortality in the national institutes of health-AARP diet and health study. *JAMA Intern Med.* 2017;177:87-95. doi:10.1001/jamainternmed.2016.7511.
20. West R, et al. Health-care interventions to promote and assist tobacco cessation: a review of efficacy, effectiveness and affordability for use in national guideline development. *Addiction.* 2015;110(9):1388-1403. doi:10.1111/add.12998.

31

NAFLD/NASH

Byron Faler, MD

A 41-year-old Hispanic male with a body mass index of 48 kg/m^2 and medical history of diabetes, hyperlipidemia, hypertension, and gastroesophageal reflux disease (GERD) is being evaluated for bariatric surgery. His surgical history is significant for a prior laparoscopic cholecystectomy. He does not smoke and drinks 1 to 2 glasses of wine per week. A recent esophagogastroduodenoscopy (EGD) showed mild reflux esophagitis but was otherwise normal. Preoperative labs showed an Hgb A1C of 6.9%, AST of 70 IU/L, ALT of 110 IU/L, normal bilirubin, normal complete blood count (CBC), and normal electrolytes and renal panel. After completing his preparatory program, he is scheduled for a laparoscopic Roux-en-Y gastric bypass (RYGB).

1. **In regards to the diagnosis of nonalcoholic fatty liver disease (NAFLD) and nonalcoholic steatohepatitis (NASH), which of the following statements is correct?**
   A. The microscopic differentiation of alcoholic liver disease from NAFLD/NASH is distinguished by the presence of Mallory–Denk bodies.
   B. In this patient, the diagnosis of NASH cannot be given even if the pathologic features are discovered by biopsy.
   C. Imaging with ultrasound and computed tomography (CT) is highly sensitive for detecting NAFLD but is not able to reliably distinguish NASH.
   D. Liver biopsy should be reserved only for those individuals with clinical and laboratory evidence of early cirrhosis due to potential complications.

2. **After entry into the abdomen for a planned gastric bypass, the liver is visualized and found to be enlarged, slightly yellow, and slightly nodular in appearance. There is no evidence of significant ascites or any gastroesophageal varices. Which of the following statements is correct?**
   A. The findings would indicate that the surgeon should cease and not proceed with the RYGB.
   B. This degree of liver disease may have higher rates of postsurgery complications, but patients can have improvement in their liver condition following metabolic surgery.
   C. Conversion from laparoscopic to an open bariatric surgery would be advised.
   D. The degree of severity of cirrhosis has no impact on the postoperative morbidity and mortality risk.

3. **Which of the following statements about perioperative management of NAFLD/NASH and cirrhosis is correct?**
   A. The model for end-stage liver disease (MELD) score utilizes serum creatinine, total bilirubin, AST, ALT, and international normalized ratio (INR) for its calculation.
   B. The lack of subjective variability in calculating the Child–Pugh score makes this the most accurate predictor of postoperative 30-day mortality.
   C. Acute hepatorenal syndrome is readily reversed with administration of high-volume crystalloid resuscitation.
   D. Hepatic encephalopathy management focuses on reversal of causative factors such as infection as

well as administration of nonabsorbable disaccharides to lower serum ammonia.

4. Which of the following statements regarding the expected outcomes of NAFLD/NASH after bariatric surgery is true?

A. Overall liver function and histological findings will progressively worsen due to the nutritional deficiencies.

B. While there is some improvement in transaminase levels, the histologic findings from NASH are not improved.

C. Sleeve gastrectomy has no impact on NAFLD/NASH while the RYGB induces significant improvement.

D. Liver biopsy results following surgery show a decreased NAFLD activity score (NAS).

ANSWERS

1. C. NAFLD is believed to be the consequence of metabolic syndrome that is classically composed of abdominal obesity, hypertriglyceridemia, low high-density lipoprotein (HDL) levels, hypertension, and elevated fasting glucose.[1,2] NAFLD is typically asymptomatic and most commonly only isolated fatty liver (IFL). These patients may be found to have a twofold to fourfold increase in AST and ALT, which typically shows an AST/ALT ratio of <1, which is in contrast to alcoholic hepatitis that has greater AST levels in comparison to ALT. Elevations in alkaline phosphatase (AP) and gamma-glutamyl-transpeptidase (GGTP) may also be seen, but the bilirubin, prothrombin time, and albumin are typically normal. The diagnosis of NAFLD can often be reliably made radiographically with both an ultrasound and CT scan, which have shown high sensitivities. However, these studies lack accuracy in identifying more advanced stages of disease including NASH or fibrosis.[1]

To date, liver biopsy remains the gold standard diagnostic modality for identifying NASH and fibrosis and should be considered in the appropriate clinical setting. Histologic findings of NAFLD include macrovesicular fat accumulation in more than 5% of hepatocytes. IFL, the most common and initial stage of NAFLD, does not have any significant necrosis, inflammation, or fibrosis. However, as the disease progresses to NASH, then hepatocyte ballooning degeneration as well as inflammatory infiltrates and Mallory–Denk bodies are seen as well as fibrosis.[3,4] A pathologic scoring system called the NAS has been developed to aid in correctly identifying liver histology with NASH versus IFL. Alcoholic steatosis and steatohepatitis are generally indistinguishable from NASH histologically. Therefore a diagnosis of NASH can only be appropriately applied to those patients without significant alcohol use (<20–40 g of alcohol/day).[1] While biopsy continues to be the standard, other emerging and less invasive methods of identifying fibrosis are showing promising results. These include transient elastography and acoustic radiation force impulse (ARFI) elastography that are ultrasound-based studies and magnetic resonance elastography.

2. B. NAFLD has been reported to be present in about one-third of adults in Westernized countries and in 60% to 90% of patients undergoing bariatric surgery. Moreover, 15% to 30% of routine liver biopsies in patients undergoing bariatric surgery have shown NASH or fibrosis.[5–7] Having an index of suspicion prior to bariatric surgery of those who are at highest risk for NASH (diabetics, Hispanics, male) may help guide the need for more intensive evaluation of cirrhosis. However, bariatric surgeons may encounter the scenario where cirrhosis is encountered at the time of a planned weight loss surgery. Wolter et al. discovered undiagnosed cirrhosis by liver biopsy in 4% of patients undergoing bariatric surgery.[8] A retrospective cohort study of bariatric surgery patients found those with cirrhosis identified during surgery did have a higher rate of overall complications but had a similar length of stay and overall improvement in their MELD score with no long-term cirrhosis-related complications. The authors concluded that bariatric surgery of various forms can be completed in well-compensate cirrhotic patients with acceptable complication risk.[9]

The degree of cirrhosis and its sequelae has direct implications to the perioperative risk as demonstrated by numerous studies. Therefore, the approach to patients with obvious varices, renal insufficiency, and large volume ascites should be altered compared to those with only a fibrotic-appearing liver.[9] Open surgery compared to laparoscopic has not demonstrated any morbidity or mortality benefit in cirrhotic patients.[10] When liver disease is suspected at the time of bariatric surgery, a liver biopsy is warranted in order to establish the degree of fibrosis present. Ultimately, the appearance of the liver alone should not warrant the surgeon from completing the planned bariatric procedure because the degree of cirrhosis in the liver cannot be determined by the gross appearance alone. Moreover, in patients with incidentally discovered but compensated cirrhosis, the planned bariatric procedure would be beneficial to the liver disease as well as the obesity. If there is evidence of uncompensated cirrhosis, large varices, abnormal bleeding, and ascites, the best option would be to perform a liver biopsy and abort the bariatric procedure.

3. **D.** The perioperative management of patients with cirrhosis can be challenging due to the numerous physiologic sequelae of their liver disease including significant volume shifts, coagulopathy, malnutrition, renal insufficiency, gastroesophageal varices, and neurologic deficits. A major component in the management of these patients begins with evaluating their degree of liver disease. The two major scoring systems that have developed are the Child–Pugh score and MELD score. The Child–Pugh score uses serum total bilirubin, INR, albumin, degree of ascites, and degree of encephalopathy while the MELD score uses serum creatinine, total bilirubin, INR, and serum sodium. Both scoring systems have demonstrated to be strong predictors of perioperative mortality and morbidity risk.[11,12] Neef et al. found patients undergoing nonhepatic general surgical operations had perioperative mortality rates of 10%, 17%, and 63% for Child's A, B, and C, respectively. These mortality rates were 9% for MELD <10, 19% for MELD 10 to 15, and 54% for MELD >15.

The subjective nature of the degree of ascites and encephalopathy involved in the Child–Pugh score have led many clinicians to favor the MELD score.[13] The data used in calculating the MELD score should be recent and should not be during periods of reversible conditions such as prerenal azotemia or spontaneous bacterial peritonitis that can significantly alter the score results. Due to alterations in splanchnic and renal vascular physiology as well as electrolyte and serum oncotic pressures, cirrhotic patients can present significant challenges in fluid management and renal injury or acute renal dysfunction are seen in 15% to 25% of hospitalized cirrhotic patients.[1] Hepatorenal syndrome is a potential renal complication in cirrhotic patients with ascites resulting from a cascade of events leading to severe renal arterial vasoconstriction and overall high mortality. This is generally treated through prompt recognition followed by medical therapy involving colloid such as albumin, vasopressors, and octreotide as well as potentially TIPS (transjugular intrahepatic portosystemic shunt) or a liver transplantation.

Hepatic encephalopathy involves a spectrum of neurological effects and also suggests a poor prognosis. The treatment is largely based on eliminating any precipitating factors (bleeding, infection, etc.), administration of nonabsorbable disaccharides (lactulose) to inhibit intestinal ammonia absorption, and oral antibiotics such as rifaximin.[1]

4. **D.** There is increasing evidence that bariatric surgery has significant beneficial effects on liver function and liver histology.[14–16] Several systematic reviews have been published and consistently demonstrated postoperative improvement in biochemical testing parameters (AST, ALT, AP, GGT) as well as liver histology for steatosis, steatohepatitis, and fibrosis.[17,18] Pooled data from Fahkry et al. showed improvement in biochemical parameters in 32% to 96% of patients. While often believed to be irreversible, liver fibrosis has been shown to improve in 12% to 30% of patients following bariatric surgery.[17,18] A study of 109 patients by Lassailly et al. found NASH resolved in 85% of patients at 1 year following both the RYGB or sleeve gastrectomy. A greater proportion of those with mild NASH had resolution compared to those with more advanced disease.[19] Several studies have also compared the impact of NAFLD by RYGB versus sleeve gastrectomy.[20–22] In general, these comparative studies have found no significant difference in these two operations with regards to their beneficial effects on NAFLD.[23]

REFERENCES

1. Torres DM, Harrison SA. Ch 87: Nonalcoholic fatty liver disease. In: Feldman M, ed. *Sleisenger and Fordtrans GI and Liver Disease*. 10th ed. Philadelphia, PA: Elsevier Inc.; 2016:1428-1441.
2. Chalasani NP. Alcoholic and nonalcoholic steatohepatitis. In: Goldman L, Schafer A, ed. *Goldman-Cecel Medicine*. 26th ed. Philadelphia, PA: Elsevier; 2020:986-989.
3. Tiniakos DG, Anstee QM, Alastair DB. Fatty liver disease. In: Burt AD, ed. *MacSweens's Pathology of the Liver*. Philadelphia, PA: Elsevier, Ltd; 2018:308-371.
4. Reddy SK, Geller DA. Hepatic steatosis, steatohepatitis, and chemotherapy-related liver injury. In: Jarnagin WR, ed. *Blumgart's Surgery of the Liver, Biliary Tract, and Pancreas*. 6th ed. Philadelphia, PA: Elsevier, Inc.; 2017:1065-1072.

5. Souto KP, Meinhardt NG, Ramos MJ, et al. Nonalcoholic fatty liver disease in patients with different baseline glucose status undergoing bariatric surgery: analysis of intraoperative liver biopsies and literature review. *Surg Obes Relat Dis*. 2018;14(1):66-73.
6. Subichin M, Clanton J, Makuszewski M, et al. Liver disease in the morbidly obese: a review of 1000 consecutive patients undergoing weight loss surgery. *Surg Obes Relat Dis*. 2015;11:137-141.
7. Udelsman BV, Corey KE, Lindvall C, et al. Risk factors and prevalence of liver disease in review of 2557 routine liver biopsies performed during bariatric surgery. *Surg Obes Relat Dis*. 2019;15:843-849.
8. Wolter S, Dupree A, Coelius C, et al. Influence of liver disease on perioperative outcome after bariatric surgery in a Northern German cohort. *Obes Surg*. 2017;27:90-95.
9. Younus H, Sharma A, Miquel R, et al. Bariatric surgery in cirrhotic patients: *is it safe*? *Obes Surg*. 2020;30:1241-1248.
10. Goh BB, Schauer PR, McCullough AJ. Considerations for bariatric surgery in patients with cirrhosis. *World J Gastroenterol*. 2018;24(28):3112-3119.
11. Northup PG, Wanamaker RC, Lee VD, et al. Model for end-stage liver disease (MELD) predicts nontransplant surgical mortality in patients with cirrhosis. *Ann Surg*. 2005;242(2):244-251.
12. Neef H, Mariaskin D, Spangenberg HC, et al. Perioperative mortality after non-hepatic general surgery in patients with liver cirrhosis: an analysis of 138 operations in the 2000s using child and MELD scores. *J Gastrointest Surg*. 2011;15:1-11.
13. Farnsworth N, Fagan SP, Berger DH, et al. Child-Turcotte-Pugh versus MELD score as a predictor of outcome after elective and emergent surgery in cirrhotic patients. *Am J Surg*. 2004;188(5):580-583.
14. Tai CM, Huang CK, Hwang JC, et al. Improvement of nonalcoholic fatty liver disease after bariatric surgery in morbidly obese Chinese patients. *Obes Surg*. 2012;22:1016-1021.
15. Schonfels W. Beckmann JH, Ahrens M, et al. Histologic improvement of NAFLD in patients with obesity after bariatric surgery based on standardized NAS (NAFLD activity score). *Surg Obes Relat Dis*. 2018;14:1607-1617.
16. Cherla DV, Rodriguez NA, Vangoitsenhoven R, et al. Impact of sleeve gastrectomy and Roux-en-Y gastric bypass on biopsy-proven non-alcoholic fatty liver disease. *Surg Endosc*. 2020;34(5):2266-2272.
17. Fakhry TK, Mhaskar R, Schwitalla T, et al. Bariatric surgery improves nonalcoholic fatty liver disease: a contemporary systematic review and meta-analysis. *Surg Obes Relat Dis*. 2019;15:502-511.
18. Bower G, Toma T, Harling L, et al. Bariatric surgery and non-alcoholic fatty liver disease: a systematic review of liver biochemistry and histology. *Obes Surg*. 2015;25:2280-2289.
19. Lassailly G, Caiazzo R, Buob D, et al. Bariatric surgery reduces features of nonalcoholic steatohepatitis in morbidly obese patients. *Gastroenterology*. 2015;149(2):379-388.
20. Nickel F, Tapking C, Benner L, et al. Bariatric surgery as an efficient treatment for non-alcoholic fatty liver disease in a prospective study with 1-year follow-up. *Obes Surg*. 2018;28:1342-1350.
21. Kalinowski P, Paluszkiewicz R, Ziarkiewicz-Wro´blewska Bogna, et al. Liver function in patients with nonalcoholic fatty liver disease randomized to Roux-en-Y gastric bypass versus sleeve gastrectomy. *Ann Surg*. 2017;266(5):738-745.
22. Froylich D, Corcelles R, Daigle C, et al. Effect of Roux-en-Y gastric bypass and sleeve gastrectomy on nonalcoholic fatty liver disease: a comparative study. *Surg Obes Relat Dis*. 2016;12:127-131.
23. Baldwin D, Chennakesavalu M, Gangemi A. Systematic review and meta-analysis of Roux-en-Y gastric bypass against laparoscopic sleeve gastrectomy for amelioration of NAFLD using four criteria. *Surg Obes Relat Dis*. 2019;15:2123-2130.

32

Renal Disease

Rahul Gupta, MBBS

A 55-year-old morbidly obese male with a body mass index (BMI) of 42 kg/m^2 presents for evaluation preceding weight loss surgery. The patient's medical history is consistent with hypertension, chronic kidney disease (CKD) stage 3 (glomerular filtration rate [GFR] category), and type 2 diabetes mellitus. Medications include insulin, amlodipine, and metoprolol. He informs that lisinopril was added a few days previously at an urgent care facility that he visited for a minor cut. He also reports a 10 pack-year history of smoking.

1. What is the expected GFR of this patient (mL/min/1.73 m^2)?

A. >90
B. 60–89
C. 30–59
D. 15–29
E. <15

2. Which of the following has a reno-protective effect?

A. Obesity
B. Hypertension
C. Diabetes
D. Lisinopril
E. Smoking

3. Dietetic-nutritional therapy is an important concept in preventing progression of CKD to end-stage renal disease (ESRD). The components of nutrition therapy in CKD include:

A. Nonmonitored intake of energy and protein
B. Weight gain
C. Increased sodium
D. Decreased phosphate
E. Increased free water intake

4. Which of the following may be present in patients with CKD?

A. Left ventricular hypertrophy
B. Decreased bleeding time
C. Metabolic alkalosis
D. Hypokalemia
E. Hypophosphatemia

5. Modifiable factor to prevent perioperative acute kidney injury include:

A. Resuscitation with hydroxy-ethyl starch
B. Dopamine as a vasopressor of choice
C. Avoidance of nonsteroidal anti-inflammatory drugs
D. Liberal use of contrast for imaging
E. Permissive hypotension

ANSWERS

1. C. CKD is defined as abnormalities of kidney structure or function, present for >3 months, with implications for health.[1] The stages of kidney disease are based on degree of impairment of renal function and defined in terms of cause, GFR categories (Table 32-1), and albuminuria.[1] Numerous studies have provided evidence independently correlating GFR category with mortality, cardiovascular events, and rate of ESRD.[2,3]

Renal dysfunction has important implications on pharmacokinetics and pharmacodynamics. Water

Table 32-1 STAGES OF CHRONIC KIDNEY DISEASE

Stage	Degree of impairment	GFR (mL/min/1.73 m^2)
1	Normal function but structural or genetic disposition to kidney disease	>90
2	Mildly reduced function with findings of stage 1	60–89
3	Moderately reduced function	30–59
4	Severely reduced function	15–29
5	End stage renal disease or dialysis dependent	<15

retention alters volume of distribution. Uremic toxins alter plasma protein binding in addition to derangements in glomerular filtration and tubular excretion.

Significant variation in GFR estimation, between methods, exist in obese patients.[4] There is no consensus on normalization of kidney parameters to body surface area (BSA) and therefore obese CKD patients require individualization of drug dosage regimens.

2. **D.** Renin-angiotensin-aldosterone system is a critical link between hypertension and CKD. Angiotensin-converting enzyme (ACE) inhibitors impart reno-protective effect independent of antihypertensive effect. In the HOPE trial (Heart Outcomes prevention evaluation), ACE inhibitors lowered the risk of overt nephropathy by 24%.[5] It is recommended that ACE-I or angiotensin II receptor blockers (ARBs) be used in CKD with urine albumin excretion >300 mg/24 hours. It may be initiated earlier in patients with diabetes mellitus.

   An increasing body of evidence suggests obesity as an independent risk factor for CKD. The risk has been suggested to be twice normal despite adjustments for other risk factors. Pathological changes in obesity-related glomerulopathy include glomerulomegaly and early changes resembling diabetic nephropathy. Glomerular hyper filtration is seen proportional to BMI due to extracellular volume expansion, which is again similar to early diabetic nephropathy.[6]

   Hypertension can be both a cause and a consequence of CKD. Targeting <130/80 has benefits for cardiovascular disease and proteinuria. Diabetes is the most common cause of renal failure accounting for 44% of new cases. Smoking increases the risk of renal dysfunction and proteinuria in both genders.

3. **D.** Dietetic-nutritional therapy is an important component in management of patients with CKD. The hallmarks of nutrition strategy are weight loss, limited protein intake, phosphate homeostasis, and control of factors that exacerbate hypertension. Positive balance in phosphate promotes hyperparathyroidism and aggravates mineral and bone derangements. Phosphate homeostasis is obtained through interplay of intestinal dietary phosphate, renal absorption of filtered phosphate, and the shift of phosphate from cellular interstitial and bone storage pools.

   Uncontrolled energy and protein intake accelerate metabolic problems and uremic status. This can contribute to obesity, dyslipidemia, and exacerbates insulin resistance. Obesity has been characterized as an independent factor contributing to CKD.[7] Protein catabolism increases fixed acid load and in presence of decreased excretion of H+ ion worsens the metabolic acidosis. Metabolic acidosis results in hyperkalemia, muscle protein catabolism, insulin resistance, and bone demineralization.[8,9] It is advised that the protein intake be limited to 0.8 g/kg/day in patients with GFR <30 mL/min/1.73m^2.

   Weight loss with diet low in calories, sodium, and fat improves glycaemia, hypertension, and cardiovascular risk.[10] The renal benefits of weight loss are related to reduction in hypertension, proteinuria and overall improvement in metabolic syndrome. Meta-analysis of six studies on impact of weight loss in patients with CKD showed a baseline improvement in systolic BP by 9 mmHg and proteinuria of 1.31 g/24 hours.[11] Excess of sodium and water worsen arterial hypertension, heart failure, and increases oxidative stress.[12]

4. **A.** CKD is associated with increased incidence of cardiovascular disease. This is the leading cause of mortality in patients with ESRD. Cardiovascular effects include accelerated atherosclerosis, vascular calcification, conduction abnormalities, left ventricular hypertrophy, and hypertension.

   Platelet dysfunction leads to prolonged bleeding time in patients with CKD. Abnormalities include anomalistic interaction of von Willebrand factor

(VWF) with platelet glycoprotein IIb-IIIa, reduced platelet ADP content, and diminished thromboxane A2.[13] DDAVP (desmopressin) shortens the bleeding time. The improvement is the result of qualitative and quantitative changes in FVIII: VWF multimers. The effect peaks at 1 to 2 hours and is expected to last about 4 hours.

Kidneys excrete fixed acids and recover HCO3 (bicarbonate) filtered in renal tubules. Net endogenous acid production is counterbalanced by urine net acid excretion to prevent progressive metabolic acidosis. Renal impairment therefore results in metabolic acidosis and not alkalosis. Oral bicarbonates are indicated if serum bicarbonate is <22 meq/L in patients with CKD.

Kidneys play a major role in homeostasis of potassium. Potassium is filtered without restriction and 90% to 95% reabsorbed in proximal tubule and loop of Henle. Excretion begins in distal convoluted tubule and is further modified by the distal nephron and collecting duct. Therefore loss of nephron function results in accumulation of potassium. Other factors also contribute to hyperkalemia seen in CKD. Metabolic acidosis shifts intracellular potassium into an extracellular compartment. Insulin deficiency in diabetes prevents the ability to disperse acute potassium load into intracellular space.[14]

Chronic kidney disease-mineral and bone disorder (CKD-MBD) is a syndrome that generally begins in stage 3. Hyperphosphatemia, hypocalcemia, elevated parathormone, abnormalities in bone turnover, and metastatic calcifications are hallmarks of this disorder. Pathophysiology of this condition is related to impaired excretion of phosphorous and diminished conversion of vitamin D to calcitriol. This leads to compensatory elevation of parathormone. Parathyroid hormone (PTH) and vitamin D3 alterations are the earliest detectable biochemical changes. Renal osteo-dystrophy is an integral part of the syndrome and is used only with respect to pathological changes in the bone.[15] The treatment involves a low-phosphate diet (800–1000 mg/day), intestinal phosphate binders, inhibition of intestinal phosphate transporters, bisphosphonates, and dialysis.

5. **C.** Minimizing exposure to nephrotoxic drugs is crucial for maintenance of renal function. The Scream Project in Sweden concluded that 18% of patients with CKD were inappropriately prescribed nephrotoxic drugs, mainly nonsteroidal anti-inflammatory drugs (NSAIDs).[20] NSAIDs (e.g. Toradol, ibuprofen) reduce renal blood flow by inhibition of cyclooxygenase and consequently decreasing prostaglandin-induced vasodilatation. This effect is especially evident in in patients with atherosclerotic disease, CKD, and state of renal hypoperfusion.

Intravascular volume depletion should be avoided by close monitoring of clinical signs, appropriate use of invasive hemodynamic monitoring, and fluid titration based on intake and output. All isotonic crystalloids except Hartmann's solution (which contains lactate and potassium) may be safely and preferentially used in patients with CKD.

The CRISTAL trial (colloids versus crystalloids for resuscitation of critically ill) showed no difference in mortality or kidney replacement use.[16] It is notable to mention that HES (hydroxyl-ethyl starch) has been proven to be associated with increased risk of acute kidney injury and need for RRT (renal replacement therapy).[17] The U.S. Food and Drug Administration issued a black box warning in 2013 against the use of HES in critically ill patients. If the patient does suffer acute kidney injury then early RRT reduces mortality in comparison to delayed RRT (ELAIN trial).[18]

Maintenance of renal perfusion is dependent upon both cardiac output and systemic arterial pressure. Initial therapeutic approach should focus on volume expansion. Inotropes and vasopressors may then be initiated to maintain renal perfusion. The *Cochrane Review* compared six different vasopressors and found no difference in mortality among vasopressors or combination of vasopressors. High-quality evidence did suggest increased incidence of arrhythmias with dopamine in comparison to norepinephrine.[19]

Contrast-induced nephropathy is defined as an increase in creatinine by 25% or 0.5 mg/dL within 3 days of administration of intravascular contrast. Iso-osmolar contrast has slightly lower risk of CIN (contrast-induced nephropathy) in comparison to LOCM (low osmolar contrast media). The decrease in risk is not clinically relevant but reaches statistical significance.[21] Contrast volume is an independent predictor of CIN.[22] Isotonic volume expansion is beneficial in prevention of radio-contrast–induced nephropathy. Low dose N acetyl cysteine and statins were reviewed recently in a meta-analysis conducted by the Agency for Healthcare Research and Quality. The benefits of these interventions were both clinically and statistically significant.[21]

REFERENCES

1. Inker LA, Astor BC, Fox CH, et al. KDOQI US commentary on the 2012 KDIGO clinical practice guideline for the evaluation and management of CKD. *Am J Kidney Dis.* 2014;63(5):713-735. doi:10.1053/j.ajkd.2014.01.416.
2. Van der Velde M, Matsushita K, Coresh J, et al. Lower estimated glomerular filtration rate and higher albuminuria are associated with all-cause and cardiovascular mortality. A collaborative meta-analysis of high-risk population cohorts. *Kidney Int.* 2011;79(12):1341-1352. doi:10.1038/ki.2010.536.
3. Gansevoort RT, Matsushita K, van der Valde M, et al. Lower estimated GFR and higher albuminuria are associated with adverse kidney outcomes. A collaborative meta-analysis of general and high-risk population cohorts. *Kidney Int.* 2011; 80(1): 93-104.
4. Hudson J, Mason D, Huch K. Estimates of kidney function in obese African Americans with chronic kidney disease. *Nephron Clin Pract.* 2011;118(2):C101-C108.
5. Heart Outcomes Prevention Evaluation Study Investigators. Effects of ramipril on cardiovascular and microvascular outcomes in people with diabetes mellitus: results of the HOPE study and MICROHOPE sub study. *Lancet.* 2000;355:253-259.
6. Kopple J, Massry S, Kalantar-Zadeh K. *Nutritional Management of Renal Disease.* 3rd ed. Baltimore: Williams & Wilkins; 2013.
7. Ritz E. Obesity and CKD: how to assess the risk? *Am J Kidney Dis.* 2008;52:1e6.
8. Reaich D, Channon SM, Scrimgeour CM, et al. Correction of acidosis in humans with CRF decreases protein degradation and amino acid oxidation. *Am J Physiol.* 1993;265(2 Pt1):E230-E235.
9. Einhorn LM, Zhan M, Hsu VD, et al. The frequency of hyperkalemia and its significance in chronic kidney disease. *Arch Intern Med.* 2009;169:1156-1162.
10. Bakris G, Vassalotti J, Ritz E, et al. National Kidney Foundation consensus conference on cardiovascular and kidney diseases and diabetes risk: an integrated therapeutic approach to reduce events. *Kidney Int.* 2010;78:726e36.
11. Navaneethan SD, Yehnert H, Moustarah F, et al. Weight loss interventions in chronic kidney disease: a systematic review and meta-analysis. *Clin J Am Soc Nephr.* 2009;4:1565e74.
12. Bradbury BD, Fissell RB, Albert JM, et al. Predictors of early mortality among incident US hemodialysis patients in the Dialysis Outcomes and Practice Patterns Study (DOPPS). *Clin J Am Soc Nephrol.* 2007;2:89-99.
13. Rabelink TJ, Zwaginga JJ, Koomans HA, Sixma JJ. Thrombosis and hemostasis in renal disease. *Kidney Int.* 1994;46:287-296.
14. Goraya, N. The physiology of metabolic acidosis in chronic kidney disease. In: Wesson DE, ed. *Metabolic Acidosis: A Guide to Clinical Assessment and Management.* Springer; 2016:76-86.
15. Silver J, Salusky IB, Olgarrd K. *The Spectrum of Mineral and Bone Disorders in Chronic Kidney Disease.* 2nd ed. Oxford: OUP; 2010.
16. Annane D, Siami S, Jaber S, et al. Effects of fluid resuscitation with colloids vs crystalloids on mortality in critically ill patients presenting with hypovolemic shock: the CRISTAL randomized trial. *JAMA.* 2013;310:1809-1817.
17. Myburgh JA, Finfer S, Bellomo R, et al. Hydroxyethyl starch or saline for fluid resuscitation in intensive care. *N Engl J Med.* 2012;367:1901-1911.
18. Zarbock A, Kellum JA, Schmidt C, et al. Effect of early vs delayed initiation of renal replacement therapy on mortality in critically ill patients with acute kidney injury: the ELAIN randomized clinical trial. *JAMA.* 2016;315(20):2190-2199. doi:10.1001/jama.2016.5828.
19. Gamper G, Havel C,Arrich J, Losert H, Pace NL, Mullner M, Herkenr H. Vasopressors for hypotensive shock. *Cochrane Database Syst Rev.* 2016;2. doi:10.1002/14651858.CD003709.pub4.
20. Gasparini A, Wettermark B, Schmidt-Mende K, et al. Inappropriate prescription of nephrotoxic drugs to individuals with chronic kidney disease: a community-based analysis from the Stockholm creatinine measurements (SCREAM) project. *Nephrol Dialysis Transplant.* 2017;32(suppl_3):iii13.
21. Eng J, Subramaniam RM, Wilson RF, et al. Contrast-Induced Nephropathy: Comparative Effects of Different Contrast Media (AHRQ publication; no. 15(16)-EHC022-EF). Rockville, MD: Agency for Healthcare Research and Quality; 2015.
22. McCullough PA. Contrast-induced acute kidney injury. *J Am Coll Cardiol.* 2008;51:1419-1428.

33

Chronic Steroid Use

Victoria Lyo, MD, MTM

A 58-year-old woman with a body mass index (BMI) of 43 kg/m^2, type 2 diabetes mellitus, hypertension, and rheumatoid arthritis who has taken prednisone 5 mg daily for the past 10 years completed her preoperative evaluation for surgical management of her obesity and weight-related comorbidities. She is felt to be a good candidate for surgery, and she desires a Roux-en-Y gastric bypass (RYGB).

1. **Which of the following is a side effect of chronic steroid use?**
   A. Purple striae
   B. Hypoglycemia
   C. Bleeding
   D. Peptic ulcer disease
   E. Leukopenia

2. **Regarding patients undergoing bariatric surgery on chronic steroids, which of the following is correct?**
   A. The patients tend to be younger.
   B. The patients tend to have more comorbid conditions.
   C. The patients make up 10% of all bariatric surgical patients.
   D. The patients tend to have similar ASA classifications.
   E. The patients tend to have a higher preoperative BMI.

3. **Regarding 30-day postoperative complications for bariatric patients on steroids, which of the following is correct?**
   A. More wound infections
   B. More intensive care unit (ICU) admissions
   C. Higher risk of reoperation
   D. Higher risk of bleeding
   E. Higher risk of leak

4. **Regarding the outcomes of the sleeve gastrectomy (SG) versus RYGB for a patient on chronic steroids, which of the following is true?**
   A. Leak rates are higher after SG.
   B. RYGB has higher rates of 30-day reoperation and reintervention.
   C. RYGB is associated with more bleeding.
   D. RYGB was associated with increased wound disruptions.
   E. SG has lower mortality.

ANSWERS

1. **A.** Prolonged steroid use has multiple adverse effects including weight gain, ulcers, increased susceptibility to infections, and osteoporosis.[1,2] Weight gain is the most common self-reported adverse effect, with up to 70% of patient reporting it.[2] Prospective trials have shown that 5 mg to 10mg/day of prednisone leads to a 4% to 8% increase in mean body weight when used for more than 2 years. The development of cushingoid features (truncal obesity, facial adipose tissue with moon face, purple striae, and dorsocervical adipose tissue) are dose-dependent and as common as 70% in patients at 12 months. Young patients with a higher baseline BMI and those with higher daily caloric intake were more at risk to develop features.[1]

The risk of hyperglycemia and diabetes also increases in a dose-dependent manner and improves with dose reduction. Although traditionally glucocorticoids have been thought to increase the risk of peptic ulcer disease, large meta-analyses of randomized controlled trials (RCTs) failed to show an association; however, the risk of ulcer formation is increased when steroids are used in combination with nonsteroidal anti-inflammatory drugs (NSAIDs), up to fourfold. Steroids lead to significant reductions in bone mineral density and increase the risk of fractures within 3 to 6 months of treatment, independent of age, gender, and underlying disease.[1]

While chronic steroid use increases the risk of infection, this is not due to leukopenia. In fact, there is normally leukocytosis with their use.[3]

2. **B.** There are four studies that compared outcomes after bariatric surgery for patients using chronic steroids and/or immunosuppressants. Three of these studies, Andalib et al.[4] (2005–2013), Kaplan et al.[5] (from 2011 to 2013), and Hefler et al.[6] (from 2015 to 2017), used NSQIP data and multivariable regression analysis, while Mazzei et al.[7] studied patients between 2015 and 2016 using NSQIP data and a propensity-score and case-control matching. All studies found that patients using chronic steroids and/or immunosuppressants were older (mean 49 vs. 45 years old) and had more comorbidities such as diabetes, hypertension, hyperlipidemia, chronic obstructive pulmonary disease (COPD), cardiac disease, chronic kidney disease, and obstructive sleep apnea (OSA).

   In the four studies that included patients undergoing primary bariatric surgery, 1.3% to 1.7% of patients were chronically immunosuppressed. Preoperative BMI was similar between the two groups, and in three studies, there were more patients with higher ASA classifications in the steroid groups.

3. **E.** In unmatched, unadjusted data across four studies, patients on steroids had higher rates of nearly all complications such as all morbidity, wound complications, readmission, reoperation, reintervention, unplanned ICU admission, and mortality (three of four studies). In Mazzei's study looking at patients undergoing sleeve and bypass only, overall risk of perioperative morbidity in patients on steroids was 8.2% versus 5.4% (relative risk 1.5, $P < 0.001$).[7] Relative risk of other complications included postoperative bleeding 1.7, postoperative infections 1.8, pulmonary complications 2.1, and anastomotic leak 2.1.

   Hefler's study without propensity-matched or case control analyses found that significantly higher rates of complications (i.e. all major complications, infectious complications, postoperative bleed or leak, but not death), using multivariable regression analysis adjusting for confounders and baseline differences in patient characteristics.[6]

   In the study by Mazzei et al,[7] analyzing propensity-matched patients (the only difference in groups was that sleeve gastrectomy rates were 6.5% higher than bypass), steroid use was no longer associated with reoperation, readmission, interventions, ICU admission, or mortality; the overall rate of significant morbidity was also not different (7.9% vs. 7.2%, $P = 0.2$). What remained significantly different was that steroid users had longer length of stays (2.7 vs. 2.4 days, $P = 0.001$) and the rate of anastomotic leak being higher (0.6% vs. 0.3%, $P = 0.03$). Similarly, case-control matched analyses in which the groups had similar rates of SG, readmission rates were also significantly greater (5.0% vs. 3.8%, $P = 0.02$) as were total morbidity (6.7% vs. 5.3%, $P < 0.01$); however, the only factor that seemed to contribute to this total increased morbidity was again, a higher anastomotic leak rate for those using steroids (0.5% vs. 0.2%, $P = 0.03$).

   The data are mixed and depend on the statistical analyses performed, but it is clear that the rate of leak is higher with chronic steroid use, and likely other complications as well. Surgeons should counsel patients accordingly and have a high index of suspicion for complications in the postoperative management of these patients.

4. **B.** In Hefler's paper,[6] when propensity-score matching was done to stratify patients taking steroids based on procedure type, the rate of major complications was higher after RYGB (9.6% vs 5%, $P < 0.001$), which included 30-day reoperation, reintervention, readmission, acute kidney injury, deep surgical site infection, longer length of stay, and longer operative time. Other outcomes such as mortality, leak rate, bleeding, wound disruption were not significantly different between RYGB and SG.

   Of the two studies using NSQIP data, only one[6] also showed that RYGB was a predictor of serious complications compared to SG with an odds ratio of 1.7 ($P = 0.03$). Andalib et al,[4] found that RYGB was associated with increased LOS >3 days, but morbidity and return to odds ratio was not significantly different. Mortality and readmissions could not be studied due to low numbers of events. The caveat of these two studies using NSQIP data is that the database includes non-MBSAQIP accredited bariatric surgery centers, which may skew outcomes by including varying surgeon and hospital volume and experience.

Thus, it may be preferable to offer SG rather than RYGB to steroid dependent patients to minimize postoperative risk, but individualized patient selection and risk assessment can still be used to tailor an optimal bariatric course for patients.

REFERENCES

1. Liu D, Ahmet A, Ward L, et al. A practical guide to the monitoring and management of the complications of systemic corticosteroid therapy. *Allergy Asthma Clin Immunol*. 2013;9(1):30.
2. Curtis JR, et al. Population-based assessment of adverse events associated with long-term glucocorticoid use. *Arthritis Rheum*. 2006;55(3):420-426.
3. Shoenfeld Y, Gurewich Y, Gallant LA, Pinkhas J. Prednisone-induced leukocytosis: influence of dosage, method and duration of administration on the degree of leukocytosis. *Am J Med*. 1981;71(5):773-778. doi:10.1016/0002-9343(81)90363-6.
4. Andalib A, Aminian A, Khorgami Z, et al. Early postoperative outcomes of primary bariatric surgery in patients on chronic steroid or immunosuppressive therapy. *Obes Surg*. 2016;26:1479-1486.
5. Kaplan JA, Schecter SC, Rogers SJ, et al. Expanded indications for bariatric surgery: should patients on chronic steroids be offered bariatric procedures? *SOARD*. 2017; 13:35-40.
6. Hefler J, Dang J, Modasi A, et al. Effects of chronic corticosteroid and immunosuppressant use in patients undergoing bariatric surgery. *Obes Surg*. 2019;29:3309-3315.
7. Mazzei M, Zhao H, Edwards MA, Perioperative outcomes of bariatric surgery in the setting of chronic steroid use: an MBSAQIP database analysis. *SOARD*. 2019;15:926-934.

34

Anesthesia Considerations

Phylicia Yorgure, MD, Lye-Yeng Wong, MD, Christopher Barton, MD, and Andrea Stroud, MD, MS

A 37-year-old female with a body mass index (BMI) of 39 kg/m^2 with a history of gastroesophageal reflux disease (GERD), postoperative nausea and vomiting (PONV), and obstructive sleep apnea (OSA) presents to the clinic for a preoperative evaluation for sleeve gastrectomy (SG).

1. In a patient with OSA, which of the following is consistent with OSA?

A. Dizziness
B. A rate of 20% in the obese population
C. Normal neck circumference
D. Rate of 30-day mortality same as individuals without OSA
E. Cognitive difficulties and sexual dysfunction

2. Which of the following tests provides physicians with the apnea hypopnea index (AHI)?

A. Pulmonary function test
B. STOP-BANG questionnaire
C. Overnight lab polysomnography
D. Ambulatory acid probe test
E. Berlin questionnaire

3. OSA is associated with which of the following medical conditions?

A. Renal artery stenosis
B. Emphysema
C. Hyperthyroidism
D. Atrial fibrillation
E. Neuropathy

4. Which of the following is true regarding patients with OSA?

A. Polypharmacy and multimodal pain management is not recommended
B. Use of neuraxial anesthesia is unsafe in patients with OSA
C. Morphine prevents hypoxia in the postanesthesia care unit (PACU)
D. Dexmedetomidine maintains respirations when used in patients with OSA
E. High doses of benzodiazepines and opioids prevent respiratory depression

5. What is the greatest physiologic difference during intubation in obese patients?

A. Shorter time to desaturation
B. Greater reflex bronchoconstriction
C. Slower glottic closure
D. Higher alveolar volume relative to weight
E. Increased compliance

6. Which one of the following are prophylaxis against PONV?

A. High volume perioperative fluid administration
B. Long-acting volatile anesthetics
C. Multimodal antiemetic premedication including dexamethasone
D. Use of intraoperative narcotics
E. Avoidance of propofol

ANSWERS

1. **E.** OSA is a syndrome associated with episodes of partial or complete upper airway obstruction during sleep. The disease results in repetitive arousal from sleep to restore airway patency, resulting in daytime hypersomnolence and other manifestations of disrupted sleep.[1] The reported signs and symptoms of OSA include fatigue, cognitive difficulties, nocturnal awakenings, nocturnal choking, insomnia, snoring, observed apnea, and sexual dysfunction. In addition, the physical exam findings may include obesity, neck circumference of >40 cm, craniofacial abnormalities, and anatomic nasal obstruction.[2] OSA in the morbidly obese population is increased and has been reported to be between 38% and 88%. OSA has been linked to increased risk of 30-day mortality, venous thromboembolism, need for reintervention, and a longer length of hospital stay.[3] Patients with OSA, even if asymptomatic, present important challenges in the perioperative period that must be addressed to minimize the risk of perioperative morbidity and mortality.[1]

2. **C.** There are multiple ways to assess the presence and severity of OSA during the preoperative workup, but overnight laboratory polysomnography is considered the gold standard for OSA diagnosis. If there exists a high pretest probability, type 3 polysomnography, or an at-home sleep study, can also be a reliable alternative.[4] The measures to note from the two listed studies include the AHI and oxygen desaturation index (ODI). In general, an AHI of <5 is normal, 5 to 15 mild sleep apnea, >15 moderate sleep apnea, and ≥30 severe sleep apnea.[3] An ODI of 95% to100% is normal and <90% is considered low, requiring external oxygen supplementation. The role of the sleep laboratory is to confirm the diagnosis, determine the degree of sleep apnea, assess its cause if possible, and make treatment recommendations.

   If these tests are unavailable or inaccessible to the patient, clinicians are recommended to use questionnaires such as the STOP-BANG or Berlin questionnaire to stratify the risk for OSA. Of note, STOP-BANG is a tool that correlates with 100% sensitivity an AHI >30, and 93% sensitive for an AHI >15.[4]

   The evidence for routine preoperative diagnosis and treatment of OSA in bariatric surgery programs is somewhat controversial, especially given that bariatric surgery is a highly effective treatment for OSA. The American Society for Metabolic and Bariatric Surgery (ASMBS) recommends screening in patients with clinical symptoms of OSA, but polysomnography does not need to be a routine test in all bariatric patients.[3] Modern enhanced recovery programs that utilize short-acting anesthesia medication, minimize sedatives, and promote early mobilization may reduce the risk of OSA in the postoperative period.[5] A recent study of over 5,000 bariatric surgery patients demonstrated that there was no difference in cardiopulmonary complications in a group without preoperative OSA screening, by utilizing continuous pulse oximetry monitoring postoperatively, compared to the group with known and adequately treated OSA.[6] Routine postoperative monitoring with continuous pulse oximetry is strongly recommended.[3,7]

3. **D.** OSA results in recurrent cardiometabolic perturbations from repetitive attempts to breathe against an occluded airway, precipitating episodes of hypoxia, sleep disturbance, and sympathetic nervous system surges. This leads to elevated blood pressure and heart rate, endothelial dysfunction, systemic inflammation, and insulin resistance.[8] Thus OSA likely contributes to or exacerbates several obesity-associated comorbidities, including hypertension, diabetes, coronary artery disease, congestive heart failure, and cardiac arrhythmias.

   Cardiac arrhythmias occur significantly more often in patients with OSA, and are directly related to the number of hypoxic episodes.[9] In the Sleep Heart Study, patients with sleep-disordered breathing (SDB) were compared to patients without SDB to assess the prevalence of atrial fibrillation.[9] When comparing patients with atrial fibrillation to the group that did not, they found that patients with atrial fibrillation had a significantly higher proportion of OSA (49% vs. 32%, $P = 0.0004$). After adjustment for risk factors, including age, BMI, hypertension, and chronic heart failure, those with atrial fibrillation had doubled the odds of OSA (odds ratio 2.19; 95% confidence interval, 1.40–3.42).[10]

   The mechanism is a combination of oxidative stress from cycles of hypoxia, reactive oxygen species, a chemo-reflexive tachycardia, renal sympathetic denervation, direct effect of negative intrathoracic pressure from obstructed upper airway, and elevated angiotensin II and aldosterone.[11,12] Additionally, there appears to be abnormal electrical remodeling of the myocardium, most commonly in the atrium.

Treatment with continuous positive airway pressure (CPAP) has been shown to improve atrial fibrillation in patients with OSA.[9]

4. **D.** Due to their propensity for airway collapse and underlying sleep deprivation, patients at increased perioperative risk from OSA are susceptible to the respiratory depressant and airway effects of sedatives. Dexmedetomidine has little depressant effects on respiratory drive unlike opioids and benzodiazepines. Multimodal analgesia is the mainstay of OSA management to avoid or minimize opioids and reduce postoperative pulmonary complications.[1] Nonsteroidal anti-inflammatory drugs (NSAIDs), in the absence of contraindications such as renal disease or excessive intraoperative bleeding, are great adjuncts in pain management, especially short-term in postoperative settings. NSAIDs have been shown to reduce the use of opiates and even PONV in the bariatric population.[13] The use of neuraxial anesthesia such as epidurals is also shown to be safe and effective in patients with OSA due to their localized effects.

5. **A.** The greatest physiologic difference in the obese population with regard to intubation is the time to desaturation. Apnea models demonstrate the rapid desaturation in obese patients following 1 mg/kg of intravenous succinylcholine, with the time to $SaO_2 =$ 80% of 3.1 min, which is shorter than the time to desaturation in a 10-kg child (3.7 min) or a moderately ill 70-kg adult (5.5 min).[14] The multifactorial explanation for this phenomenon includes higher baseline oxygen consumption, lower alveolar volume relative to weight, and de-recruiting of lung from a restrictive component of chest wall and abdominal weight.[2] Both reflex bronchoconstriction and glottic closure are mediated by the parasympathetic system; the former by irritant receptors in the upper airways, while the latter by the superior laryngeal nerve.

   Intraoperative ventilation strategies include preoxygenation, use of positive end-expiratory pressure (PEEP), and low tidal volume ventilation.[4] A ramped position is optimal for induction, intubation, and ventilation, improving oxygenation as well as the laryngoscopic view; while supine position should always be avoided.[4] Additionally, in patients with an expected difficult airway, video laryngoscopy should be available. During the procedure, maintenance of low tidal volumes reduces the risk of postoperative pulmonary complications.[4] Intraoperative positioning such as Trendelenburg also plays a role because it can significantly increase airway pressures, which may lead to further postoperative atelectasis and prolonged hypoxia.[2] At the time of extubation, considerations should include awake extubation in patients at increased perioperative risk from OSA, confirmation of full reversal of neuromuscular blockade, and extubation in lateral, semi-upright, or other nonsupine positions.[3]

6. **C.** Preoperatively, the patient should be assessed for PONV. Patients who are female, nonsmokers, have a history of motion sickness or PONV, and are undergoing laparoscopic procedures greater than 1 hour are at risk. The frequency of PONV is demonstrated to be as high as 70% after laparoscopic surgery.[15] After assessing the risk of PONV, a multimodal approach should be enacted. This includes avoidance of volatile gases, narcotics, and fluid overload, use of total intravenous anesthesia (TIVA), antiemetics, and corticosteroids.[16-21] In a randomized control trial, Ziemann-Gimmel et al. compared opioid-free TIVA to volatile and opioid anesthesia and they demonstrated that TIVA led to lower rates of early PONV.[22] The recommended antiemetics include "5-hydroxytryptamine receptor antagonists, corticosteroids, butyrophenones, neurokinin-1 receptor antagonists, antihistamines and anticholinergics."[23] Bataille et al. discussed the pathophysiology that drives PONV in morbidly obese patients during surgery and linked failure of antiemetics in treating PONV to the enhanced release of 5-hydroxytryptamine postoperatively. This hormone is produced and stored in the enterochromaffin cells of the GI tract and in the central nervous system and its release can be provoked by surgical trauma such as after a gastric sleeve or bypass surgery.[24]

REFERENCES

1. Practice guidelines for the perioperative management of OSA: an updated report by the American Society of Anesthesiologist task force on perioperative management of patients with OSA. *Anesthesiology*. 2014;120 (2): 268-286.
2. Roetman KJ, Bernards C. Perioperative implications of obstructive sleep apnea. *Adv Anesthes*. 2010;28:245-267.
3. ASMBS Clinical Issues Committee. Peri-operative management of obstructive sleep apnea. *Surg Obes Relat Dis*. 2012;8(3):e27-e32.
4. de Raaff CAL, et al. Obstructive sleep apnea and bariatric surgical guidelines: summary and update. *Curr Op Anaesthesiol*. 2018;31(1):104-109.

5. Berends F, Aarts E. Preoperative screening and treatment of OSA is like using a sledgehammer for cracking nuts. *Obes Surg.* 2020;30:1140-1142.
6. van Veldhuisen S.L. Arslan I, Denden LN, et al. Safety of continuous postoperative pulse oximetry monitoring without obstructive sleep apnea screening in >5000 patients undergoing bariatric surgery. *Obes Surg.* 2020;30:1079-1085.
7. de Raaff CAL, Gorter-Stam MAW, de Vries N, et al. Perioperative management of obstructive sleep apnea in bariatric surgery: a consensus guideline. *Surg Obes Relat Dis.* 2017;13(7):1095-1109.
8. Yacoub M, Youssef I, Salifu MO, McFarlane SI. Cardiovascular disease risk in obstructive sleep apnea: an update. *J Sleep Disord Ther.* 2017;7(1):283.
9. Mehra R, Benjamin EJ, Shahar E, et al. Association of nocturnal arrhythmias with sleep-disordered breathing: the sleep heart health study. *Am J Respir Crit Care Med.* 2006;173(8):910-916.
10. Gami AS, Pressman G, Caples SM, et al. Association of atrial fibrillation and obstructive sleep apnea. *Circulation.* 2004;110(4):364-367.
11. Youssef I, Kamran H, Yacoub M, et al. Obstructive sleep apnea as a risk factor for atrial fibrillation: a meta-analysis. *J Sleep Disord Ther.* 2018;7(1):282.
12. Shawon MS, Perret JL, Senaratna CV, et al. Current evidence on prevalence and clinical outcomes of co-morbid obstructive sleep apnea and COPD: a systematic review. *Sleep Med Rev.* 2017;32:58-68.
13. Apfel CC, Heidrich FM, Jukar-Rao S, et al. Evidence-based analysis of risk factors for postoperative nausea and vomiting. *Br J Anaesth.* 2012;109:742-753.
14. Benumof JL, Dagg R, Benumof R. Critical hemoglobin desaturation will occur before return to an unparalyzed state following 1 mg/kg intravenous succinylcholine. *Anesthesiology.* 1997;87(4):979-982.
15. Thune A, Appelgren L, Haglind E. Prevention of postoperative nausea and vomiting after laparoscopic cholecystectomy. A prospective randomized study of metoclopramide and transdermal hyoscine. *Eur J Surg.* 1995;161:265-268.
16. Gan TJ, Diemunsch P, Habib AS, et al. Consensus guidelines for the management of postoperative nausea and vomiting. *Anesth Analg.* Jan 2014;118:85-113.
17. Strum EM, Szenohradszki J, Kaufman WA, et al. Emergence and recovery characteristics of desflurane versus sevoflurane in morbidly obese adult surgical patients: a prospective, randomized study. *Anesth Analg.* 2004;99:1848-1853.
18. Juvin P, Vadam C, Malek L, et al. Postoperative recovery after desflurane, propofol, or isoflurane anesthesia among morbidly obese patients: a prospective, randomized study. *Anesth Analg.* Sept 2000;91:714-719.
19. Bilotta F, Doronzio A, Cuzzone V, et al. Early postoperative cognitive recovery and gas exchange patterns after balanced anesthesia with sevoflurane or desflurane in overweight and obese patients undergoing craniotomy: a prospective randomized trial. *J Neurosurg Anesthesiol.* 2009;21:207-213.
20. Kaur A, Jain AK, Sehgal R, et al. Hemodynamics and early recovery characteristics of desflurane versus sevoflurane in bariatric surgery. *J Anaesthesiol Clin Pharmacol.* 2013;29:36-40.
21. Apfel CC, Kranke P, Katz MH, et al. Volatile anaesthetics may be the main cause of early but not delayed postoperative vomiting: a randomized controlled trial of factorial design. *Br J Anaesth.* 2002;88:659-668.
22. Ziemann-Gimmel P, Goldfarb AA, Koppman J, et al. Opioid-free total intravenous anaesthesia reduces postoperative nausea and vomiting in bariatric surgery beyond triple prophylaxis. *Br J Anaesth.* 2014;112:906-911.
23. Benevides ML, Oliveira SS, de Aguilar-Nascimento JE. The combination of haloperidol, dexamethasone, and ondansetron for prevention of postoperative nausea and vomiting in laparoscopic sleeve gastrectomy: a randomized double-blind trial. *Obes Surg.* 2013;23:1389-1396.
24. Bataille A, Letourneulx JF, Charmeau A, et al. Impact of a prophylactic combination of dexamethasone-ondansetron on postoperative nausea and vomiting in obese adult patients undergoing laparoscopic sleeve gastrectomy during closed-loop propofol-remifentanil anaesthesia: a randomised double-blind placebo-controlled study. *Eur J Anaesthesiol.* 2016;33:898-905.

35

Psychiatric Stability of Axis I and Axis II Disorders

Michael Logan Rawlins, MD

A 38-year-old female with a body mass index (BMI) of 51.3 kg/m^2 presents for initial evaluation for bariatric surgery. In considering her candidacy for surgery, you perform a focused mental and behavioral health screening. The next series of questions relate to your psychological screening of this patient.

1. **Which of the following situations would be considered an absolute contraindication to bariatric surgery at this time?**
   A. An alcohol use history of 1 to 2 drinks per week
   B. Suicidal ideation 4 months ago from a failed relationship
   C. A history of bulimia in high school
   D. Current use of sertraline for depression
   E. A history of childhood sexual abuse

2. **Which of the following has the most successful weight loss compared to the others?**
   A. Alzheimer's disease
   B. Prader–Willi syndrome
   C. Severe cognitive impairment
   D. Inability or complete lack of motivation to ambulate
   E. Attention deficit hyperactivity disorder

3. **Which of the following is the most common psychological diagnosis in morbidly obese patients?**
   A. Anorexia nervosa
   B. Tobacco use disorder
   C. Bipolar disorder
   D. Depression
   E. Schizoaffective personality disorder

4. **Which of the following "weight history" admissions from the patient is MOST concerning regarding their appropriateness for surgical intervention?**
   A. No previous dieting attempts for weight loss
   B. Able to lose 20 pounds with diet but then regained all of it back
   C. Drinks high-calorie liquids at least once per day
   D. Eats food despite not feeling hungry
   E. Been overweight for 15 years

5. **Which of the following is a contraindication to bariatric surgery?**
   A. Currently homeless, not sure where they are sleeping each night
   B. Does not have money to purchase liquid protein shakes needed after surgery
   C. Mother-in-law does not feel bariatric surgery is necessary to lose weight
   D. Recent separation/divorce in the last few months, patient tearful when discussing
   E. Lives alone, geographically separated, no friend or family support to assist after surgery

ANSWERS

1. **B.** The presence of Axis I and II psychological disorders is common in weight loss surgery patients. Many of these conditions are typically under control and do not represent absolute contraindications to surgery, such as history of childhood sexual abuse, current use of SSRI antidepressants for depression, and distant but not current history of bulimia. Alcohol use history is important to gauge in the weight

loss surgery patient because it represents a large source of empty calories and represents a source of addition that should be addressed before surgery. Those patients who drink rarely or only occasionally, such as less than or equal to 1 to 2 drinks per week are not necessarily at increased risk for inadequate weight loss. However, those with current alcohol abuse disorder (3–4 drinks per day, every day) or frequent binge drinking should be encouraged to quit drinking completely because the rate of relapse is high if use is merely temporarily decreased. Some programs advocate for a period of complete alcohol abstinence for 6 to 12 months to demonstrate stability. However, there are certain conditions that are considered absolute contraindications to surgery and should be further investigated by a professional and licensed mental health professional or psychiatrist.[1] Many of those conditions typically require a period of stability for 6 to 12 months and active counseling before consideration of approval for surgery should be given. Those conditions include active suicidal or homicidal ideation, untreated major depressive disorder, active substance abuse disorder, active eating disorder such as bulimia or binge eating, untreated schizophrenia, or recent psychiatric hospitalizations, to name just a few.

2. **E.** There are many psychosocial conditions or factors that may affect weight loss surgery outcome. The presurgery psychological evaluation should certainly focus on the patient's ability (mental and motivational) to comprehend and understand the postsurgery recommendations regarding diet, exercise, and behavior modification. Conditions with severe cognitive impairment (including Alzheimer's disease) will negatively impact the patients understanding and adherence.[1] However, mild cognitive impairment (as what is seen with some Down syndrome patients) is not necessarily a contraindication to surgery, especially if they have appropriate understanding and good social support. Psychological conditions such as Prader–Willi, where the patient cannot control their urges to eat even with appropriate counseling, have been viewed as absolute contraindications to surgery. Motivation or ability to perform physical activity does have impact on the amount of weight lost after surgery. Patients should be carefully screened to determine if they absolutely cannot ambulate or will refuse to ambulate after surgery. They should be counseled that they will likely not lose as much weight as other similarly matched patients who would ambulate, and some consideration should be given to their appropriateness for surgery because exercise is considered a core component to successful weight loss after surgery. Attention deficit hyperactivity disorder, in and of itself, is not likely to lead to a poor weight loss outcome.[2]

3. **D.** Depression is present in more than 40% of morbidly obese patients and is the most common mental health diagnosis encountered prior to bariatric surgery.[3] Depression is not a contraindication to surgery if it is mild and controlled, with or without medication. In fact, depression should be viewed as an obesity-related medical comorbidity and an indication for surgery because it is likely contributing to the patient's weight gain and/or is a result of weight gain, and would likely improve with weight loss and improved overall health.

4. **A.** When taking a weight history, it is important to ask the patient all of the following: How long have you felt that you have had a weight problem? At what age did you first feel that you were overweight? What ways have you tried to lose weight? What is the maximum number of pounds that you were able to lose with a weight loss attempt? How long were you able to maintain that weight loss? How many meals per week do you feel that you have eaten too much and feel stuffed? How many times in the last month have you felt the need to purge the food you ate (vomiting, laxatives, fasting, or excessive exercise)? How many times per week do you find yourself eating during non-mealtime periods? Have you felt the need to eat even when you don't feel hungry? Do you wake up at night to eat? How many times per week do you drink high-calorie liquids (sodas, milkshake, alcohol, etc.)? Do you turn to food when you are sad or stressed? The MOST concerning weight history questionnaire answers from those listed is having had no previous dieting attempts for weight loss.[4] This indicates that the patient has never tried to lose weight on their own and has no experience with diet, exercise, and behavior modification. Almost all bariatric surgery candidates have had or should have had previous attempts at weight loss. If they have not, they are likely in the wrong office to start. The patient's motivation should be focused on diet before surgery. Weight yo-yos are common in weight loss attempts and should not be viewed as negative. The period

of time that a patient has been overweight does not affect their candidacy for surgery but will give you an idea of how long they have been struggling with their weight and how that may affect their psyche. Poor eating behaviors that are not seriously maladaptive, such as eating despite not being hungry and eating some high-calorie liquid foods, are simply behaviors that need to be recognized and modified to be the most successful weight loss surgery patient.

5. **A.** In evaluating the patient's psychosocial barriers and support systems, it is important to identify situations that will impair the candidate's ability to be successful due to lack of appropriate resources and support. Homelessness should be viewed as an absolute contraindication to surgery;[4] if the patient does not have a reliable home situation, they will not be reliable for required diet, follow-up care, vitamins, and so on. Furthermore, lack of money to purchase the necessary supplies such as liquid diet protein source and vitamins should raise concern. Additionally, no family or friend support to aid after surgery should raise significant concern for ability to follow-up. A recent separation or divorce where the patient is still clearly depressed and grieving should be addressed prior to surgery because it would be considered an untreated mental health disorder. Nonimmediate family member disapproval of bariatric surgery as a weight loss method is not a major concern. With that said, it would still be prudent to help educate that family member through attending an information session, support group, or in office visit one on one with the bariatric surgeon to help educate that family member and dispel any false myths that they might believe.

SECTION 7

Outcomes-Medical

36

Stampede Trial

Michael Mulcahy, MD, and Eric Ahnfeldt, DO

A 49-year-old female with hypertension, type 2 diabetes, and a body mass index (BMI) of 38 kg/m^2 is evaluated for bariatric surgery. Her main goal for having bariatric surgery is for better control of her type 2 diabetes. She is currently on lisinopril, metformin, and insulin glargine nightly. Her current hemoglobin A1c (HgbA1c) level is 8.4%. She chooses to undergo Roux-en-Y gastric bypass (RYGB).

1. **What is the most appropriate statement in regards to expected changes to her medications postoperatively?**
   A. RYGB leads to a sustained reduction in insulin requirements.
   B. Ten percent of patients will not require any diabetes medications after RYGB.
   C. No decrease in diabetes medication requirements is seen for BMIs less than 35.
   D. RYGB is not likely to alter her hypertensive medication regiment.

2. **Regarding the choice of RYGB for this patient, which of the following is correct?**
   A. She can expect to require more diabetes medications than patients who have had SG.
   B. She would be equally likely to sustain an HgbA1c level <6% regardless of having SG or RYGB.
   C. Her weight loss in the first year after RYGB is not related to her expected 5-year HgbA1c levels.
   D. She would be equally likely to sustain an HgbA1c level <6% regardless of having RYGB or biliopancreatic diversion (BPD).

3. **Regarding lifestyle modification and medical management of diabetes, which of the following is most accurate?**
   A. Patients older than 75 are less likely to maintain an appropriate HgbA1c level.
   B. Mexican Americans are more likely to maintain an appropriate HgbA1c level compared to non-Hispanic blacks.
   C. 10% of patients achieve resolution of their diabetes with intensive lifestyle management.
   D. Average weight loss is <10% with lifestyle modification.

4. **Regarding the physiology of diabetes after bariatric surgery, which of the following is correct?**
   A. Leptin levels increase after RYGB.
   B. The improvement of diabetes or complete resolution of diabetes after bariatric surgery often occurs prior to significant weight loss.
   C. Gastric inhibitor polypeptide (GIP) levels increase after BPD.
   D. Postprandial glucagon-like peptide 1 (GLP-1) levels decrease after SG.

ANSWERS

1. **A.** RYGB leads to a sustained reduction in insulin requirements and the need for diabetes medications. The STAMPEDE trial showed that at 5 years postoperatively, only 12% of patients who required insulin preoperatively did so postoperatively. This was significantly lower than in the medical therapy group

where 40% still required insulin at 5 years. Forty-five percent of patients did not require any medications after RYGB at 5 years in the STAMPEDE trial.[1] In another randomized control trial, 75% of patients who had RYGB did not require medications for diabetes at 2 years.[2]

The 5-year results of the STAMPEDE trial showed that BMIs greater than 35 and lower BMIs (27–34) had a postoperative reduction in the use of diabetes medications for the surgical group in comparison to medical therapy alone.[3]

The STAMPEDE trial also showed that there was a significant decrease in the percentage of patients on an angiotensin-converting enzyme inhibitor (ACEi). Before RYGB, 36% were on an ACEi and after 23% were on an ACEi ($P < 0.01$). The number of hypertensive medications also decreased after RYGB. Prior to surgery, the patients in the RYGB group were on an average of 2.73 medications and after they were on 0.96 ($P < 0.001$).[3]

2. **B.** The STAMPEDE trial showed at 5 years those who had RYGB or SG were more likely to maintain HgbA1c <6% in comparison to medical management ($P < 0.03$ for both). Although when comparing the surgeries, there was no difference between RYGB and SG to maintain an HgbA1c <6% ($P = 0.53$). Those who underwent RYGB did have significantly more weight loss and less diabetes medications requirements than SG.[3] Using the same data from the STAMPEDE trial, Zhou et al.[4] showed having lower weight loss in the first year was positively correlated to having higher 5-year glycated hemoglobin levels for both RYGB and SG.

   The biliopancreatic diversion seems to be the most effective option for type 2 diabetes control as it is more likely to improve glycated hemoglobin levels in comparison to RYGB. In a single-center randomized control trial at 2 years, patients undergoing biliopancreatic diversion had an HgbA1c of 4.95% while those who underwent RYGB had an HgbA1c of 6.35% ($P = 0.001$).[2]

3. **D.** The Look Ahead trial showed an average weight loss of 6.0% of the total weight with lifestyle modification, while the average excess weight loss when considering all bariatric surgeries together is 61%.[5,6] The STAMPEDE trial showed that 25% and 45% of patients did not require medications for their diabetes at 5 years after SG and RYGB, respectively. In the medical management group, only 2% did not require medications for their diabetes at 5 years. Twenty percent of the medical group had hemoglobin A1cs of <7%.[3] According to National Health and Nutrition Examination Survey (NHANES) data from 2011 to 2014, 50.8% of patients with diabetes achieved an HgbA1c of less than 7%. This percentage was lower for patients less than 75 years old and Mexican Americans.[7]

4. **B.** The return to normal insulin and glucose levels has been shown in RYGB and BPD prior to significant weight loss.[8,9] These studies suggest etiologies other than weight loss may be important in the resolution of type 2 diabetes after bariatric surgery.

   Multiple studies have been published showing that bariatric surgery has a significant impact on gut hormones, including leptin, GLP-1, and GIP, which may contribute to the resolution of type 2 diabetes. Leptin is a hormone that typically increases in response to fat deposition causing a subsequent decrease in neuropeptide Y in the ventromedial nucleus. Consequently, appetite is decreased (leptin) and metabolism is increased (neuropeptide Y). However, Leptin levels have been shown to decrease postoperatively in RYGB and BPD before a significant change in BMI is seen[8,9]; so how this affects insulin control is not clear.

   GLP-1 and GIP are hormones that impact a patient's insulin response to glucose ingestion. Alterations of the effect of GLP-1 and GIP are apparent in those with diabetes.[10] Fasting GIP levels decrease in diabetic patients after undergoing RYGB at 3 weeks postoperatively.[8] One week after BPD, fasting GIP was also found to significantly decrease.[9] Conversely, GLP-1 levels have been shown to increase after BPD, SG, and RYGB.[9,11,12] The relationship of leptin, GLP-1, and GIP and the resolution of diabetes after bariatric surgery is also not clear and continues to be studied.

   In addition to hormone changes, alterations in gut microbiota may also contribute to the resolution of type 2 diabetes after bariatric surgery. For example, *Roseburia* species have been shown to be increased in those who have had RYGB or SG and also achieved remission of diabetes.[13]

REFERENCES

1. Schauer PR, Bhatt DL, Kirwan JP, et al. Bariatric surgery versus intensive medical therapy for diabetes—5-year outcomes. *NEJM*. 2017;376(7):641-651.

2. Mingrone G, Panunzi S, De Gaetano A, et al. Bariatric surgery versus conventional therapy for type 2 diabetes. *NEJM*. 2012;366(17):1577-1585.
3. Schauer PR, Bhatt DL, Kirwarn JP, et al. Bariatric surgery versus intensive medical therapy for diabetes—3-year outcomes. *NEJM*. 2014;370(21):2002-2013.
4. Zhou K, Wolski K, Malin SK, et al. Impact of weight loss trajectory following randomization to bariatric surgery on long-term diabetes glycemic and cardiometabolic parameters. *Endocr Pract*. 2019;25(6):572-579.
5. Wing RR, Bolin P, Brancati FL, et al. The Look Ahead Research Group. Cardiovascular effects of intensive lifestyle intervention in type 2 diabetes. *NEJM*. 2013; 369(2):145-154.
6. Buchwald H, Avidor Y, Brauwald E, et al. Bariatric Surgery: systematic review and meta-analysis. *JAMA* 2004. 292(14): 1724-28.
7. Cowie CC. Diabetes diagnosis and control: missed opportunities to improve health. *Diabetes Care*. 2019;42(6):994-1004.
8. Rubino F, Gagner M, Gentileschi P, et al. The early effect of the Roux-en-Y gastric bypass on hormones involved in body weight regulation and glucose metabolism. *Ann Surg*. 2004;240(2):236-242.
9. Guidone C, Manco M, Valera-Mora E, et al. Mechanisms of recovery from type 2 diabetes after malabsorptive bariatric surgery. *Diabetes*. 2006;55(7):2025-2032.
10. Batterham RB, Cummings DE. Mechanisms of diabetes improvement following bariatric/metabolic surgery. *Diabetes Care*. 2016;39:893-901.
11. Tsoli M, Chronaiou A, Kehagia I, Kalfarentzos F, Alesandrides TK. et al. Hormone changes and diabetes resolution after biliopancreatic diversion and laparoscopic sleeve gastrectomy: a comparative prospective study. *Surg Obes Relat Dis*. 2013;9(5):667-677.
12. Umeda LM, Silva EA, Carneiro G, Arasaki CH, Geloneze B, Zanella MT et al. Early improvement in glycemic control after bariatric surgery and its relationships with insulin, GLP-1, and glucagon secretion in type 2 diabetic patients. *Obes Surg*. 2011;21:896-901.
13. Murphy R, Tsai P, Jullig M, Liu A, Plank L, Booth M. et al. Differential changes in gut microbiota after gastric bypass and sleeve gastrectomy bariatric surgery vary according to diabetes remission. *Obes Surg*. 2017;27:917-925.

37

Diabetes Summit: BMI 30 to 35

Andrew M. Brown, MD, and Aurora D. Pryor, MD

A 29-year-old female with a body mass index (BMI) of 33 kg/m^2 along with newly diagnosed type 2 diabetes mellitus presents to your office for an initial evaluation. She is interested in weight loss, but is very worried about her diabetes because her HgbA$_{1c}$ was recently found to be 7.4%. She would like to discuss her surgical options. She has heard of "gastric bands" but would also like to know if there are other procedures that can help her given her BMI.

1. **With regards to safety and efficacy of laparoscopic adjustable gastric banding (LAGB), what is the expected long-term excess weight loss?**
   A. 25% to 35%
   B. 35% to 45%
   C. 45% to 55%.
   D. 55% to 65%.
   E. >65%

2. **Regarding her therapeutic options, which procedure is she eligible for based on National Institutes of Health (NIH) and U.S. Food and Drug Administration (FDA) criteria?**
   A. LAGB
   B. Sleeve gastrectomy (SG)
   C. Roux-en-Y gastric bypass (RYGB)
   D. Biliopancreatic diversion with duodenal switch (BPD/DS)
   E. None

3. **Regarding the effectiveness of bariatric surgery in patients with BMI ≤35, which of the following is correct compared to preoperative values?**
   A. There is a postop increase in Glucagon-like peptide 1 (GLP-1) response, serum insulin, and gastric emptying time.
   B. There is a postop decrease in GLP-1 response, serum insulin, and in gastric emptying time.
   C. There is a postop decrease in GLP-1 response and serum insulin, and an increase in gastric emptying time.
   D. There is a postop increase in GLP-1 response and serum insulin, and a decrease in gastric emptying time.
   E. There is no change in GLP-1 but resection or bypass anatomy decreases gastric emptying time.

4. **Regarding the effectiveness of laparoscopic RYGB in patients with BMI ≤35, long-term remission of type 2 diabetes mellitus for RYGB is:**
   A. <30%
   B. 30% to 40%
   C. 40% to 50%
   D. 50% to 60%
   E. >60%

ANSWERS

1. **C.** Long-term excess weight loss (EWL) with LAGB has been tracked out as far as 20 years. Single-site EWL at 20 years showed 48.9% EWL, and meta-analysis of 17 reports showed 45.9% EWL.[1] A smaller review, in patients with BMI <35, showed EWL of 48.7% in long-term follow-up.[2] By contrast, long-term weight loss with an SG was 55% to 60% at 5 years, and in

head-to-head matched comparison, SG had superior total weight loss (TWL) in long-term follow-up (27.7 ± 11.7% vs. 19.4 ± 11.1% [SG vs. LAGB, $P < 0.001$]).[3,4]

There is inconsistency in the literature as to the clear benefit of LAGB over best medical therapy in terms of diabetes improvement and remission. Some data show an increased relative risk of remission with LAGB of up to 5.5, while other data show similar reductions in HgbA1c at 3 and 12 months as compared to medical therapy (1.2 ± 0.3 vs. −1.0 ± 0.3%; $P = 0.496$).[5,6] However, it is clear that LAGB is at least equal to, if not superior to, medical therapy in terms of improvement in diabetes.

Bariatric surgery as a whole is safe in patients with class I obesity. Including all bariatric procedures, composite morbidity was 3.8%, and 30-day mortality was 0.5%.[7] The mortality following LAGB is nonnegligible, and at least partially related to technique and band position. At least 9% of surgeons report at least one operative mortality, and systematic review shows an early mortality rate of around 0.5%.[8,9] Most of these deaths were cardiopulmonary in nature, but 18.7% of all deaths were directly related to position of the band.[9]

2. **A.** The eligibility criteria for metabolic and bariatric surgery were laid in 1992 by the NIH, and are still widely used. Patients are eligible with a BMI ≥40, or a BMI between 35 and 40, with high-risk comorbidities. These include type 2 diabetes mellitus, obstructive sleep apnea, or certain cardiovascular risk factors.[10,11] These criteria are generally used for the primary bariatric procedures, such as SG, RYGB, and BPD/DS. As of early 2011, the FDA changed the eligibility criteria for gastric banding to include patients with a BMI of 30 to 40 with eligible comorbidities, and those with a BMI above 40 without comorbidities.[12] Given our patient's BMI of 33 with diabetes, she would be eligible for only LAGB, based on NIH/FDA criteria.

   Compared to bariatric surgery, medical treatment of type 2 diabetes mellitus in patients with a BMI less than 35 provides negligible benefit. In 5-year follow-up of 299 patients undergoing medical treatment for their diabetes, there was no significant change in their $HgbA_{1c}$.[13] Similarly, in short-term follow-up at 6 months, a group of medical weight management patients had no diabetes remission and had a relative paucity of weight loss. These patients did significantly worse than their matched surgical cohort.[14] Multiple studies have looked at the failure rates of LAGB, with one Swedish 10-year experience showing failure rates at 32%.[15] Similar rates were seen in a different 10-year experience, with 21.7% of patients requiring reoperation, and the failure rate being up to 36.9% at 7 years follow-up.[16]

   Revisional surgery rates following LAGB are unacceptably high, ranging from 7% to 60%.[17] As a result, there is a plethora of data regarding the effectiveness of additional weight loss and improved outcomes with conversion to another bariatric procedure. There appears to be increased excess weight loss with conversion to salvage RYGB or BPD/DS, but all are acceptable options.[18] In review of MBSAQIP data, single stage conversion to RYGB does seem to have greater morbidity and higher complication rates than conversion to SG.[19]

   Conversion from failed LAGB to any other bariatric surgery leads to improvement in type 2 diabetes mellitus. Specifically, conversion from LAGB to RYGB improved diabetes in 72% of patients, and conversion from LAGB to SG improved diabetes in 65% of patients.[20]

3. **D.** SG has been shown to be effective for both weight loss and comorbidity reduction in patients with an initial BMI between 30 and 35 kg/m^2. Berry et al. showed that excess weight loss percentage (EWL%) was 83.2% at 2 years, and 75.8% at 3-year follow-up.[21] Similarly, Noun et al. showed equally impressive outcomes, with 24.1% total weight loss at 1 year, and at 5 years, 76% of patients had achieved ≥50% of excess BMI lost.[22] Diabetes remission has been shown to be up to rates of 50% to 60% at 1 to 3 years following SG in the class I obese population.[21,23] Compared to RYGB in patients with a BMI of 30 to 35, SG is inferior in terms of reduction of HgbA1c (−3.1% vs. −2.1%, $P = 0.008$), and rates of complete remission of diabetes (46.9% vs. 16.7%, $P = 0.03$).[13]

   As compared to preoperatively, following surgery, there is a significant increase in meal-stimulated GLP-1 response and serum insulin at 30 minutes, and a significant decrease in gastric emptying time. These are some of the proposed mechanisms by which laparoscopic SG positively impacts diabetic status.[24] In a head-to-head comparison, SG is significantly better than medical therapy alone in terms of diabetes resolution. Furthermore, SG is superior in terms of control of hypertension and dyslipidemia.[25] GLP-1 is a hormone released from intestinal cells after enteral nutrient exposure, which leads to a glucose-dependent insulin response. As a result of the significant glucose role, GLP-1 stimulates insulin secretion. Additionally, GLP-1 acts as an enterogastrone, meaning it slows gastric emptying time and stimulates gastric acid secretion. This is result of the exposure of the small intestine to nutrients, which then stimulates a powerful inhibitory feedback reflex to slow gastric emptying and small intestinal transit. GLP-1, in addition to peptide YY, are potent mediators of this "ileal brake."[26]

4. E. There are few randomized controlled trials that look at RYGB in patients with type 2 diabetes mellitus and a BMI ≤35. However, on systematic review and meta-analysis, data show remission rates of 63.6% (95% confidence interval, 52.1%–73.8%).[24] This rate was lower than that of BPD and ileal transposition, but greater than LAGB, SG, and mini-gastric bypass. Complication rates for RYGB in BMI ≤35 patients are actually the highest of any bariatric surgery procedure type. The rate for bypass is 8.6%, compared to 6.7% in BPD and 0% of SG in the meta-analysis by Parikh et al.[27] Feng et al., with MBSAQIP data showed rates of morbidity of 7.83% with RYGB, 2.87% with SG, and 17.65% with BPD.[7]

At 5-year follow-up, there is significantly improved weight loss and change in BMI between RYGB and SG in patients who are nonmorbidly obese. Mean BMI change at 5 years was –7.4 versus –5.1 in the RYGB versus the SG group ($P = 0.001$), respectively.[13] Coinciding with the fact that there are higher rates of morbidity with RYGB than SG, there is also higher length of stay with the RYGB than with the SG (2.0 versus 1.6, $P < 0.001$).[7]

Certain biomarkers have been investigated to determine their role in preoperative predicting of surgical success in terms of diabetes improvement and better weight loss outcomes. Elevated baseline soluble form of receptor for advanced glycated end products (sRAGE), and elevated preoperative fasting C-peptide can help predict diabetes remission in low-BMI patients after RYGB.[24,28]

REFERENCES

1. O'Brien PE, Hindle A, Brennan L, et al. Long-term outcomes after bariatric surgery: a systematic review and meta-analysis of weight loss at 10 or more years for all bariatric procedures and a single-centre review of 20-year outcomes after adjustable gastric banding. *Obes Surg.* 2019;29(1):3-14.
2. Angrisani L, Cutolo PP, Formisano G, et al. Long-term outcomes of laparoscopic adjustable silicone gastric banding (LAGB) in moderately obese patients with and without co-morbidities. *Obes Surg.* 2013;23(7):897-902.
3. Deitel M, Gagner M, Erickson AL, et al. Third International Summit: Current status of sleeve gastrectomy. *Surg Obes Relat Dis.* 2011;7(6):749-759.
4. Johari Y, Ooi G, Burton P, et al. Long-term matched comparison of adjustable gastric banding versus sleeve gastrectomy: weight loss, quality of life, hospital resource use and patient-reported outcome measures. *Obes Surg.* 2020;30(1):214-223.
5. Dixon JB, O'Brien PE, Playfair J, et al. Adjustable gastric banding and conventional therapy for type 2 diabetes: a randomized controlled trial. *JAMA.* 2008;299(3):316-323.
6. Ding SA, Simonson DC, Wewalka M, et al. Adjustable gastric band surgery or medical management in patients with type 2 diabetes: a randomized clinical trial. *J Clin Endocrinol Metab.* 2015;100(7):2546-2556.
7. Feng X, Andalib A, Brethauer SA, et al. How safe is bariatric surgery in patients with class I obesity (body mass index 30-35 kg/m^2)? *Surg Obes Relat Dis.* 2019;15(2):253-260.
8. Gagner M, Milone L, Trelles N. Mortality after laparoscopic adjustable gastric banding: results from an anonymous questionnaire to ASBS members. *Obes Surg.* 2009;19(12):1657-1663.
9. Gagner M, Milone L, Yung E, et al. Causes of early mortality after laparoscopic adjustable gastric banding. *J Am Coll Surg.* 2008;206(4):664-669.
10. Sjoholm K, Anveden A, Peltonen M, et al. Evaluation of current eligibility criteria for bariatric surgery: diabetes prevention and risk factor changes in the Swedish obese subjects (SOS) study. *Diabetes Care.* 2013;36(5):1335-1340.
11. Gastrointestinal surgery for severe obesity: National Institutes of health Consensus Development Conference Statement. *Am J Clin Nutr.* 1992;55(2 Suppl):615S-619S.
12. Summary of safety and effectiveness – Adjustable silicone gastric band, implanted. *FDA Advisory Board.* 2011. http://accessdata.fda.gov.
13. Hsu CC, Almulaifi A, Chen JC, et al. Effect of bariatric surgery vs medical treatment on type 2 diabetes in patients with body mass index lower than 35: five-year outcomes. *JAMA Surg.* 2015;150(12):1117-1124.
14. Parikh M, Chung M, Sheth S, et al. Randomized pilot trial of bariatric surgery versus intensive medical weight management on diabetes remission in type 2 diabetic patients who do NOT meet NIH criteria for surgery and the role of soluble RAGE as a novel biomarker of success. *Ann Surg.* 2014;260(4):617-622.
15. Mittermair RP, Obermuller S, Perathoner A, et al. Results and complications after Swedish adjustable gastric banding-10 years experience. *Obes Surg.* 2009;19(12):1636-1641.
16. Suter M, Calmes JM, Paroz A, et al. A 10-year experience with laparoscopic gastric banding for morbid obesity: high long-term complication and failure rates. *Obes Surg.* 2006;16(7):829-835.

17. Pujol Rafols J, Al Abbas AI, Devriendt S, et al. Roux-en-Y gastric bypass sleeve gastrectomy, or one anastomosis gastric bypass as rescue therapy after failed adjustable gastric banding: a multicenter comparative study. *Surg Obes Relat Dis*. 2018;14(11):1659-1666.
18. Elnahas A, Graybiel K, Farrokhyar F, et al. Revisional surgery after failed laparoscopic adjustable gastric banding: a systematic review. *Surg Endosc*. 2013;27(3):740-745.
19. Janik MR, Rogula TG, Mustafa RR, et al. Safety of revision sleeve gastrectomy compared to roux-y gastric bypass after failed gastric banding: analysis of the MBSAQIP. *Ann Surg*. 2019;269(2):299-303.
20. Yan J, Cohen R, Arminian A. Reoperative bariatric surgery for treatment of type 2 diabetes mellitus. *Surg Obes Relat Dis*. 2017;13(8):1412-1421.
21. Berry MA, Urrutia L, Lamoza P, et al. Sleeve gastrectomy outcomes in patients with BMI between 30 and 35 – 3 years of follow-up. *Obes Surg*. 2018;28(3):649-655.
22. Noun R, Slim R, Nasr M, et al. Results of laparoscopic sleeve gastrectomy in 541 consecutive patients with low baseline body mass index (30-35 kg/m^2). *Obes Surg*. 2016;26(12):2824-2828.
23. Lee WJ, Ser KH, Chong K, et al. Laparoscopic sleeve gastrectomy for diabetes treatment in nonmorbidly obese patients: efficacy and change in insulin secretion. *Surgery*. 2010;147(5):664-669.
24. Vigneshwaran B, Wahal A, Aggarwal S, et al. Impact of sleeve gastrectomy on type 2 diabetes mellitus, gastric emptying time, glucagon-like peptide 1 (GLP-1), ghrelin and leptin in non-morbidly obese subjects with BMI 30-35.0 kg/m^2: a prospective study. *Obes Surg*. 2016;26(12):2817-2823.
25. Abbatini F, Capoccia D, Casella G, et al. Type 2 diabetes in obese patients with body mass index of 30-35 kg/m^2: sleeve gastrectomy versus medical treatment. *Surg Obes Relat Dis*. 2012;8(1):20-24.
26. Marathe CS, Rayner CK, Jones KL, et al. Effects of GLP-1 and incretin-based therapies on gastrointestinal motor function. *Exp Diabetes Res*. 2011;2011:279530.
27. Parikh M, Issa R, Vieira D, et al. Role of bariatric surgery as treatment for type 2 diabetes in patients who do not meet current NIH criteria: a systematic review and met-analysis. *J Am Coll Surg*. 2013;217(3):527-532.
28. Zhao L, Li W, Su Z, et al. Preoperative fasting C-peptide predicts type 2 diabetes mellitus remission in low BMI Chinese patients after Roux-en-Y gastric bypass. *J Gastrointest Surg*. 2018;22(10):1672-1678.

38

Cardiac

Linda P. Zhang, MD

A 55-year-old female with a past medical history of type 2 diabetes mellitus, hypertension, atrial fibrillation, and morbid obesity (body mass index [BMI] 58 kg/m^2) is interested in bariatric surgery for weight loss. She has tried various weight loss programs in the past, but has been unable to have sustained weight loss. She has difficulty walking up one flight of stairs due to shortness of breath. She is concerned that her heart isn't strong enough to tolerate surgery and would like to know more about her operative risk and long-term postoperative cardiovascular benefits.

1. **Regarding preoperative evaluation for surgical management of her obesity, which of the following is correct?**
   A. Patients should undergo a cardiac evaluation including an electrocardiogram, stress echo, and evaluation by a cardiologist.
   B. Placement of an inferior vena cava (IVC) filter should be routinely done for BMI >50 kg/m^2.
   C. Oral hormonal contraceptives should be stopped at least 3 months prior to surgery.
   D. A lower BMI threshold (BMI <35) for bariatric surgery should be considered for certain ethnicities.
   E. Bariatric surgery is contraindicated in patients with coronary artery disease and heart failure.

2. **Which of the following is true regarding this patient's perioperative cardiovascular risk?**
   A. For prophylaxis against deep vein thrombosis (DVT), subcutaneously administered unfractionated heparin or low-molecular-weight heparin is preferred.
   B. Extended chemoprophylaxis after hospital discharge.
   C. Patients with high perioperative risk for myocardial infarction should be managed in an ICU.
   D. Pulmonary embolism accounts for 40% of all deaths within 30 days of surgery.
   E. Cardioprotection from a decrease in blood pressure postoperatively occurs after significant weight loss.

3. **Regarding postoperative cardiovascular events for patients undergoing bariatric surgery, which of the following statement is true?**
   A. Metabolic surgery is associated with lower usage of insulin, noninsulin diabetes medication, and renin-angiotensin system inhibitors.
   B. Metabolic surgery is not associated with significantly lower risk of atrial fibrillation.
   C. All injectable insulin and oral insulin regimes can be continued until the patient follows up with their primary care provider 2 weeks postoperatively.
   D. The risk of cardiac event within 90 days after metabolic surgery is approximately 4%.
   E. Antihypertensive medications should be stopped postoperatively to minimize risk of hypotension.

4. **Which of the following statements is TRUE regarding adverse cardiovascular events for patients after metabolic surgery versus nonsurgical weight loss?**
   A. Metabolic surgery does not affect the incidence of heart failure.

B. Intensive lifestyle intervention can reduce the rate of cardiovascular events in overweight or obese adults with type 2 diabetes.
C. Five percent nonsurgical weight loss can alter the incidence of atrial fibrillation.
D. For obese patients, metabolic surgery is associated with significantly lower overall long-term mortality than nonsurgical treatment.
E. The risk of a cardiac event is greater in patients who've had bariatric surgery is a function of the amount of weight lost.

ANSWERS

1. **D.** A lower threshold for screening, diagnosis, and treatment of obesity is recommended for patients of certain ethnicities, including South Asians, Southeast Asians, and East Asians. These ethnic groups are at increased risk for type 2 diabetes mellitus, cardiometabolic disease, and mortality at a lower BMI. Various organizations, including the American Diabetes Association, the WHO Expert Consult Group, and the Working Group on Obesity in China, recommend screening for diabetes for all Asian American adults with a BMI of >23 kg/m^2.[1–3]

The need for extensive cardiac testing and cardiology evaluation should be based on individual risk factors. Findings on history and physical exam should guide surgeons on the need to refer patients for cardiac optimization. Perioperative cardiovascular evaluation should follow the latest American College of Cardiology/American Heart Association guidelines.[4] Patients with known cardiac disease must have a cardiology consultation prior to bariatric surgery.

Routine preoperative placement of an IVC filter should not be done for prophylaxis against pulmonary embolism. It may be considered in individuals with history of DVT, pulmonary embolism, or clotting disorder.[5]

Oral contraceptives should be discontinued 1 cycle prior to bariatric procedure to minimize the risk of thromboembolic events postoperatively. For postmenopausal women, hormone replacement therapy should be discontinued 3 weeks prior to surgery.[6]

Having coronary artery disease and heart failure does not preclude a patient from having bariatric surgery. Preoperatively, each patient should be risk stratified based on their history and functional status. Several risk assessment tools can be used, including the Revised Cardiac Risk Index[7] or Cardiac Arrest Calculator.[8] These tools take into account the patient's age, ASA class, history of coronary disease, history of heart failure, stroke, insulin-dependent diabetes, renal function, and functional status.[9]

2. **D.** Pulmonary embolism is the leading cause of death after bariatric surgery, with an incidence of about 1%. It accounts for 40% of all deaths within 30 days postoperatively.[10] Laparoscopic bariatric surgery has less risk of pulmonary embolism compared to open surgery.

Prophylaxis against DVT includes both sequential compression devices and pharmacological regimes such as unfractionated heparin or low-molecular-weight heparin given within 24 hours after bariatric surgery.[5] Early ambulation within 24 hours postoperatively is also recommended for every patient.

For high-risk patients (history of DVT, known hypercoagulable state, or limited ambulation), chemoprophylaxis after hospital discharge should be considered. Studies show that more than 80% of DVT events occur postoperatively after hospital discharge.[11]

For patients with a high risk of perioperative myocardial infarction, it is recommended that they stay in a telemetry-capable setting for at least the first 24 hours after their bariatric surgery. Routine admission to an ICU is not necessary as long as there is adequate monitoring on a telemetry floor.[6]

A decrease in blood pressure is cardioprotective and results in reduction of cardiovascular events and mortality. However, this decrease can occur even before appreciable weight loss, especially in patients with orthostatic intolerance and possible dysautonomia. Studies show a 12% reduction in the use of antihypertensive medications at just 1 month postoperatively, and 25% reduction at 6 months.[12]

3. **A.** Multiple studies in the past have shown that metabolic surgery can improve glucose and blood pressure control, resulting in lower use of cardiovascular and diabetic medications. This, in turn, can lower the incidence of other cardiovascular events, such as myocardial infarction and atrial fibrillation.[13]

There is a significant reduction in risk of atrial fibrillation after metabolic surgery. This is in contrast to nonsurgical weight loss in the Look AHEAD trial, which did not find a lower risk of developing atrial fibrillation after intensive lifestyle changes.[11,14]

For patients with type 2 diabetes, all insulin secretagogues, thiazolidinediones, and sodium-glucose cotransporter-2 inhibitors should be discontinued in the immediate postoperatively period to reduce the risk of hypoglycemia. These medications should be dose adjusted to take into account the postoperative lower calorie intake.[6] This should be discussed with the patient in the preoperative period and should include input from the patient's primary care provider or endocrinologist.

For patients with obesity and diabetes, the 90-day postoperative risk of a cardiac event is approximately 1%.[11]

Various studies have shown that bariatric surgery is effective in lowering blood pressure. However, the effect of weight loss blood pressure is variable and unpredictable. Antihypertensive medications should not be immediately stopped after surgery unless clearly indicated.[11] Instead, blood pressure should be evaluated frequently and repeatedly during the first 2 years, and dosages should be titrated as blood pressure improves.[15]

4. D. Numerous studies have shown a reduction in cardiovascular disease risk after metabolic surgery, which results in a reduced number of cardiovascular deaths after surgery. Compared to nonsurgical control groups, the incidence of first-time myocardial infarction or stroke are also lower in the surgery group. Futhermore this reduced risk is not due to weight loss but rather the metabolic effects of surgery.[16]

By improving glucose level and blood pressure, metabolic surgery lowers the incidence of adverse cardiovascular events, which results in decrease incidence of heart failure. It has been suggested that the mechanism for this benefit may be due to change in cardiac metabolism, hemodynamic function, and workload.[11]

The Look AHEAD study showed that despite intensive lifestyle interventions and early signs of improved fitness, there was no significant reduction in risk of major adverse cardiovascular event such as myocardial infarction, stroke, hospitalization for angina, and death[17] in overweight and obese patients.

Recent meta-analysis studies showed that a small-to-moderate amount of weight loss does not alter the incidence of atrial fibrillation.[14] Substantial weight loss in metabolic surgery, as seen in the Swedish Obese Subjects study, is needed to significantly lower the risk of atrial fibrillation.[18,19]

REFERENCES

1. World Health Organization Regional Office for the Western Pacific, International Association for the Study of Obesity, International Obesity Task Force. *The Asia-Pacific Perspective: Redefining Obesity and Its Treatment.* Australia: Health Communications Australia Pty Limited; 2000.
2. Razak F, Anand SS, Shannon H, et al. Defining obesity cut points in a multiethnic population. *Circulation.* 2007;115:2111-2118.
3. Zheng W, McLerran DF, Rolland B, et al. Association between body-mass index and risk of death in more than 1 million Asians. *N Engl J Med.* 2011;364:719-729.
4. Fleisher LA, Fleischmann KE, Auerbach AD, et al. 2014 ACC/AHA guideline on perioperative cardiovascular evaluation and management of patients undergoing noncardiac surgery: executive summary: a report of the American College of Cardiology/American Heart Association Task Force on Practice Guidelines. *Circulation.* 2014;130:2215-2245.
5. American Society for Metabolic and Bariatric Surgery Clinical Issues Committee. ASMBS updated position statement on prophylactic measures to reduce the risk of venous thromboembolism in bariatric surgery patients. *Surg Obes Relat Dis.* 2013;9:493-497.
6. Mechanick JI, Apovian C, Brethauer S, et al. Clinical practice guidelines for the perioperative nutrition, metabolic, and nonsurgical support of patients undergoing bariatric procedures - 2019 update: Cosponsored by American Association of Clinical Endocrinologists/American College of Endocrinology, The Obesity Society, American Society for Metabolic and Bariatric Surgery, Obesity Medicine Association, and American Society of Anesthesiologists. *Obesity (Silver Spring).* 2020;28(4):O1-O58.
7. Davis C, Tait G, Carroll J, Wijeysundera DN, Beattie WS. The revised cardiac risk index in the new millennium: a single-centre prospective cohort re-evaluation of the original variables in 9,519 consecutive elective surgical patients. *Can J Anaesth.* 2013;60:855-863.
8. Gupta PK, Gupta H, Sundaram A, et al. Development and validation of a risk calculator for prediction of cardiac risk after surgery. *Circulation.* 2011;124:381-387.
9. Roshanov PS, Walsh M, Devereaux PJ, et al. External validation of the Revised Cardiac Risk Index and update of its renal variable to predict 30-day risk of major cardiac complications after non-cardiac surgery: rationale and plan for analyses of the VISION study. *BMJ Open.* 2017;7:e013510.
10. Helm MC, Simon K, Higgins R, Kindel TL, Gould JC. Perioperative complications increase the risk of venous thromboembolism following bariatric surgery. *Am J Surg.* 2017;214:1135-1140.
11. Aminian A, Andalib A, Khorgami Z, et al. Who should get extended thromboprophylaxis after bariatric surgery? A risk assessment tool to guide indications for post-discharge pharmacoprophylaxis. *Ann Surg.* 2017;265:143-150.

12. Ponnusamy V, Owens AP, Purkayastha S, Iodice V, Mathias CJ. Orthostatic intolerance and autonomic dysfunction following bariatric surgery: a retrospective study and review of the literature. *Auton Neurosci*. 2016;198:1-7.
13. Aminian A, Zajichek A, Arterburn DE, et al. Association of metabolic surgery with major adverse cardiovascular outcomes in patients with type 2 diabetes and obesity. *JAMA*. 2019. doi:10.1001/jama.2019.14231
14. Alonso A, Bahnson JL, Gaussoin SA, et al.; Look AHEAD Research Group. Effect of an intensive lifestyle intervention on atrial fibrillation risk in individuals with type 2 diabetes: the Look AHEAD randomized trial. *Am Heart J*. 2015;170(4):770-777.e5.
15. Puzziferri N, Roshek TB 3rd, Mayo HG, Gallagher R, Belle SH, Livingston EH. Longterm follow-up after bariatric surgery: a systematic review. *JAMA*. 2014;312: 934-942.
16. Sjöström L, Peltonen M, Jacobson P, et al. Bariatric surgery and long-term cardiovascular events. *JAMA*. 2012;307:56–65.
17. Wing RR, Bolin P, Brancati FL, et al.; Look AHEAD Research Group. Cardiovascular effects of intensive lifestyle intervention in type 2 diabetes. *N Engl J Med*. 2013;369(2):145-154.
18. Jones NR, Taylor KS, Taylor CJ, Aveyard P. Weight change and the risk of incident atrial fibrillation: a systematic review and meta-analysis. *Heart*. 2019. doi:10.1136/heartjnl-2019-314931
19. Jamaly S, Carlsson L, Peltonen M, Jacobson P, Sjöström L, Karason K. Bariatric surgery and the risk of new onset atrial fibrillation in Swedish obese subjects. *J Am Coll Cardiol*. 2016;68(23):2497-2504.

39

The Impact of Metabolic and Bariatric Surgery on the Risk and Outcomes of Malignancies

Samantha Terranella, MD, and Philip Omotosho, MD

A 45-year-old female with a body mass index (BMI) of 39 kg/m^2 and medical history significant for type 2 diabetes mellitus, hypertension, and hyperlipidemia presents to your clinic to undergo initial evaluation for bariatric surgery. She has a family history of breast cancer in her mother and pancreatic cancer in her father. She heard that obesity increases her risk for cancer and therefore the patient has several questions in regards to cancer risk as it relates to bariatric surgery.

1. **Which of the following is a proposed mechanism underlying the relationship between obesity and cancer?**
   A. Hyperinsulinemia and elevated insulin-like growth factor 1 (IGF-1); elevated IGF-1 promoting a change in the cellular environment resulting in prohibition of apoptosis.
   B. Decreased levels of circulating estrogen. Decreased levels of estrogen leading to the inactivation of pathways that prevent uninhibited cell division.
   C. Decreased bioavailability of steroid hormones. Decreased leptin levels that increase cell division.
   D. Chronic obesity-related inflammation excess IL-2 causing chronic inflammation leading to cellular change.

2. **The patient tells you that she has read that being overweight can actually reduce her risk of death from cancer and she is concerned having weight loss surgery will actually increase her risk of cancer-related death. Which answer choice best describes the phenomenon to which the patient refers and its associated definition?**
   A. The Obesity Paradox—The observation that overweight and obese states appear to be protective and have been associated with improved survival in cancer compared to normal weight patients.
   B. The Obesity–Cancer Link—The inverse relationship between the physiologic and metabolic changes observed in overweight and obese states and cancer incidence.
   C. The Cancer Paradox—The dichotomy between the theoretical increased risk of cancer in obese patients, secondary to the higher number of cells at risk for mutations, and what is actually observed in clinical practice.
   D. The Fed State Theory—The idea that the increased nourished state of an obese patient improves their outcomes in metabolically active conditions, such as cancer.

3. **After bariatric surgery, which factor has been linked to a relative decrease in cancer incidence and mortality?**
   A. Male sex
   B. Sleeve gastrectomy
   C. The percentage of total body weight loss after undergoing bariatric surgery
   D. Colon and lung cancers

4. Obesity is associated with an increased risk of colorectal cancer (CRC). Which of the following most accurately reflects the current understanding of the relationship between obesity and CRC?

A. Bariatric surgery has been clearly shown to reduce this risk long term.
B. The impact of bariatric surgery on CRC incidence is conflicting.
C. Bariatric surgery has no impact on CRC incidence.
D. Patients who have undergone bariatric surgery are actually found to have a higher incidence of CRC.

ANSWERS

1. A. There is strong epidemiologic evidence linking overweight and obese states to an increased risk of cancer incidence and mortality.[1,2] One large prospective study found that an estimated 14% to 20% of cancer deaths were attributed to overweight and obese status.[3] While the connection between obesity and the promotion of tumorigenesis likely varies by cancer type, several mechanisms have been proposed to explain this link.[2] The most commonly described factors linking obesity to cancer are the activation of the insulin-IGF-1 axis, elevated sex hormones, adipokines, and obesity-related inflammation (Figure 39-1).[1] Excess calorie intake and weight gain cause insulin resistance and a hyperinsulin state. Increased circulating insulin leads to activation of the insulin-IGF-1 pathway. IGF-1, in turn, promotes a change in the cellular environment resulting in prohibition of apoptosis and promotion of cellular proliferation and tumor growth.[1,4]

Similarly, aromatase is produced in excess amounts in the adipose tissue of obese and overweight individuals. Aromatase acts to convert andro gens to estrogens leading to increased circulating estrogen, particularly observed in overweight postmenopausal females.[1] Increased estrogen binds to estrogen receptors leading to the activation of intracellular pathways that stimulate cell division and activate IGF to promote tumor progression through the inhibition of apoptosis.[4] Adipose tissue also produces specific adipocyte-derived cytokines, termed adipokines. Leptin is one of the most well studied of these hormones.[4] Leptin levels rise in obese states and are thought to be involved in the dysregulation of cancer growth through the inhibition of apoptosis and the stimulation of cell division.[1]

Adiponectin, another obesity-related adipokine, is actually found in low levels in obese and overweight individuals and has been shown to be associated with

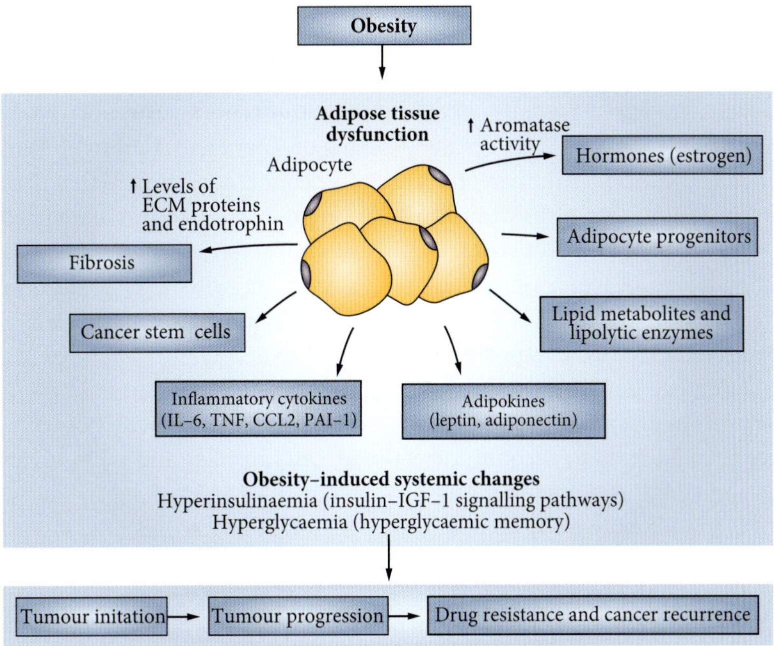

Figure 39-1 Obesity and cancer-mechanisms underlying tumour progression and recurrence. (Reproduced with permission from Park J, Morley TS, Kim M, et al: Obesity and cancer–mechanisms underlying tumour progression and recurrence. *Nat Rev Endocrinol.* 2014;10(8):455–465)

elevated cancer risks in several prospective and epidemiological studies.[1] Finally, obesity has been found to be associated with chronic inflammation and elevations in IL-6 and TNF.[1] This chronic inflammatory state is correlated with the promotion of cancer in several organs including the liver and colon.

2. **A.** The observed relationship between overweight and obese patients and improved health outcomes in a variety of disease states has been described. In the cancer literature, numerous studies have suggested that overweight and obese states are associated with improved survival compared to normal weight patients.[5] This is called the Obesity Paradox. However, the general implication of a direct causal relationship between obesity and improved cancer survival can be misleading. Important caveats in interpreting the results of these studies are to note the timing of when BMI was determined along with the age of the participants in the study.[5] Studies in the colorectal cancer population have demonstrated poor prognostication with elevated prediagnosis BMI but improved survival with elevated posttreatment BMI.[6] In regards to age, studies have shown improved cancer-related outcomes with obese and overweight states in individuals over 60 years with no improvement in outcomes in younger patient populations.[7] The apparent obesity paradox may be further explained by methodological limitations, such as confounding, detection bias, reverse causality, and collider bias.[5,8] One such theory is that "opportunistic surveillance" happens in obese patients who have earlier pre-illness healthcare that can result in detection of earlier staged cancer.[9] Another proposed explanation is that weight loss of previously obese patients due to high metabolic demands of the disease state creates the illusion of worse outcomes in normal weight patients.[5] Moreover, BMI is a poor measure of true adiposity and body composition because it does not differentiate between lean mass and fat mass.[5] BMI varies by age, sex and gender, yet no specific norms have been adopted to account for these differences. When other anthropometric measures are used that better approximate body composition, such as waist to hip ratio, skinfolds, or body composition analysis software, the obesity paradox has not been observed.[9] The current findings suggest that increase in body fat should not be encouraged to promote survival benefits in cancer. Rather, an increase in fat mass is likely of benefit only when it is accompanied by normal or increased lean mass as a potential marker of nutritional reserve.[9]

3. **D.** The Swedish Obese Subjects (SOS) study was one of the first and largest prospective studies to compare mortality outcomes in obese patients who underwent bariatric surgery with matched controls who were treated with conservative weight management strategies.[10] The study found that cancer-related mortality was significantly lower in the population of patients that underwent bariatric surgery compared to those who were managed with conservative weight loss strategies.[10] On subsequent analysis, the research team found that cancer incidence was reduced in obese females who underwent bariatric surgery, but there was no difference in cancer incidence between groups of male patients.[11] Reductions in cancer incidence and cancer-related mortality may be observed in females due to several factors. First, a higher proportion of patients undergoing bariatric surgery are female sex.[12] Second, the most prevalent obesity-related cancers tend to be either exclusively or more commonly observed in females, such as endometrial and breast cancer, respectively.[12] The findings from the SOS study have been echoed in numerous large cohort studies, which have since demonstrated that the type of surgery and the percentage of weight loss are also significantly associated with reduction in cancer incidence.[13,14] One large retrospective cohort study demonstrated a risk reduction for hormone-related cancers in patients that underwent gastric bypass, but not gastric banding or sleeve gastrectomy.[15] Another large retrospective cohort study found that percentage of total body weight loss $>10\%$ was associated with a reduced risk of cancer.[12] Larger reductions in cancer incidence were seen with every additional 10% increase in weight loss (Figure 39-2).

4. **B.** Epidemiologic studies have found a link between obesity and CRC incidence with a 24% increased risk of CRC in men and a 9% increased risk of CRC in women for every 5 kg/m^2 increase in BMI.[16,17] This finding underscores the importance of investigating the impact of intentional weight loss strategies, such as bariatric surgery, on mitigating the risk of CRC. However, to date, the research on the association between bariatric surgery and incidence of CRC has been widely variable. One large retrospective study by Schauer et al. found that the incidence of

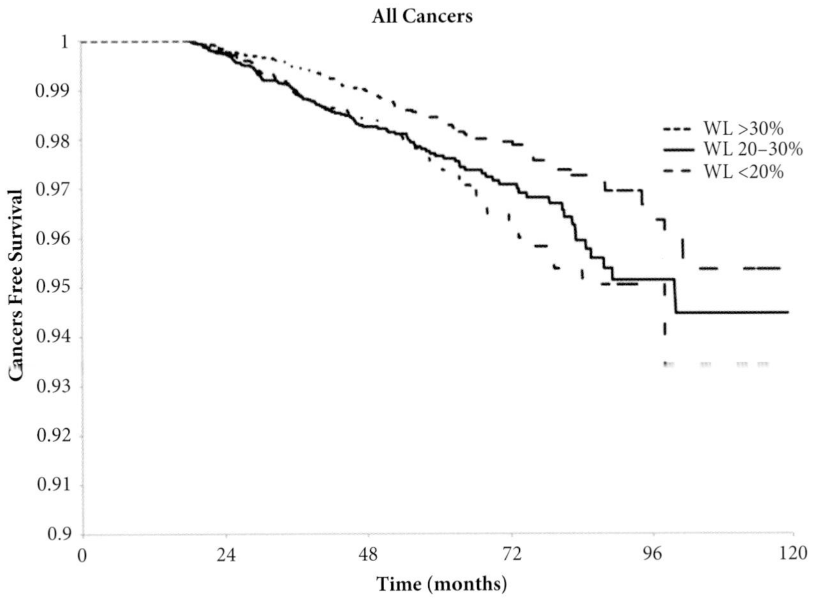

Figure 39-2 Kaplan–Meier estimated cancer-free survival for all cancer in patients who underwent bariatric surgery by percentage weight loss at 1 year. (Reproduced with permission from Schauer DP, Feigelson HS, Koebnick C, et al: Association between weight loss and the risk of cancer after bariatric surgery. *Obesity (Silver Spring)* 2017;25 Suppl 2(Suppl 2):S52–S57).

CRC was significantly lower in the population who underwent bariatric surgery when compared to a matched nonsurgical cohort.[18] Another large retrospective study by Bailly et al. reported similar findings with a 34% increased risk of developing CRC in obese patients who did not undergo bariatric surgery compared to a matched bariatric surgery cohort.[19] In contrast to the previously highlighted findings, other studies comparing the bariatric surgery population with a matched nonsurgical cohort found that the risk of CRC was actually higher in the surgery population after 10 years following bariatric surgery, and furthermore, they found that patients who underwent bariatric surgery had a higher standardized incidence ratio of CRC when compared to the general population.[20] Other studies, such as that by Mackenzie et al., found that patients who underwent gastric bypass had an increased risk of CRC, but those that underwent sleeve gastrectomy or gastric banding saw no increase in CRC incidence.[15] Several hypotheses have been proposed to explain a possible correlation between bariatric surgery and the increased incidence of CRC over time, including changes to the intestinal mucosa and microbiota, increased exposure to bile salts, and increased protein consumption leading to a pro-tumorigenic and carcinogenic environment.[21] Ultimately, while there is a clear consensus regarding the correlation between obesity and CRC, the data is highly conflicted as to the true impact that bariatric surgery has on CRC incidence and therefore remains the subject of ongoing research.

REFERENCES

1. Park J, Morley TS, Kim M, Clegg DJ, Scherer PE. Obesity and cancer–mechanisms underlying tumour progression and recurrence. *Nat Rev Endocrinol.* 2014;10(8):455-465. doi:10.1038/nrendo.2014.94
2. Calle EE, Thun MJ. Obesity and cancer. *Oncogene.* 2004;23(38):6365-6378. doi:10.1038/sj.onc.1207751
3. Calle EE, Rodriguez C, Walker-Thurmond K, Thun MJ. Overweight, obesity, and mortality from cancer in a prospectively studied cohort of U.S. adults. *N Engl J Med.* 2003;348(17):1625-1638. doi:10.1056/NEJMoa021423
4. Basen-Engquist K, Chang M. Obesity and cancer risk: recent review and evidence. *Curr Oncol Rep.* 2011;13(1):71-76. doi:10.1007/s11912-010-0139-7
5. Lennon H, Sperrin M, Badrick E, Renehan AG. The obesity paradox in cancer: a review. *Curr Oncol Rep.* 2016;18(9):56. doi:10.1007/s11912-016-0539-4.
6. Wu S, Liu J, Wang X, Li M, Gan Y, Tang Y. Association of obesity and overweight with overall survival in colorectal cancer patients: a meta-analysis of 29 studies. *Cancer Causes Control.* 2014;25(11):1489-1502. doi:10.1007/s10552-014-0450-y

7. Navarro WH, Agovi MA, Logan BR, et al. Obesity does not preclude safe and effective myeloablative hematopoietic cell transplantation (HCT) for acute myelogenous leukemia (AML) in adults. *Biol Blood Marrow Transplant.* 2010;16(10):1442-1450. doi:10.1016/j.bbmt.2010.04.009
8. Lee DH, Giovannucci EL. The obesity paradox in cancer: epidemiologic insights and perspectives. *Curr Nutr Rep.* 2019 Sep;8(3):175-181. doi:10.1007/s13668-019-00280-6
9. Gonzalez MC, Pastore CA, Orlandi SP, Heymsfield SB. Obesity paradox in cancer: new insights provided by body composition. *Am J Clin Nutrit.* 2014;99(5):999-1005. doi:10.3945/ajcn.113.071399
10. Sjöström L, Narbro K, Sjöström CD, et al. Effects of bariatric surgery on mortality in Swedish obese subjects. *N Engl J Med.* 2007;357(8):741-752. doi:10.1056/NEJMoa066254
11. Sjöström L, Gummesson A, Sjöström CD, et al. Effects of bariatric surgery on cancer incidence in obese patients in Sweden (Swedish Obese Subjects Study): a prospective, controlled intervention trial. *Lancet Oncol.* 2009;10(7):653-662. doi:10.1016/S1470-2045(09)70159-7
12. Schauer DP, Feigelson HS, Koebnick C, et al. Association between weight loss and the risk of cancer after bariatric surgery. *Obesity (Silver Spring).* 2017;25(Suppl 2):S52-S57. doi:10.1002/oby.22002
13. Adams TD, Hunt SC. Cancer and obesity: effect of bariatric surgery. *World J Surg.* 2009;33(10):2028-2033. doi:10.1007/s00268-009-0169-1
14. Christou NV, Lieberman M, Sampalis F, Sampalis JS. Bariatric surgery reduces cancer risk in morbidly obese patients. *Surg Obes Relat Dis.* 2008;4(6):691-695. doi:10.1016/j.soard.2008.08.025
15. Mackenzie H, Markar SR, Askari A, et al. Obesity surgery and risk of cancer. *Br J Surg.* 2018;105(12):1650-1657. doi:10.1002/bjs.10914
16. Afshar S, Kelly SB, Seymour K, et al. The effects of bariatric surgery on colorectal cancer risk: systematic review and meta-analysis. *Obes Surg.* 2014;24:1793-1799. doi:10.1007/s11695-014-1359-y
17. Bardou M, Barkun AN, Martel M. Obesity and colorectal cancer. *Gut.* 2013;62:933-947.
18. Schauer DP, Feigelson HS, Koebnick C, et al. Bariatric surgery and the risk of cancer in a large multisite cohort. *Ann Surg.* 2019;269(1):95-101. doi:10.1097/SLA.0000000000002525
19. Bailly L, Fabre R, Pradier C, Iannelli A. Colorectal cancer risk following bariatric surgery in a nationwide study of French individuals with obesity. *JAMA Surg.* 2020. doi:10.1001/jamasurg.2020.0089
20. Tao W, Artama M, von Euler-Chelpin M, et al. Colon and rectal cancer risk after bariatric surgery in a multicountry Nordic cohort study. *Int J Cancer.* 2019. doi:10.1002/ijc.32770
21. Derogar M, Hull MA, Kant P, et al. Increased risk of colorectal cancer after obesity surgery. *Ann Surg.* 2013;258:983-988.

40

Weight Loss—Long Term

John R. Romanelli, MD, and Brittany Kern, MD

A 55-year-old female with a body mass index (BMI) of 44 kg/m^2 with the associated comorbidities of obstructive sleep apnea, diabetes mellitus, hypertension, and arthritis is found to be an appropriate candidate for surgical weight loss after thorough preoperative evaluation. She has had no previous abdominal surgeries. She is inquiring about the long-term weight loss outcomes for each of the major surgical options.

1. Which of the following is true regarding long-term weight loss outcomes for sleeve gastrectomy (SG)?

A. Percentage excess weight loss (%EWL) with SG is equal to Roux-en-Y gastric bypass (RYGB) at 5 years.
B. %EWL with SG is ~55% at 5 years.
C. Weight loss is usually sustained with SG.
D. Size of the gastric sleeve correlates to the %EWL at 5 years.
E. Rate of %EWL peaks at 5 years but continues to increase slowly in the years following.

2. In regards to long-term weight loss outcomes after RYGB, which of the following is true?

A. The clinical significance of its superior weight loss remains unclear.
B. The %EWL continues to increase after 5 years.
C. RYGB and biliopancreatic diversion with duodenal switch (BPD/DS) have equivalent %EWL in patients with a BMI of 45 to 55 kg/m^2.
D. In those patients with a BMI ≥50 kg/m^2, RYGB has overall failure rates of ≤40%.
E. The resolution of obesity-related comorbidities is greater with RYGB at 5 years than SG.

3. Comparing BPD/DS to SG or RYGB, which of the following is true?

A. Long-term effects on overall nutritional status are similar to that of the RYGB.
B. The %EWL at 5 years for BPD/DS is equal to RYGB at 5 years
C. The %EWL for BPD/DS continues to increase after 2 years.
D. There is no difference in the %EWL seen with BPD/DS versus BPD alone.
E. BPD/DS has a greater %EWL in patients with a BMI ≥50 kg/m^2 than those with a BMI ≤50 kg/m^2.

4. Which of the following is true regarding long-term weight loss outcomes for laparoscopic adjustable gastric band placement (AGB)?

A. The %EWL of laparoscopic AGB is equal to that of laparoscopic SG at 5 years.
B. The long-term data (>5 years) shows overall %EWL is greater for AGB than SG.
C. SG has a higher revision rate when compared to AGB.
D. The %EWL for AGB at 10 years is maintained for up to 20 years.
E. AGB explantation has little effect on long-term weight loss.

ANSWERS

1. B. The SLEEVEPASS randomized clinical equivalence trial published in 2018 showed nonequivalence of %EWL at 5 years for laparoscopic SG versus laparoscopic RYGB, with %EWL for SG of 49%, whereas

%EWL for RYGB was 57% (A).[1] Interestingly, the SLEEVEPASS trial showed overall lower %EWL for both procedures compared to other studies, with most studies showing a 5 year %EWL ranging from 51% to 65% for SG (B).[2,3] In a retrospective outcome study beyond 5 years, a failure rate defined as %EWL <50% occurred in nearly half of the SG patients at 7 years (C).[4] This same study showed the peak weight loss following SG is seen at 1 and 2 years and this number continues to decrease slowly in the years following (E).[4] Several studies have correlated volume of the gastric sleeve to initial %EWL; however, looking at longer-term results, the inverse relationship of sleeve volume to %EWL disappears (D).[5]

2. **A.** Multiple meta-analyses looking at the long-term weight loss outcomes of laparoscopic RYGB have shown that the 5-year %EWL is greater compared to SG, and conflicting data exists regarding the initial and midterm, defined as 3 to 5 years, %EWL (C).[2,6] The SLEEVEPASS trial assessed the clinical significance of this difference in %EWL and concluded that although the difference exists, it failed to meet their parameters for clinical significance, which was supported by similar findings in the SM-BOSS randomized clinical trial (A).[1,7] Multiple randomized controlled trials have shown that the 5-year %EWL for RYGB ranges from 57% to 77%, although the mean is closer to ~71% (B).[1-3,6] In patients with a BMI ≥50 kg/m^2, RYGB has shown to have inferior results with the majority of patients resulting with a final BMI ≥35 kg/m^2 and an overall failure rate ≥40%, thus failing to cure the obesity and obesity related comorbidities. For these patients, duodenal switch is suggested for superior results (D).[8] Regarding the resolution and improvement of obesity-related comorbidities such as type 2 diabetes, dyslipidemia, obstructive sleep apnea, and hypertension, multiple studies have resulted in inconclusive data, with some studies showing superior rates of resolution with RYGB while others showed no significant difference in comorbidity resolution (E).[2,6]

3. **C.** In a retrospective review looking at the long-term outcomes of BPD/DS, the %EWL seen at 5 years was higher than both SG and RYGB and this was consistent with all periods of evaluation, even out to 10 years (B). The %EWL with BPD/DS continues to increase even after the first 2 years, whereas the %EWL with SG and RYGB decreases after the first two years (C).[9] It was also seen that BPD/DS has greater %EWL in patients with a BMI ≤50 kg/m^2 versus those with a BMI ≥50 kg/m^2. It still remains the recommended procedure of choice for those patients with a BMI ≥50 kg/m^2 because it provides superior results compared to RYGB (E).[9] In comparing BPD alone to BPD/DS, studies have shown that although both achieve excellent long-term weight loss results, BPD/DS remains superior with %EWL being 10% to 25% greater at 10 years (D).[10,11] Multiple studies have shown that BPD/DS results in multiple nutritional deficiencies requiring long-term supplementation, most importantly protein malnutrition, vitamin D, vitamin K, zinc, as well as anemia, which tends to be seen more frequently with BPD alone (A).[10]

4. **D.** In a prospective case-matched study, it was shown that SG has a greater %EWL when compared to laparoscopic AGB at 5 years and multiple other studies have supported this finding (A).[12] The initial rate of weight loss for SG is greater than for AGB and this relationship persists even in the long-term data, with the %EWL with AGB tending to range between 45% and 55% at 10 years (B).[9,13] When extending the follow-up to 20 years, published data showed that the %EWL is maintained, although in clinical practice, this statistic seems somewhat variable (D).[13] AGB tends to have a higher revision rate between 20% and 50% over the longer term when compared to SG, although this rate has been shown to decrease as operative experience increased (C).[13,14] Band explantation is a fairly common occurrence, with rates found to be between 30% and 50%. The reasons for explantation include erosion, slippage, port site infection, weight loss failure, and intolerance. As previously mentioned, 20% to 50% of these patients undergo revision because no durable weight loss is seen after explantation (E).[14-16]

REFERENCES

1. Salminen P, Helmio M, Ovaska J, et al. Effect of laparoscopic sleeve gastrectomy vs laparoscopic Roux-en-Y gastric bypass on weight loss at 5 years among patients with morbid obesity: the SLEEVEPASS randomized clinical trial. *JAMA*. 2018;319:241-254.
2. Shoar S, Saber AA. Long-term and midterm outcomes of laparoscopic sleeve gastrectomy versus Roux-en-Y gastric bypass: a systematic review and meta-analysis of comparative studies. *Surg Obes Relat Dis*. 2017;13:170-180.
3. Sharples AJ, Mahawar K. Systematic review and meta-analysis of randomised controlled trials comparing

long-term outcomes of Roux-En-Y gastric bypass and sleeve gastrectomy. *Obes Surg.* 2019;30(2):664-672. doi:10.1007/s11695-019-04235-2

4. Sepulveda M, Alamo M, Saba J, Astorga C, Lynch R, Guzman H. Long-term weight loss in laparoscopic sleeve gastrectomy. *Surg Obes Relat Dis.* 2017;13(10):1676-1681.
5. Pañella C, Busto M, González A, et al. Correlation of gastric volume and weight loss 5 years following sleeve gastrectomy. *Obes Surg.* 2020. doi:10.1007/s11695-020-04445-z
6. Gu L, Huang X, Li S, et al. A meta-analysis of the medium- and long-term effects of laparoscopic sleeve gastrectomy and laparoscopic Roux-en-Y gastric bypass. *BMC Surg.* 2020;20(1):30. doi:10.1186/s12893-020-00695-x
7. Peterli R, Wölnerhanssen BK, Peters T, et al. Effect of laparoscopic sleeve gastrectomy vs laparoscopic roux-en-Y gastric bypass on weight loss in patients with morbid obesity: the SM-BOSS randomized clinical trial. *JAMA.* 2018;319:255-265.
8. Skogar ML, Sundbom M. Duodenal switch is superior to gastric bypass in patients with super obesity when evaluated with the bariatric analysis and reporting outcome system (BAROS). *Obes Surg.* 2017;27(9):2308-2316.
9. Zilberstein B, Santo MA, Carvalho MH. Critical analysis of surgical treatment techniques of morbid obesity. *Arq Bras Cir Dig.* 2019;32(3):e1450. doi:10.1590/0102-672020190001e1450
10. Sethi M, Chau E, Youn A, et al. Long-term outcomes after biliopancreatic diversion with and without duodenal switch: 2-, 5-, and 10-year data. *Surg Obes Relat Dis.* 2016;12(9):1697-1705.
11. Marceau P, Biron S, Hould FS, et al. Duodenal switch improved standard biliopancreatic diversion: a retrospective study. *Surg Obes Relat Dis.* 2009;5(1):43-47.
12. Johari Y, Ooi G, Burton P, et al. Long-term matched comparison of adjustable gastric banding versus sleeve gastrectomy: weight loss, quality of life, hospital resource use and patient-reported outcome measures. *Obes Surg.* 2020:30:214-223. doi:10.1007/s11695-019-04168-w
13. O'Brien PE, Hindle A, Brennan L, et al. Long-term outcomes after bariatric surgery: a systematic review and meta-analysis of weight loss at 10 or more years for all bariatric procedures and a single-centre review of 20-year outcomes after adjustable gastric banding. *Obes Surg.* 2019;29(1):3-14. doi:10.1007/s11695-018-3525-0
14. Froylich D, Abramovich-Segal T, Pascal G, et al. Long-term (over 10 years) retrospective follow-up of laparoscopic adjustable gastric banding. *Obes Surg.* 2017;28(4):976-980. doi:10.1007/s11695-017-2952-7.
15. Khoraki J, Moraes MG, Neto APF, Funk LM, Greenberg JA, Campos GM. et al. Long-term outcomes of laparoscopic adjustable gastric banding. *Am J Surg.* 2018; 215(1):97-103. doi:10.1016/j.amjsurg.2017.06.027.
16. Cho EJ, Seong MK. Explantation of adjustable gastric bands: an observation study of 10 years of experience at a tertiary center. *Yonsei Med J.* 2019;60(8):782. doi:10.3349/ymj.2019.60.8.782.

41

Obstructive Sleep Apnea

Derek T. Dirks, MD, and Kevin Reavis, MD

A 61-year-old male with a body mass index (BMI) of 41 kg/m^2 with a history of hypertension and type 2 diabetes mellitus reports having symptoms of daytime sleepiness and snoring at night. On exam, he is noted to have a thick neck and a short mandible. He is undergoing preoperative workup for bariatric surgery.

1. Which of the following is the most significant risk factor for obstructive sleep apnea (OSA) in this patient?

A. Age
B. Diabetes
C. Obesity
D. Male sex
E. Short mandible

2. What is the most accurate test for diagnosis of OSA?

A. Type 3 portable sleep monitoring
B. STOP-BANG questionnaire
C. Berlin questionnaire
D. Epworth Sleepiness Scale
E. Overnight polysomnography (PSG)

3. Regarding perioperative management in patients with OSA undergoing bariatric surgery, which of the following is correct?

A. Perioperative continuous positive airway pressure (CPAP) use is only recommended in patients with severe OSA.
B. Patients should start using their CPAP machine 48 hours before surgery.
C. Patients should not bring their own CPAP machine and mask to reduce the risk of contamination in the hospital.
D. Positional therapy is appropriate for patients with positional OSA who do not tolerate CPAP.
E. Nasal CPAP systems are inadequate for bariatric surgery patients.

4. Regarding postoperative outcomes in OSA after bariatric surgery, which of the following is correct?

A. Roux-en-Y gastric bypass (RYGB) results in resolution or improvement of OSA in 50% of patients.
B. Average reduction in apnea hypopnea index (AHI) about 12 months after bariatric surgery is around 30 events per hour.
C. There are several validated screening tools for resolution of OSA after bariatric surgery.
D. Purely restrictive procedures are significantly more efficacious than procedures with a malabsorptive component.
E. Despite improvement in OSA after bariatric surgery, obesity-hypoventilation syndrome (OHS) severity is unaffected by weight loss.

ANSWERS

1. C. The prevalence of OSA in the bariatric surgery population is 35% to 94%, with over 75% of studies reporting a prevalence >60%.[1] The prevalence of OSA in the general population appears to be increasing along with the increased prevalence of obesity.[2]

The most significant risk factor for OSA is obesity because over 70% of people with OSA are obese. Other risk factors associated with OSA include older age (plateauing in the sixth to seventh decades), male gender (2–3 times more common in males), and craniofacial and upper airway abnormalities.[3] There are many conditions that are associated with OSA; however, they are not considered risk factors. These include diabetes, OHS, congestive heart failure, hypertension, cardiovascular disease, atrial fibrillation, pulmonary hypertension, chronic lung disease, stroke, hypothyroidism, and polycystic ovary syndrome.

2. **E.** The gold standard for diagnosis of OSA is overnight PSG. PSG determines the frequency and duration of apneas and hypopneas, which is used to determine the AHI. An AHI of ≥5 events per hour is diagnostic of OSA in adults. OSA is further categorized as mild (AHI of 5–14.9), moderate (AHI of 15–29.9), and severe (AHI of ≥30).[1]

   Due to several factors (cost, limited sleep laboratory capacity, time management, etc.), routine PSG is an impractical screening tool and there are several options for preoperative OSA screening prior to bariatric surgery. Type 3 portable sleep monitoring devices measure fewer variables than PSG; however, their use is less costly and more convenient for patients because it can be used at home. Type 3 portable monitoring may be used to screen for OSA in preoperative bariatric surgery patients and is most reliable when moderate-to-severe OSA is suspected.[4]

   Validated preoperative OSA screening questionnaires include the STOP-BANG and Berlin questionnaires. The Epworth Sleepiness Scale measures sleepiness in ordinary life situations and is used to screen for excessive sleepiness. It is neither sensitive or specific for OSA, so it should not be used as a screening tool.[5]

   Elevated $PaCO_2$ has been investigated and is not an accurate predictor of OSA; however, it may be used as part of the diagnosis of OHS in patients with OSA.[1]

3. **D.** Perioperative use of CPAP in patients with OSA is effective in reducing perioperative pulmonary complications, and as a result it is the most prescribed treatment.[1] It is recommended that patients with moderate-to-severe OSA (defined as AHI ≥15/hour) be treated with CPAP in the perioperative period.[6] It is advised that patients start using their CPAP machines at least a few weeks prior to surgery, so that they can become accustomed to it and ensure that the fit is tolerable and effective. Patients should also bring their home CPAP machine with them for use in the hospital so that its efficacy can be assessed by continuously monitoring vital signs and SaO_2.[1]

   The decision to use a full facemask or nasal CPAP is based on patient comfort and efficacy. Patients with positional OSA who do not tolerate CPAP may be managed with the use of positional therapy. Positional OSA is diagnosed when the patient only experiences symptoms while lying on their back, which may be treated with various devices that encourage the patient to sleep on their side. These devices include commercial waistbands and homemade constructions that mimic the "tennis ball technique" (using a physical device to avoid the supine position).[7]

4. **B.** Bariatric surgery has been shown to be efficacious in symptomatic improvement and resolution of OSA. In the first 1 to 2 postop years, OSA has been objectively shown to improve by about 30 events per hour.[8] RYGB and sleeve gastrectomy show significant reduction in AHI by 78% and 81%, respectively.[9] A 2013 meta-analysis comparing OSA outcomes after bariatric surgery showed comparable rates of resolution/improvement of OSA after RYGB (79%), sleeve gastrectomy (86%), and adjustable gastric banding (77%).[10] A 2016 review showed significant postoperative reductions in AHI across all procedures; however, it showed a trend toward greater improvement after procedures with a malabsorptive component compared to purely restrictive procedures.[9]

   There are no validated screening tools for resolution of OSA postoperatively, so a polysomnogram is recommended to document resolution prior to discontinuing OSA treatment. The weight loss achieved after bariatric surgery not only improves OSA severity, but it also improves the severity of OHS.[1]

REFERENCES

1. Christel AL, de Raaff MD, Marguerite AW, et al. Perioperative management of obstructive sleep apnea in bariatric surgery: a consensus guideline. *Surg Obes Relat Dis.* 2017;13(7):1095-1109.
2. Peppard PE, Young T, Barnet JH, Palta M, Hagen EW, Hla KM. Increased prevalence of sleep-disordered breathing in adults. *Am J Epidemiol.* 2013;177(9):1006.

3. Young T, Skatrud J, Peppard PE. Risk factors for obstructive sleep apnea in adults. *JAMA*. 2004;291(16):2013.
4. Chesson AL, Berry RB, Pack A. Practice parameters for the use of portable monitoring devices in the investigation of suspected obstructive sleep apnea in adults. *Sleep*. 2003;26:907-913.
5. Kapur VK, Auckley DH, Chowdhuri S, et al. Clinical practice guideline for diagnostic testing for adult obstructive sleep apnea: an American Academy of Sleep Medicine clinical practice guideline. *J Clin Sleep Med*. 2017;13(3):479.
6. Kang SA, Kim GW, Yoon YS, Lee CS, Song JH. Airway management of patients undergoing laparoscopic gastric bypass surgery: a single center analysis. *Korean J Anesthesiol*. 2013;65:S117-S118.
7. de Vries GE, Hoekema A, Doff MH, et al. Usage of positional therapy in adults with obstructive sleep apnea. *J Clin Sleep Med*. 2015;11(2):131.
8. Ashrafian H, Toma T, Rowland SP, et al. Bariatric surgery or non-surgical weight loss for obstructive sleep apnoea? a systematic review and comparison of meta-analyses. *Obes Surg*. 2015;25:1239-1250.
9. Quintas-Nerves M, Preto J, Drummond M. Assessment of bariatric surgery efficacy on obstructive sleep apnea (OSA). *Sociedade Portuguesa de Pneumologia*. 2016;22(6): 331-336.
10. Sarkhosh K, Switzer NJ, El-Hadi M, et al. The impact of bariatric surgery on obstructive sleep apnea: a systematic review. *Obes Surg*. 2013;23:414-423.

42

Osteoarthritis

Derek T. Dirks, MD, and Kevin Reavis, MD

A 47-year-old female with a body mass index (BMI) of 46 kg/m^2 and a history of chronic osteoarthritis is undergoing preoperative evaluation for bariatric surgery. She reports chronic pain in her back and lower extremity joints. She is concerned that she may need to have joint replacement surgery in the future and would like to salvage the function that she has.

1. **The association between obesity and osteoarthritis is strongest with which joint?**

   A. Hip
   B. Sacroiliac
   C. Knee
   D. Intervertebral
   E. Ankle

2. **Which of the following is true about outcomes related to osteoarthritis after bariatric surgery?**

   A. Forty percent of patients with knee pain have improvement after successful bariatric surgery.
   B. Surgical weight loss can improve pain in non–weight-bearing joints with osteoarthritis.
   C. Initial improvement in knee and hip pain after bariatric surgery is not sustained long term.
   D. Gait is not improved after successful bariatric surgery.
   E. Bariatric surgery consistently improves outcomes for subsequent joint replacement surgery.

3. **Regarding inflammation, arthritis, and obesity, which of the following is correct?**

   A. Adipose tissue acts as an organ in the immune system by releasing leukocytes that can lead to joint damage.
   B. Proinflammatory cytokines do not change significantly after bariatric surgery.
   C. Obesity is not a significant risk factor for psoriatic arthritis.
   D. Surgical weight loss improves rates of remission of rheumatoid arthritis.
   E. Osteoarthritis is primarily due to mechanical "wear and tear" with little involvement of inflammation.

ANSWERS

1. **C.** The strongest association between osteoarthritis (OA) and obesity is at the knee joint. For women with high BMI, the relative risk of unilateral knee OA is increased 2- to 7-fold and 18-fold for bilateral knee OA. Obesity has been shown to increase the risk of knee OA through increased joint loading, low-grade meta-inflammation, reduced physical activity, and subsequent loss of protective muscle strength.[1] The relationship between OA and obesity is well established, and obesity is recognized as the main modifiable risk factor for OA of weight-bearing joints.[2] Figure 42-1 shows plain films that highlight the changes that occur with obesity on weight-bearing joints to include loss of joint space.

2. **B.** Surgical weight loss has been shown to significantly improve symptoms of osteoarthritis.[1] A systematic review of 3,837 patients showed that 73% of patients with knee pain had improvement after undergoing bariatric surgery. These patients also showed significant improvement in physical function and stiffness in the knees.[3] An observational study of 2,000 patients followed 3 years after bariatric surgery showed that

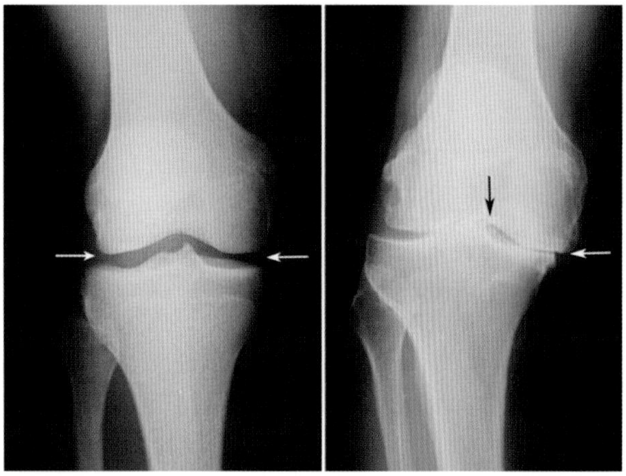

Figure 42-1 Knee joint changes that result from obesity. (Reproduced with permission from OrthoInfo. © American Academy of Orthopaedic Surgeons. https://orthoinfo.org/)

between 50% and 75% reported improvement in knee and hip pain at 1 year that was sustained out to 3 years postoperatively. Patients also had improvement in body pain and physical function at 1 year, but this improvement was not sustained at 3 years.[4] Surgical weight loss also improves gain with increased swing time, stride length, gait speed, and lower extremity range of motion.[5] Surgically induced weight loss results in improvement of health-related quality of life scores that are comparable with those of patients without joint pain. Interestingly, patients with osteoarthritis of non–weight-bearing joints do show improvement in pain at those sites. This is attributed to a decrease in the low-grade inflammation typically associated with obesity.[1] It is notable that despite the improvements in symptomatic outcomes described above, there is not a clear indication for bariatric surgery prior to joint replacement surgery. A recent systematic review that included over 11,000 patients who underwent bariatric surgery prior to total joint arthroplasty (TJA) showed no clear positive impact on early, short-term, or long-term complications after TJA.[6]

3. **D.** The relationships between obesity, metabolic syndrome, and chronic inflammation have been shown in several studies. Metabolic syndrome is associated with an increased inflammatory state, and the increased adipose tissue characteristic of it is one of the contributors. Adipose tissue acts as an endocrine and paracrine organ, releasing inflammatory cytokines, such as TNF-alpha, interleukin 6, C-reactive protein, and others.[2,7] Consequently, these proinflammatory cytokines have been shown to decrease after successful bariatric surgery.[8] While mechanical factors have a role in OA, proinflammatory cytokines also play a significant role in the production of proteolytic enzymes responsible for the degradation of the extracellular matrix of joint tissues.[9] Given these findings, it is not surprising that rheumatoid arthritis and psoriatic arthritis can have significant improvement after bariatric surgery. A cohort study of obese patients with rheumatoid arthritis showed improvement in the rate of moderate-to-high disease activity at 12 months postoperatively from 54% to 4%. Additionally, remission rates of rheumatoid arthritis improved from 26% to 74% postoperatively.[10] Obesity has been shown to be a significant risk factor for development of arthritis in patients with psoriasis. Loss of >5% baseline body weight increases the rate of achieving minimal disease activity in postoperative bariatric patients with psoriatic arthritis.[10]

REFERENCES

1. Nguyen, TN, Blackstone, RP, Morton JM, Ponce, J, Rosenthal, RJ. Chapter 33: Effects of bariatric surgery on non-metabolic disease. *The ASMBS Textbook of Bariatric Surgery*. Vol 1. Springer; 2015:378.
2. Gill RS, Al-Adra DP, Shi X, Sharma AM, Birch DW, Karmali S. The benefits of bariatric surgery in obese patients with hip and knee osteoarthritis: a systematic review. *Obes Rev*. 2011;12:1083-1089.
3. Groen VA, van de Graaf VA, Scholtes VA, Sprague S, van Wagensveld BA, Poolman RW. Effects of bariatric surgery for knee complaints in (morbidly) obese adult patients: a systematic review. *Obes Rev*. 2015;16(2):161.
4. King WC, Chen JY, Belle SH, et al. Change in pain and physical function following bariatric surgery for severe obesity. *JAMA*. 2016;315(13):1362.
5. Springer BD, Carter JT, McLawhorn AS, et al. Obesity and the role of bariatric surgery in the surgical management of osteoarthritis of the hip and knee: a review of the literature. *Surg Obes Relat Dis*. 2017;13(1):111.
6. Gu A, Cohen JS, Malahias MA, Lee D, Sculco PK, McLawhorn AS. The effect of bariatric surgery prior to lower-extremity total joint arthroplasty: a systematic review. *HSS J*. 2019;15(2):190-200. doi:10.1007/s11420-019-09674-2
7. Norata GD, Ongari M, Garlaschelli K, Raselli S, Grigore L, Catapano AL. Plasma resistin levels correlate with determinants of the metabolic syndrome. *Eur J Endocrinol*. 2007;156(2):279.
8. Richette P, Poitou C, Garnero P, et al. Benefits of massive weight loss on symptoms, systemic inflammation and cartilage turnover in obese patients with knee osteoarthritis. *Ann Rheum Dis*. 2011;70(1):139.
9. Liu-Bryan R, Terkeltaub R. Emerging regulators of the inflammatory process in osteoarthritis. *Nat Rev Rheumatol*. 2015;11(1):35-44.
10. Lespessailles E, Hammoud E, Toumi H, Ibrahim-Nasser N. Consequences of bariatric surgery on outcomes in rheumatic diseases. *Arthritis Res Ther*. 2019;21(1):83. doi:10.1186/s13075-019-1869-z

SECTION 8

Complications

43

Band Prolapse

Alex Clem, MD, and Pamela Masella, MD

1. A 35-year-old female with a history of a laparoscopic adjustable gastric band (LAGB) 3 years prior, who recently had fluid added to her band, presents to your clinic for evaluation of progressive postprandial nausea associated with intermittent regurgitation of undigested food. Her vital signs are HR 98, BP 123/80, RR 16, SpO2 99% on room air.

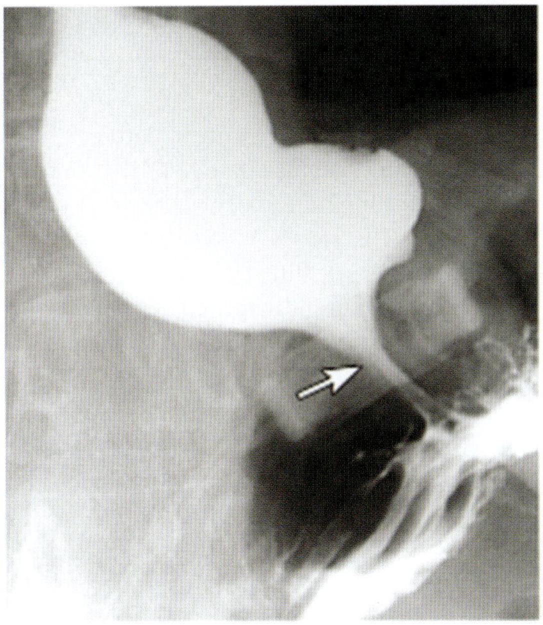

Figure 43-1 (Reproduced with permission from Levine MS, Carucci LR. Imaging of bariatric surgery: normal anatomy and postoperative complications. *Radiology.* 2014;270(2):327-341.)

You order an upper gastrointestinal (UGI) study (Figure 43-1). What is the next best step in management?

A. LAGB removal
B. Removal of fluid from band with repeat UGI evaluation
C. Endoscopic removal
D. Laparoscopic detorsion of the stomach

2. Two years later, this patient returns to the ER with oral (PO) intolerance and vomiting. She has been otherwise doing well with a current body mass index (BMI) of 29 kg/m^2. Her vital signs are a HR 120 bpm, BP 110/70, RR 18, and SpO2 on room air is 97%. Two liters of crystalloid are given in the ER with improvement of her HR to 100 bpm. Her initial labs show WBC 8k. Na+ 135. K+ 3.0. Cl 90. UA demonstrates a urine pH of 4.8.

You obtain an abdominal x-ray and the band is noted to have a phi angle of 75. What is the likely diagnosis?

A. Stomal stenosis
B. Band slippage
C. Band erosion
D. Malpositioned band

3. Her previous pathology was surgically corrected and 5 years later, this same patient presents with acute onset on nausea, vomiting, and epigastric pain. Her presurgery BMI was 40 and her current BMI is 32. She is tender in her epigastrium with peritonitis. Her vital signs are HR 130, BP 80/40 after 30 mL/kg of crystalloid fluid resuscitation,

temperature 38.7°C, RR 24, SaO2 94% on room air. Norepinephrine was initiated to maintain mean arterial pressure (MAP) of 65 mmHg.

What is the next best step in management of this patient?

A. Computed tomography (CT) scan with PO and intravenous (IV) contrast
B. Exploratory laparotomy
C. Diagnostic laparoscopy
D. Remove all fluid from the band

4. **A 45-year-old female with a history of an LAGB 2 years ago presents to the ER with nausea, vomiting, and epigastric pain. Her vital signs are HR 110, BP 100/70, RR 20, SpO2 94% on room air, and temperature 38.4°C. On physical exam, she is tender in the epigastrium and she has some erythema surrounding her port site incision. A plain film of her abdomen shows a phi angle of 42°. Labs show a WBC of 15.5.**

Which of the following is the most concerning complication?

A. Band slippage
B. Stomal stenosis
C. Band erosion
D. Port and tubing disruption

ANSWERS

1. **B.** Stomal stenosis/obstruction in gastric banding is the most common complication occurring in up to 14% of LAGB patients.[1-3,7] It most commonly occurs after a recent fill. This complication occurs when the band is too tight causing luminal narrowing or obstruction. Patients usually present with nausea, vomiting, abdominal pain, and inability to handle secretions. A UGI study may reveal dilation of the proximal stomach, narrowing at the site of the band, reflux into the esophagus, and slow transit to the distal stomach (see Figure 43-1). First-line treatment is to remove the fluid from the band to increase the luminal diameter. Most recommend removing all of the fluid initially and then refilling slowly after resolution of symptoms. In an LAGB, some degree of stomal stenosis is required to induce satiety and subsequent weight loss, so some utilize a more tailored approach, by removing small amounts of fluid. A UGI study after fluid removal can be done to confirm luminal diameter has increased sufficiently to allow passage of food. If the patient's symptoms do not resolve with complete removal of fluid from the band, removal may be necessary (Figure 43-2). Prolonged stomal stenosis and/or obstruction can result in pouch dilation, band slippage, or gastric volvulus.

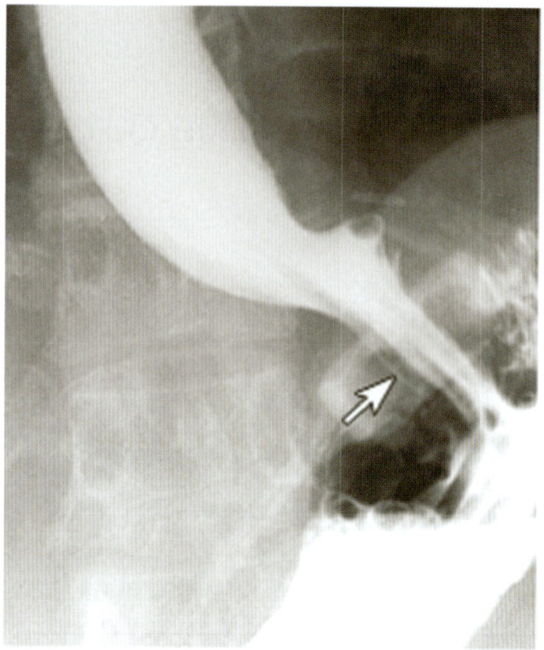

Figure 43-2 UGI demonstrating improved contrast progression after removal of fluid from band. (Reproduced with permission from Levine MS, Carucci LR. Imaging of bariatric surgery: normal anatomy and postoperative complications. Radiology. 2014;270(2):327-341.)

2. **B.** Gastric band slippage is one of the most common complications of LAGB occurring in 1% to 24% of patients.[5] The causes of slippage include recurrent vomiting, overfilling of the band, poor dietary habits, or poor surgical technique. Slippage often results in prolapse of the stomach fundus above the band, luminal narrowing, and/or obstruction. Symptoms include nausea, vomiting, and PO intolerance. In severe cases, band slippage can result in gastric volvulus, ischemia, and perforation. Some have utilized protocolized filling techniques under fluoroscopy and dietary education to reduce the incidence of band slippage. Diagnosis is routinely made by obtaining a plain abdominal film or UGI study and calculating the phi angle. The phi angle is measured between a vertical angle oriented with the spine and one along the long axis of the band. Normal is between 4 and 58 degrees (see Figure 43-3).[8] Additionally, the band should appear as a straight line, not as an "O," confirming that it is not rotated

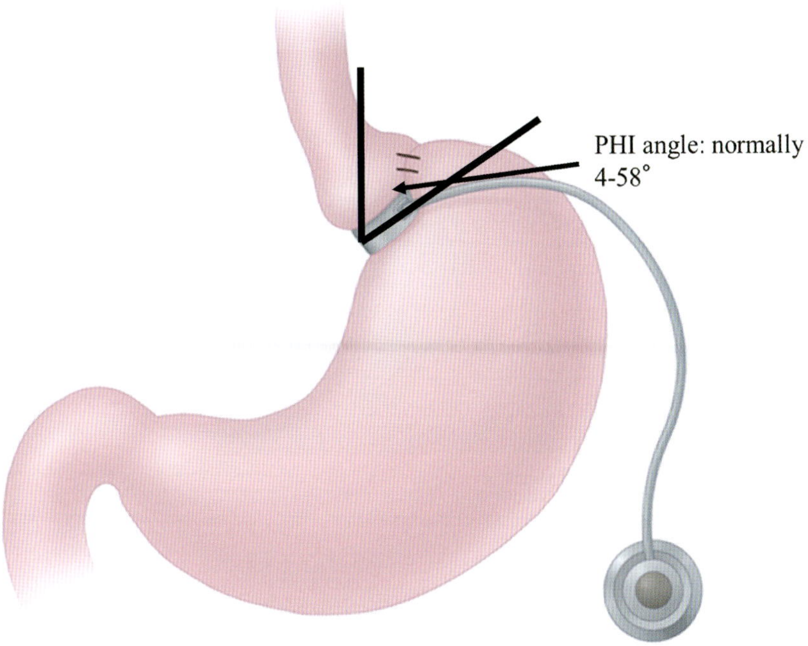

Figure 43-3 Normal band position and phi angle. (Modified with permission from Molmenti EP, de Santibañes M, de Santibañes E. *Liver Transplantation: Operative Techniques and Medical Management.* New York, NY: McGraw Hill; 2021.)

anteriorly or posteriorly (see Figures 43-4 and 43-5). In this patient, his symptoms and imaging demonstrating a phi angle >58 degrees are concerning for band slippage. There is no evidence of infection, hematemesis, or failure of weight loss that might indicate band erosion. Band malpositioning, which occurs by poor surgical technique and placement of the band around the gastric fat pad or more distal stomach, would be seen clearly on a UGI study or abdominal x-ray and may not cause nausea or vomiting. Treatment includes removal of fluid within the band, removal of the band if no resolution of symptoms, or repositioning of the band, although this has questionable utility.

3. **B.** This patient is hemodynamically unstable. Given her hemodynamic instability, she is unlikely to tolerate pneumoperitoneum necessary for diagnostic laparoscopy. A portable, upright film may confirm the diagnosis, but sending an unstable patient to the CT scanner is inappropriate. The patient has symptoms of gastric volvulus and possible ischemia likely from distal band slippage. Given her hemodynamic instability with failure to respond with fluid resuscitation and current vasopressor requirements, the patient should undergo exploratory laparotomy with removal of adjustable gastric band. If the stomach is obviously necrotic, then resection should be performed. If the stomach is of questionable viability, then the patient should be left open with a temporary abdominal closure and plans for re-look once stable.

4. **C.** This patient has clinical symptoms of obstruction and also infection, which is concerning for band erosion. Band erosion can cause infection symptoms at the port site as well. Additional symptoms include cessation of weight loss, weight regain, lack of satiety, abscess, and free perforation. Hematemesis can indicate erosion into the left gastric artery. In a systematic review of band erosion, rates have been reported from 0.23% to 32.65% with the majority of studies report rates <5%.[6] Median time for erosion was 22 months.[6] This is typically caused by high pressures generated by the inflated band causing pressure necrosis. Typically, the band only partially erodes; however, it can completely erode and cause intraluminal obstruction from distal migration. If the band is noted incidentally to be eroded, it should be removed due to risk of obstruction or GI bleeding. Diagnosis is usually made by upper endoscopy and visualization of the eroded band (see Figure 43-6). It can also be visualized on a CT or UGI scan by noting barium passage around the intraluminal portion of the eroded band. Treatment is to remove the band (see Figure 43-7). This can be done laparoscopically or endoscopically.

A

B

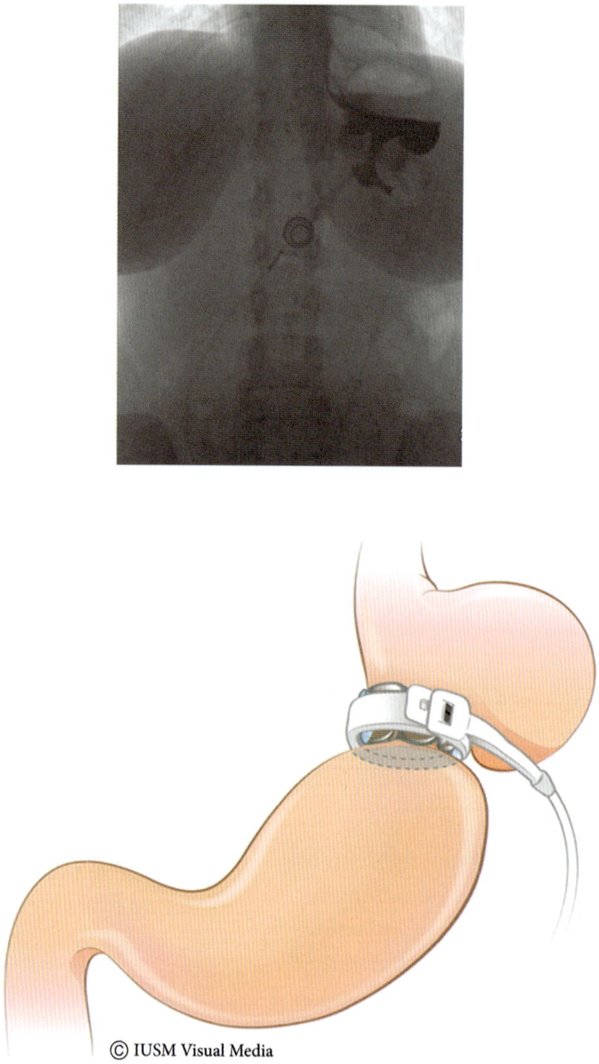

Figure 43-4 Anterior slippage. (A: Reproduced with permission from Zinner MJ, Ashley SW, Hines OJ: Maingot's Abdominal Operations, 13th ed. New York, NY: McGraw Hill; 2019. B: ©IUSM Visual Media.)

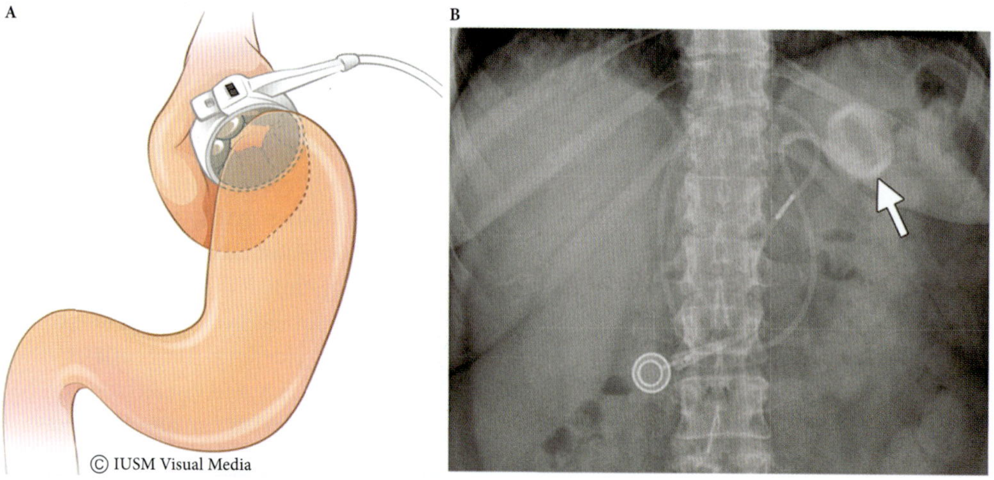

Figure 43-5 Posterior slippage. (A: ©IUSM Visual Media. B: Reproduced with permission from Sonavane SK, Menias CO, Kantawala KP, et al. Laparoscopic adjustable gastric banding: what radiologists need to know, *Radiographics*. 2012;32(4): 1161-1178.)

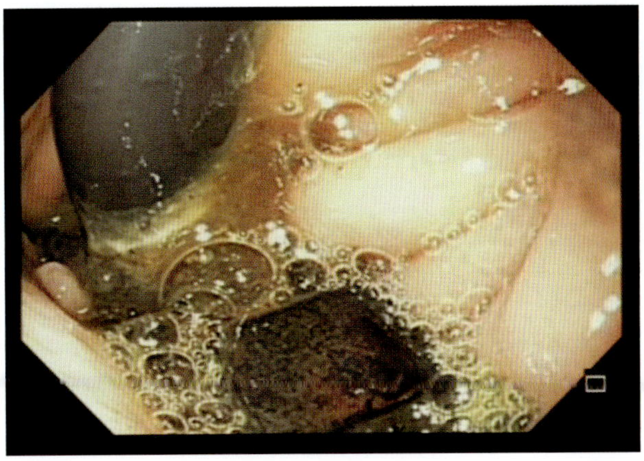

Figure 43-6 Band erosion. (Reproduced with permission from Dr. Eric Pauli.)

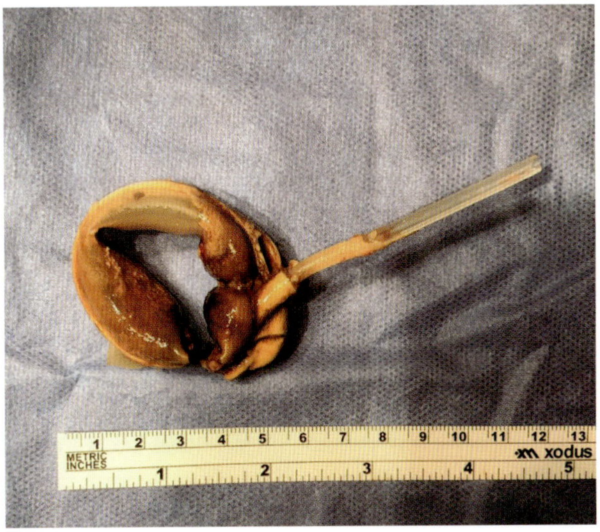

Figure 43-7 Band removal. (Reproduced with permission from Dr. Eric Pauli.)

A PHI angle between 4 and 58 degrees indicates that slippage, while worrisome, is not likely. Stromal stenosis can occur but given that she has had the band in for 2 years without issue and has not had a recent fill, this diagnosis is also unlikely. The silicone port and tubing can fracture or be injured, especially during fill attempts, resulting in erythema near the port site but this is unlikely to be painful or cause nausea, vomiting, and abdominal pain. Patients who present with tenderness and erythema near the port site have to have an erosion ruled out. An esophagogastroduodenoscopy (EGD) is diagnostic, and a CT may be suggestive with intraluminal portion of band.

REFERENCES

1. Blachar A, Blank A, Gavert N, Metzer U, Fluser G, Abu-Abeid S. Laparoscopic adjustable gastric banding surgery for morbid obesity: imaging of normal anatomic features and postoperative gastrointestinal complications. *AJR Am J Roentgenol.* 2007;188(2):472-479.
2. Gravante G, Araco A, Cervelli V. Laparoscopic adjustable gastric bandings. *Surg Endosc.* 2008;22:259-260. doi:10.1007/s00464-007-9574-4
3. Levine MS, Laura R. Carucci imaging of bariatric surgery: normal anatomy and postoperative complications. *Radiology.* 2014;270(2):327-341. doi:10.1148/radiol.13122520.
4. Blachar A, Blank A, Gavert N, Metzer U, Fluser G, Abu-Abeid S. Laparoscopic adjustable gastric banding surgery for morbid obesity: imaging of normal anatomic features and postoperative gastrointestinal complications. *AJR Am J Roentgenol.* 2007;188(2):472-479.
5. Egan RJ, Monkhouse SJ, Meredith HE, Bates SE, Morgan JD, Norton SA. The reporting of gastric band slip and related complications; a review of the literature. *Obes Surg.* 2011;21(8):1280-1288.
6. Egberts K, Brown WA, O'Brien PE. Systematic review of erosion after laparoscopic adjustable gastric banding. *Obes Surg.* 2011;21:1272-1279.
7. Spivak H, Favretti F. Avoiding postoperative complications with the LAP-BAND system. *Am J Surg.* 2002;184 (6B):31S-37S.
8. Mehanna MJ, Birjawi G, Moukaddam HA, Khoury G, Hussein M, Al-Kutoubi A. Complications of adjustable gastric banding, a radiological pictorial review. *Am J Roentgenol.* 2006;186(2):522–534. Crossref, Medline, Google Scholar.

44

Bypass Stricture

Carl M. Pesta, DO

A 42-year-old female with a body mass index (BMI) of 42 kg/m^2 is 5 weeks post Roux-en-Y gastric bypass (RYGB) via medical tourism in South America. The operative note that she carries states a 21-mm circular stapler was used for the gastrojejunostomy anastomosis. Five days prior to her presentation at your emergency department, she developed progressive intolerance to soft foods, and now to liquids to the point that she "cannot keep anything down." She complains of confusion, and difficulty walking.

1. On physical exam, the patient has horizontal nystagmus on lateral gaze, and an ataxic gait. After starting an intravenous (IV) infusion and administering hydration, which of the following is the most appropriate initial step in patient care?

A. Insta-glucose 40% gel 15 grams orally
B. Thiamine 100 mg IV
C. B12 1000 mcg intramuscular (IM)
D. Dextrose 5% in water 50 mL/hour
E. Calcium chloride IV

2. In regards to the gastrojejunostomy anastomosis in gastric bypass, which is correct?

A. A 21-mm circular stapler has better weight loss and a higher stricture rate than a 25-mm circular stapler.
B. There is a decreased anastomotic stricture rate in the linear stapled technique versus the circular stapled one.
C. A 21-mm circular stapler has equivalent weight loss and a higher stricture rate than a 25-mm circular stapler.
D. A retrocolic Roux limb has a higher stricture rate than an antecolic one.
E. The handsewn technique takes significantly longer time to create.

3. In regards to endoscopic dilation of a gastro-jejunostomy stricture, which of the following is correct?

A. Gastric perforation is a complication in 10% of attempts.
B. Balloon dilation is recommended to 20 mm for best results.
C. Eighty-eight percent of strictures are resolved with one dilation.
D. Treatments prior to 90 days have better results than after 90 days.
E. A marginal ulcer is a contradiction to dilation.

4. Regarding marginal ulcers, strictures, and perforation, which of the following is correct?

A. Proton pump inhibitors decrease the incidence of marginal ulcers and therefore stricture formation.
B. The incidence of perforation is inversely proportional to the number of dilations performed.
C. An ischemic segment (2-cm stricture) decreases the incidence of successful endoscopic balloon dilation.
D. Abdominal pain is a rare complaint in patients with a marginal ulcer.
E. Heavy smokers have 2 times greater incidence of marginal ulcers than light smokers.

ANSWERS

1. **B.** This patient has evidence of Wernicke's encephalopathy. Wernicke's encephalopathy is a well-known central nervous system complication of thiamine (vitamin B_1) deficiency. It is classically manifested by the triad of confusion, ophthalmoplegia, and ataxia.[1] With prolonged vomiting after bariatric surgery, Wernicke's encephalopathy usually occurs within 2 to 8 months postoperatively, especially in patients with a weight loss >7 kg per month.[2] Wernicke's encephalopathy has occurred as early as 2 weeks after bariatric surgery and as late as 20 years later.[3] Treatment is specific to the replacement of thiamine (B_1) 50 mg to 100 mg given parenterally before starting infusions is recommended. Glucose administered prior to giving thiamine can precipitate or worsen the encephalopathy. Recovery begins promptly starting with visual symptoms during the first day with return of normal gait and confusion within the next few days to weeks.[4] Failure to treat a thiamine deficiency aggressively can result in permanent neurologic deficits. Bariatric patients presenting with vomiting and oral (PO) intolerance should have a thorough neurologic exam. A diagnosis of a stricture can be made with an upper gastrointestinal swallow series and a small amount of contrast (100cc max). The contrast used should be thin barium and not gastrograffin because the aspiration of gastrograffin can be fatal.

2. **C.** Creation of the gastrojejunostomy for gastric bypass surgery has many techniques including handsewn and stapled methods. In the stapled category, there is a linear stapled technique with a handsewn closure and a circular stapled technique. Finally, the circular stapled method has the variety of different sized diameters, most commonly 21 mm and 25 mm. A metanalysis of these different techniques has shown that the highest stricture rate occurs with the 21-mm circular stapler. With this, there has been no statistical difference in weight loss associated with the 21 mm versus 25 mm stapler.[5] There have been multiple studies showing variable results of a linear stapler compared to circular stapled anastomosis in regards to stricture, weight loss, and operative time. No consensus has occurred in regards to any of those outcomes.[6] Additionally, the ante colic versus retro colic nature of the Roux limb has a bearing on outcomes. The retrocolic placement shows a significantly decreased rate of stricture formation most likely attributed to the reduction in tension by placing the limb in this anatomic position versus ante colic.[7]

3. **D.** Gastric stricture is a well-known complication following gastric bypass. It has a reported incidence of around 6% but it can be as high as 18% in a 21-mm circular stapled technique.[8,9] Through the scope balloon dilation is a well-documented intervention for this complication. Endoscopic dilation has an overall success rate of approximately 60% with the first dilation, meaning approximately 40% of patients require more than one dilation.[8] Timing of dilation is also important to overall successful management of strictures. We know that stenosis diagnosed and treated in the first 90 days has a success rate of 98% resolution without surgery, whereas those after 90 days have a 40% incidence of revisional surgery to correct. The risk of perforation during a single dilation is 2% to 4%.[9–11] The dilation is performed up to 15 mm initially.[12] A marginal ulcer is not a contraindication to dilation; however, it does increase the risk of perforation.

4. **C.** While endoscopic dilations are safe and mostly successful, the rate of perforation positively correlates with the number of dilation sessions.[13] An ischemic segment, defined as a stricture greater than 2 cm in the jejunum, has a strong correlation with the failure of endoscopic therapy and thus may warrant surgical revision.[13] Strictures caused by marginal ulcers can also be due to smoking, *helicobacter pylori* infection, and a gastric fistula to the remnant stomach. This fistulous connection allows more stomach acid to brought to the anastomosis resulting in an ulcer and possibly a stricture. Use of a proton pump inhibitor has not proven to decrease the formation of marginal ulcers.[14] Light, moderate, and heavy smokers have the same rate of marginal ulcer formation, 17.4%, 17.1%, and 17.9%, respectively. It is imperative that patients must stop smoking prior to surgery and refrain from smoking afterward.[15] Patients should also avoid nonsteroidal anti-inflammatory drug (NSAID) medications and be tested for *helicobacter pylori* infection. If a gastro-gastric fistula is the cause of the stricture, the fistula must be removed, which usually requires a revision of the gastric pouch and gastro-jejunal anastomosis. Abdominal pain is one of the most common complaints when it comes to marginal ulcers (n = 35/59).[16] This complaint alone warrants initiation

of treatment and workup. Patients may also present with hematemesis, melena, and if the ulcer results in a stricture, heartburn, and regurgitation.

REFERENCES

1. Victor M, Adams RD, Collins GH, eds. *The Wernicke-Korsakoff Syndrome and Related Neurologic Disorders Due to Alcoholism and Malnutrition*. Philadelphia: FA Davis; 1989.
2. Toth C, Voll C. Wernicke's encephalopathy following gastroplasty for morbid obesity. *Can J Neurol Sci*. 2001;28: 89-92.
3. Shuster MH, Vazquez JA. Nutritional concerns related to Roux-en-Y gastric bypass: what every clinician needs to know. *Crit Care Nurs Q*. 2005;28:227-260.
4. Diamond I. Nutritional disorders of the nervous system. In: Wyngaarden JB, Smith LH, eds. *Cecil Textbook of Medicine*. 19th ed. Harcourt Brace Jovanovich, Inc; 1992:2125.
5. Markar SR, Penna M, Venkat-Ramen V, Karthikesalingam A, Hashemi M. Influence of circular stapler diameter on postoperative stenosis after laparoscopic gastrojejunal anastomosis in morbid obesity. *Surg Obes Relat Dis*. 2012;8(2):230-235. doi:10.1016/j.soard.2011.03.016.
6. Jiang HP, Lin LL, Jiang X1, Qiao HQ. Meta-analysis of hand-sewn versus mechanical gastrojejunal anastomosis during laparoscopic Roux-en-Y gastric bypass for morbid obesity. *Int J Surg*. 2016;32:150-157. doi:10.1016/j.ijsu.2016.04.024.
7. Ribeiro-Parenti L, Arapis K, Chosidow D, Dumont JL, Demetriou M, Marmuse JP. Gastrojejunostomy stricture rate: comparison between antecolic and retrocolic laparoscopic Roux-en-Y gastric bypass. *Surg Obes Relat Dis*. 2015;11(5):1076-1084. doi:10.1016/j.soard.2015.01.019.
8. Baumann AJ, Mramba LK, Hawkins RB, et al. Endoscopic dilation of bariatric RNY anastomotic strictures: a systematic review and meta-analysis. *Obes Surg*. 2018;28(12):4053-4063. doi:10.1007/s11695-018-3491-6.
9. Carrodeguas L, Szomstein S, Zundel N, Lo Menzo E, Rosenthal R. Gastrojejunal anastomotic strictures following laparoscopic Roux-en-Y gastric bypass surgery: analysis of 1291 patients. *Surg Obes Relat Dis*. 2006;2(2): 92-97.
10. Yimcharoen P, Heneghan H, Chand B, et al. Successful management of gastrojejunal strictures after gastric bypass: is timing important? *Surg Obes Relat Dis*. 2012;8(2):151-157. doi:10.1016/j.soard.2011.01.043.
11. Almby K, Edholm D. Anastomotic strictures after Roux-en-Y gastric bypass: a cohort study from the Scandinavian obesity surgery registry. *Obes Surg*. 2019;29(1):172-177. doi:10.1007/s11695-018-3500-9.
12. Peifer KJ, Shiels AJ, Azar R, Rivera RE, Eagon JC, Jonnalagadda S. Successful endoscopic management of gastrojejunal anastomotic strictures after Roux-en-Y gastric bypass. *Gastrointest Endosc*. 2007;66(2):248-252.
13. de Moura EGH, Orso IRB, Aurélio EF, de Moura ETH, de Moura DTH, Santo MA. Factors associated with complications or failure of endoscopic balloon dilation of anastomotic stricture secondary to Roux-en-Y gastric bypass surgery. *Surg Obes Relat Dis*. 2016;12(3):582-586. doi:10.1016/j.soard.2015.11.006.
14. Wennerlund J, Gunnarsson U, Strigård K, Sundbom M. Acid-related complications after laparoscopic Roux-en-Y gastric bypass: risk factors and impact of proton pump inhibitors. *Surg Obes Relat Dis*. 2020;S1550-7289(20):30014-9. doi:10.1016/j.soard.2020.01.005.
15. Dittrich L, Schwenninger MV, Dittrich K, Pratschke J, Aigner F, Raakow J. Marginal ulcers after laparoscopic Roux-en-Y gastric bypass: analysis of the amount of daily and lifetime smoking on postoperative risk. *Surg Obes Relat Dis*. 2020;16(3):389-396. doi:10.1016/j.soard.2019.11.022.
16. Moon RC, Teixeira AF, Goldbach M, Jawad MA. Management and treatment outcomes of marginal ulcers after Roux-en-Y gastric bypass at a single high volume bariatric center. *Surg Obes Relat Dis*. 2014;10(2):229-234. doi:10.1016/j.soard.2013.10.002.

45

Gastric Bypass Leaks

Keitaro Nakamoto, MD

A 45-year-old morbidly obese female presents 7 days after undergoing a laparoscopic Roux-en-Y gastric bypass complaining of epigastric pain and low-grade fever. She has been tolerating a full liquid diet. A computed tomography (CT) scan performed with intravenous (IV) contrast and upper gastrointestinal (GI) contrast study are both negative. Vital signs show a heart rate of 123 and a systolic blood pressure of 110.

1. Which of the following is the next best course of action?

A. Discharge home
B. Esophagogastroduodenoscopy (EGD)
C. Diagnostic laparoscopy
D. Admit, nothing by mouth (NPO), IV fluids

2. What is the most commonly reported location for a leak after gastric bypass?

A. Gastric pouch staple line
B. Jejunojejunostomy
C. Remnant stomach staple line
D. Gastrojejunal anastomosis

3. Which of the following is true about the data to decrease the incidence of leaks from a gastric bypass?

A. Favors the use of staple line reinforcement
B. Favors the use of fibrin sealants
C. Intraoperative endoscopy shows benefit
D. There is no difference in leak rates amongst methods of creating the gastrojejunostomy

4. Which statement is true regarding imaging patients post-gastric bypass?

A. CT with PO contrast should be performed.
B. CT scan with IV and PO contrast has a high level of sensitivity to diagnose leaks.
C. Upper GI studies should be performed in the upright position.
D. Contrast filling of the excluded stomach is normal.

ANSWERS

1. C. Surgeons should have a low threshold for exploration in post-gastric bypass patients because bariatric patients may decompensate and succumb to sepsis due to their comorbidities. An upper GI study and CT scan can be negative in up to one-third of patients with a leak, even when combined.[1] Heart rate exceeding 120 bpm may be the most reliable sign of leak.[2] The patient's workup should evaluate for a pulmonary embolism, a myocardial infarction, bleeding, hypovolemia, and a leak. The hemodynamically unstable patient needs operative intervention. Hemodynamically stable patients with a persistent tachycardia also need a surgical exploration to make sure that a leak is not missed. Of the options given, surgical exploration is the best choice.

2. D. Leaks after gastric bypass can happen in any location but are most commonly reported at the gastrojejunostomy.[1,3–5] The majority of leaks at the gastrojejunostomy can be treated conservatively, especially if the patient is not tachycardic and hemodynamically normal. This may be due to low acid production in the gastric pouch and a lack of biliopancreatic reflux from the long Roux limb.[6] Conversely, leaks from the jejunojejunostomy are discovered later and result in higher mortality rates. In one study, jejunojejunostomy leaks were associated with a 40% mortality rate, with a longer median detection time compared to gastrojejunostomy leaks (4 vs. 2 days, $P = 0.037$).[7]

3. **D.** There have been several studies comparing circular stapler, linear stapler, and handsewn anastomosis for the gastrojejunostomy and they have shown no significant differences in leak rates. However, circular staplers have shown to be associated with higher incidence of wound infections and strictures, especially with the 21-mm diameter circular stapler.[8–13]

   There is no high level evidence that proves effectiveness of staple line reinforcement, fibrin sealant, or intraoperative endoscopy in reducing the risk of leak.[5] While there is some data that suggests intraoperative endoscopy can find leaks earlier and reduce postoperative complications,[14] more comprehensive studies do not confirm this.[15] Staple line reinforcement does help reduce bleeding but not leaks.[16]

4. **A.** A CT scan does not have a consistently high level of sensitivity in diagnosing leaks in this patient population. Even when upper GI study and CT scan is combined, up to one-third of patients will have both studies interpreted as negative despite them having a leak.[1] Thus, if clinical suspicion remains, surgeons should have a low threshold to take the patient for a surgical exploration even if imaging is negative. When a CT scan is performed, PO contrast should ideally be given, to differentiate the gastric pouch and Roux limb from the excluded stomach and biliopancreatic limb that typically do not fill with contrast. The volume of given oral contrast material will depend on the patient's tolerance and symptoms; however, in general, 100 to 300 cc is sufficient. The collapsed excluded stomach should be identified, because failure to do so may could result in the misdiagnosis of this structure as an abscess.[17] Distention or contrast filling of the excluded stomach may signify reflux due to distal obstruction, jejunojejunostomy swelling, or gastro-gastric fistula, and is abnormal.[18] Upper GI studies should be performed in the supine position, to facilitate adequate distention of the gastric pouch. The left posterior oblique (LPO) position allows the most optimal assessment of the proximal anastomosis.[19]

REFERENCES

1. Gonzalez R, Sarr MG, Smith CD, et al. Diagnosis and contemporary management of anastomotic leaks after gastric bypass for obesity. *J Am Coll Surg*. 2007;204(1):47-55.
2. Buckwalter JA, Herbst CA Jr. Leaks occurring after gastric bariatric operations. *Surgery*. 1988;103(2):156-160.
3. Marshall JS, Srivastava A, Gupta SK, Rossi TR, DeBord JR. Roux-en-Y gastric bypass leak complications. *Arch Surg*. 2003;138(5):520-523; discussion 523-524.
4. Csendes A, Burgos AM, Braghetto I. Classification and management of leaks after gastric bypass for patients with morbid obesity: a prospective study of 60 patients. *Obes Surg*. 2012;22(6):855-862.
5. Kim J, Azagury D, Eisenberg D, et al. ASMBS position statement on prevention, detection, and treatment of gastrointestinal leak after gastric bypass and sleeve gastrectomy, including the roles of imaging, surgical exploration, and nonoperative management. *Surg Obes Relat Dis*. 2015;11(4):739-748.
6. Csendes A, Burdiles P, Burgos AM, Maluenda F, Diaz JC. Conservative management of anastomotic leaks after 557 open gastric bypasses. *Obes Surg*. 2005;15(9):1252-1256.
7. Lee S, Carmody B, Wolfe L, et al. Effect of location and speed of diagnosis on anastomotic leak outcomes in 3828 gastric bypass cases. *J Gastrointest Surg*. 2007;11(6):708-713.
8. Finks JF, Carlin A, Share D, et al. Effect of surgical techniques on clinical outcomes after laparoscopic gastric bypass—results from the Michigan Bariatric Surgery Collaborative. *Surg Obes Relat Dis*. 2011;7(3):284-289.
9. Giordano S, Salminen P, Biancari F, Victorzon M. Linear stapler technique may be safer than circular in gastrojejunal anastomosis for laparoscopic Roux-en-Y gastric bypass: a meta-analysis of comparative studies. *Obes Surg*. 2011;21(12):1958-1964.
10. Burla L, Weibel P, Baum C, Huber M, Gurtler T, Weber M. Linear versus circular stapler for gastrojejunal anastomosis in laparoscopic Roux-en-Y gastric bypass: an analysis of 211 cases. *Surg Res Pract*. 2020;2020:4090797.
11. Leyba JL, Llopis SN, Isaac J, Aulestia SN, Bravo C, Obregon F. Laparoscopic gastric bypass for morbid obesity-a randomized controlled trial comparing two gastrojejunal anastomosis techniques. *JSLS*. 2008;12(4):385-388.
12. Bohdjalian A, Langer FB, Kranner A, Shakeri-Leidenmuhler S, Zacherl J, Prager G. Circular- vs. linear-stapled gastrojejunostomy in laparoscopic Roux-en-Y gastric bypass. *Obes Surg*. 2010;20(4):440-446.
13. Suggs WJ, Kouli W, Lupovici M, Chau WY, Brolin RE. Complications at gastrojejunostomy after laparoscopic Roux-en-Y gastric bypass: comparison between 21- and 25-mm circular staplers. *Surg Obes Relat Dis*. 2007;3(5):508-514.

14. Valenzuela-Salazar C, Rojano-Rodriguez ME, Romero-Loera S, et al. Intraoperative endoscopy prevents technical defect related leaks in Roux-en-Y gastric bypass: a randomized control trial. *Int J Surg*. 2018;50:11-17.
15. Minhem MA, Safadi BY, Tamim H, Mailhac A, Alami RS. Does intraoperative endoscopy decrease complications after bariatric surgery? Analysis of American College of Surgeons national surgical quality improvement program database. *Surg Endosc*. 2019;33(11): 3629-3634.
16. Ichter ZA, Voeller L, Rivas H, Khoury H, Azagury D, Morton JM. Buttressing of the EEA stapler during gastrojejuncal anastomosis decreases rate of bleeding-related complications for laparoscopic gastric bypass. *Surg Obes Relat Dis*. 2017;13(5):802-806.
17. Levine MS, Carucci LR. Imaging of bariatric surgery: normal anatomy and postoperative complications. *Radiology*. 2014;270(2):327-341.
18. Bassiouny RH, Chalabi NaM. Value of contrast-enhanced multidetector computed tomography in imaging of symptomatic patients after laparoscopic Roux-en-Y gastric bypass and laparoscopic sleeve gastrectomy. *Egypt J Radiol Nucl Med*. 2020;51(1):25.
19. Carucci LR, Turner MA, Yu J. Imaging evaluation following Roux-en-Y gastric bypass surgery for morbid obesity. *Radiol Clin North Am*. 2007;45(2):247-260.

46

Sleeve Leak

Amy Rosenbluth, MD and Daniel J. Scott, MD

A 48-year-old male with a body mass index (BMI) of 50 kg/m^2 and a medical history significant for obstructive sleep apnea (OSA) presents to your office with an interest in bariatric surgery. After a complete preoperative workup and counseling, he has elected to undergo a sleeve gastrectomy. The procedure is completed without incident and his postoperative stay is uncomplicated. However, he presents back to your office on postoperative day 7 complaining of worsening epigastric pain, nausea, and vomiting. On intake, the triage nurse notes that he is afebrile but tachycardic to 120.

1. For the described patient, what about their presentation is most concerning and predictive for a leak?

A. Afebrile
B. Epigastric pain
C. Nausea
D. Tachycardia

2. Regarding the risk of staple line leak after sleeve gastrectomy, which of the following is correct?

A. Bougie size does affect the risk of staple line leaks.
B. Buttressing material reduces the risk of staple line leaks.
C. Oversewing the staple line reduces the risk of staple line leaks.
D. Sleeve gastrectomy has a higher leak risk as compared to gastric bypass.

3. Where is the most common location to have a sleeve leak and what is its likely anatomic cause?

A. Staple line leaks occur most frequently at the incisura as a result of a narrowed region at the incisura.
B. Staple line leaks occur most frequently at the incisura as a result of a large retained fundus.
C. Staple line leaks occur most frequently just below the gastroesophageal (GE) junction as a result of a narrowed region at the incisura.
D. Staple line leaks occur most frequently just below the GE junction as a result of a large retained fundus.

4. Which of the following is most likely to prevent a late occurring sleeve leak from healing?

A. Poor vascular supply in the area of the leak
B. Suboptimal patient nutrition
C. Excess inflammation
D. A sleeve that is twisted around its longitudinal axis

ANSWERS

1. D. Sustained tachycardia in a sleeve gastrectomy patient should be considered a leak until proven otherwise. One review of patients found that tachycardia was a presenting symptom in 100% of their leak patients. Other findings associated were a leukocytosis and elevated C-reactive protein. None of the patients in that study presented with abdominal pain or nausea.[1] While tachycardia can be a marker of other pathologies (bleeding, cardiac event, pneumonia, pulmonary embolism, etc.), sustained tachycardia is one of the most commonly associated finding with a sleeve leak. Epigastric pain and nausea may or may not be present. Additionally, if present, the pain may not be confined to the epigastric region, it may be diffused or radiating from the back or shoulder. And abdominal pain may represent a pathological finding or be present as a normal part of the postoperative course.[2] If a sleeve leak is suspected based on clinical findings, further workup can be considered with imaging or operative exploration based on the stability of the patient.[3] Certainly, hemodynamically unstable patients need operative intervention, but patients with persistent tachycardia >120, hemodynamic stability, and a negative workup should also undergo surgical exploration.

2. **A.** A bougie size of >40 Fr is associated with a lower leak rate. One review analyzing risk factors for sleeve leaks found that a bougie size >40 Fr was associated with a leak rate of 0.92%, whereas a smaller bougie size had a rate of 2.67%.[4]

   There have been many reviews analyzing the use of buttressing material and its relation to bleeding and leaks. Many of these studies have been underpowered, and frequently their interpretation can be made difficult by multiple products and techniques. However, most reviews show that buttressing does not reduce the risk of staple line leaks.[5,6] Similarly, oversewing the staple line has not shown to have a benefit of reducing leaks.[7] There is a similar risk of staple line leaks between bypasses and sleeves; a large review revealed the leak rate after laparoscopic gastric bypass to be 0.8% and the leak rate of sleeve gastrectomy to be 0.7%.[8] The ASMBS quotes the range between 0.1% and 8.3% for laparoscopic and open gastric bypasses and between 0% and 7% for sleeve gastrectomies.[3]

3. **C.** Most sleeve gastrectomy leaks (up to 85%) occur just below the GE junction. While there can be many causes for a leak, the anatomical cause would be a narrow incisura angularis. The sleeve, unlike the gastric bypass, can create a high intraluminal pressure due to its long, narrowed anatomy. Further narrowing at the incisura can cause radial force at the GE junction that surpasses the staple line.[3,9] A retained fundus can lead to lower than expected weight loss, but is not an anatomical cause of leaks.

4. **D.** There are many different algorithms for management of sleeve leaks, and management should be tailored to the presentation of the patient. Certainly, a patient presenting septic with peritonitis warrants a return to the operating room for washout and drainage. More stable patients can often have less invasive management. In stable but symptomatic patients, there are several endoscopic options including stenting, suturing, clipping, and endovac therapies that have proven useful in management of sleeve leaks. Some delayed leaks or mircroperforation may have self-sealed at time of presentation, and they may present only with an abscess requiring interventional radiology (IR) drainage. When evaluating these patients, it is important to remember that management should include fluid resuscitation, antibiotics, source control (either by drainage, or operative/endoscopic intervention), and nutritional support.[3]

   Treating sleeve leaks can be challenging due to the high pressure within the lumen of the sleeve configuration. This is because there are sphincters at both ends of the sleeve. Leaks that occur in sleeves that have a distal stenosis, kink, or twist are particularly difficult to manage.[10] These leaks are less likely to heal by endoscopic or primary repair means only.[11] The lesions seem to raise the intraluminal pressure even more making a repair less likely to be successful. These patients would require a conversion to a RYGB to, in part, reduce the intraluminal pressure, which would allow a better chance for healing.[12]

REFERENCES

1. Jurowich C, Thalheimer A, Seyfried F, et al. Gastric leakage after sleeve gastrectomy—clinical presentation and therapeutic options. *Langenbecks Arch Surg.* 2011;396:981. doi:10.1007/s00423-011-0800-0
2. Burgos AM, Braghetto I, Csendes A, et al. gastric leak after laparoscopic-sleeve gastrectomy for obesity. *Obes Surg.* 2009;19:1672-1677. doi:10.1007/s11695-009-9884-9
3. Kim J, Azagury D, Eisenberg D, et al. ASMBS position statement on prevention, detection, and treatment of gastrointestinal leak after gastric bypass and sleeve gastrectomy, including the roles of imaging, surgical exploration, and nonoperative management. *Surg Obes Relat Dis.* 2015;11(4):739-748.

4. Yuval JB, Mintz Y, Cohen MJ, et al. The effects of bougie caliber on leaks and excess weight loss following laparoscopic sleeve gastrectomy. Is there an ideal bougie size? *Obes Surg.* 2013;23:1685-1691. doi:10.1007/s11695-013-1047-3
5. Chen B, Kiriakopoulos A, Tsakayannis D, et al. Reinforcement does not necessarily reduce the rate of staple line leaks after sleeve gastrectomy. a review of the literature and clinical experiences. *Obes Surg.* 2009;19:166-172. doi:10.1007/s11695-008-9668-7
6. Giannopoulos GA, Tzanakis NE, Rallis GE, et al. Staple line reinforcement in laparoscopic bariatric surgery: does it actually make a difference? A systematic review and meta-analysis. *Surg Endosc.* 2010;24:2782-2788. doi:10.1007/s00464-010-1047-5
7. Musella M, et al. Laparoscopic sleeve gastrectomy. Do we need to oversew the staple line? *Ann Ital Chir.* 2011;82(4):273-277.
8. Hutter MM, et al. First report from the American College of Surgeons–Bariatric Surgery Center Network: laparoscopic sleeve gastrectomy has morbidity and effectiveness positioned between the band and the bypass. *Ann Surg.* 2011;254(3):410.
9. Nguyen NT, Armstrong C. Management of gastrointestinal leaks and fistula. In: Nguyen N, Blackstone R, Morton J, Ponce J, Rosenthal R, eds. *The ASMBS Textbook of Bariatric Surgery.* New York: Springer; 2015.
10. Vilallonga R, Himpens J, van de Vrande S., Laparoscopic management of persistent strictures after laparoscopic sleeve gastrectomy. *Obes Surg.* 2013; 23(10):1655-1661.
11. Curro G, Komaei I, Lazzara C, et al. Management of staple line leaks following laparoscopic sleeve gastrectomy for morbid obesity. *Surg Technol Int.* 2018;33:111-118.
12. Smith ZL, Park KH, Llano EM, et al. Outcomes of endoscopic leaks and fistulae after sleeve gastrectomy: results from a large multicenter US cohort. *Surg Obes Relat Dis.* 2019;15(6):850-855.

47

Reflux after Sleeve

Morgan Bresnick, MD

A 50-year-old female presents for evaluation for weight loss surgery. Her initial body mass index (BMI) is 45 kg/m^2 and she additionally suffers from the weight-related comorbidities of type 2 diabetes mellitus, hypertension, and gastroesophageal reflux disease (GERD). Her GERD has been mild and well controlled with H2 blockers as needed. She was evaluated for surgery in a multidisciplinary bariatric clinic and found to be a good candidate. After careful review of the surgical options, she opted for a laparoscopic sleeve gastrectomy (LSG).

1. **Given her history of GERD you opted to perform an endoscopy as part of her preoperative workup. Which of the following represents an absolute contraindication to sleeve gastrectomy?**
   A. Presence of a 4-cm sliding hiatal hernia
   B. Bile reflux gastritis
   C. LA grade D esophagitis
   D. Short-segment Barrett's esophagus without dysplasia
   E. Long-segment Barrett's esophagus

2. **Which of the following is a predictor of developing worsened or de novo postoperative GERD symptoms following LSG?**
   A. Female sex
   B. Class III obesity
   C. Increased neck circumference
   D. Presence of hiatal hernia, repaired at time of LSG
   E. There are no defined patient predictors for developing worsened or do novo GERD after LSG

3. **Which of the following may decrease the development of post sleeve gastrectomy reflux?**
   A. Increased gastric compliance
   B. Increased intraluminal pressure with intact pylorus
   C. A shortened abdominal length of esophagus
   D. Missed hiatal hernia
   E. Use of a 34-French bougie size

4. **At her 3-month postoperative visit following LSG, your patient complains of regular heartburn symptoms. Which of the following is the appropriate next step in management?**
   A. Lifestyle changes and medications
   B. Conversion to laparoscopic Roux-en-Y gastric bypass (RYGB)
   C. Manometry
   D. 24-hour pH probe monitoring
   E. Upper endoscopy

5. **Unfortunately, despite maximal medical therapy and lifestyle changes, your patient continues to experience daily GERD symptoms, which are interfering with her quality of life. Upper gastrointestinal series and endoscopy did not show any reversible cause for her symptoms. Which of the following is considered the best option for revision due to GERD?**
   A. Duodenal switch-biliopancreatic diversion (DS-BPD).
   B. RYGB.
   C. LES augmentation (i.e. LINX).
   D. Single anastomosis duodeno-ileal bypass with sleeve (SADI-S).
   E. Re-sleeve procedure (rSG).

ANSWERS

1. **E.** The effect of LSG on GERD remains controversial. Many studies have shown increased incidence of worsened or de novo GERD following LSG, while others have shown minimal risk of increase, or even improvement or remission of GERD symptoms following LSG. The RYGB remains the preferred procedure, by expert consensus, for patients with severe reflux, especially in the setting of Barrett's esophagus (BE). However, due to the perceived ease and overall lower risks, the LSG remains the most commonly selected weight loss surgical procedure performed today. While all of the above may be considered relative contraindications to performing an LSG, only the presence of long-segment BE or the presence of dysplasia are currently considered absolute contraindications.[1]

 The presence of BE is of particular concern due to the risk of possible evolution to carcinoma. Short-segment disease indicates that the intestinal metaplasia extends <3 cm above the LES, while long-segment disease indicates that intestinal metaplasia extends 3 cm or more above the LES (Figure 47-2). The development of esophageal carcinoma tends to follow a path from BE without dysplasia, to BE with low-grade dysplasia, to BE with high-grade dysplasia and finally to adenocarcinoma (Figure 47-1).

 While short-segment BE without dysplasia shows a relatively low risk of progression to adenocarcinoma, the continued irritation from ongoing acid reflux can contribute to that progression.

 Therefore, there is a strong recommendation that should a patient be adamant about selection of a sleeve gastrectomy in the presence of a relative contraindication, such as preexisting GERD, esophagitis, or junctional/short-segment BE without dysplasia, then the patient should be extensively counseled on the risks of worsening symptoms and the importance of postoperative follow-up.[2]

2. **E.** Unfortunately, despite the high incidence of both preoperative and postoperative GERD, there are no good predictive factors as to who will develop worsened or de novo GERD symptoms. In this relatively small study, Althuwaini et al. found a trend toward decreased incidence of new-onset or worsened GERD in patients with higher preoperative BMIs as well as those with more severe heartburn symptoms while standing. However, none of the variables could strongly predict which patients would develop new onset or worsening of symptoms postoperatively.[3] Furthermore, sleeve gastrectomy with concomitant hiatal hernia repair has been shown to be safe, without increase in mortality and only slight increase in morbidity risks.[4] Early studies had demonstrated improvement in both preoperative GERD and in development of de novo GERD when crural repair was added to sleeve gastrectomy.[5,6] Some of the more recent studies are more mixed on this effect, with some randomized studies showing minimal to no difference in GERD symptoms with concurrent crural repair.[7,8] However, the size of hernia was poorly defined, and the concurrent evaluation and

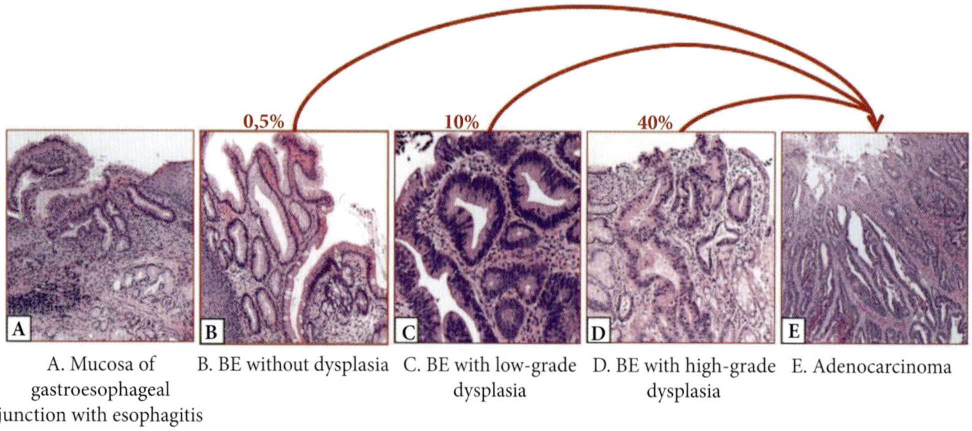

Figure 47-1 Histopathologic features of the natural history of BE. Progressive transition from squamous epithelium to intestinal metaplasia, dysplasia, and adenocarcinoma. A: normal stratified squamous epithelium. B: BE without dysplasia, with the presence of goblet cells. C: BE with low-grade dysplasia. D: BE with high-grade dysplasia. E: Adenocarcinoma. (Reproduced with permission from Conteduca V, Sansonno D, Ingravallo G, et al: Barrett's esophagus and esophageal cancer: an overview. *Int J Oncol.* 2012;41(2):414-424.)

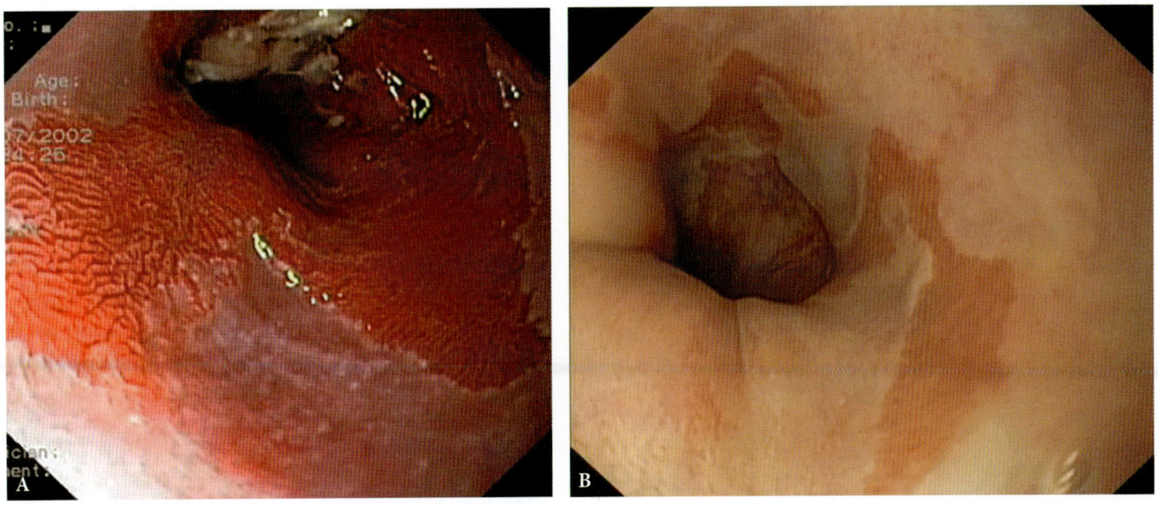

Figure 47-2 A: High grade dysplasia in Barrett's esophagus – endoscopic view. B: Uncomplicated Barrett's esophagus – endoscopic view. (Reproduced with permission from Brunicardi F, Andersen DK, Billiar TR, et al: *Schwartz's Principles of Surgery, 11th ed*. New York, NY: McGraw Hill; 2019.)

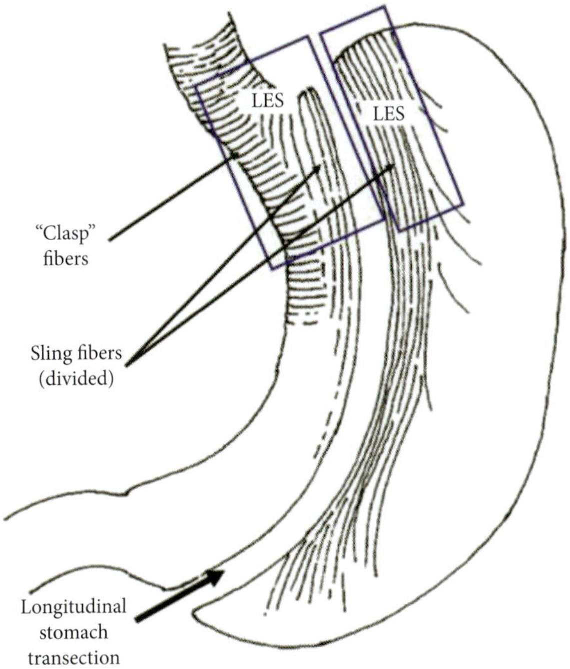

Figure 47-3 Diagrammatic representation of pathway of sling and clasp fibers which can be disrupted by longitudinal gastric transection. (Reproduced with permission from Braghetto I, Lanzarini E, Korn O, et al: Manometric changes of the lower esophageal sphincter after sleeve gastrectomy in obese patients. *Obes Surg*. 2010;20(3):357-362.)

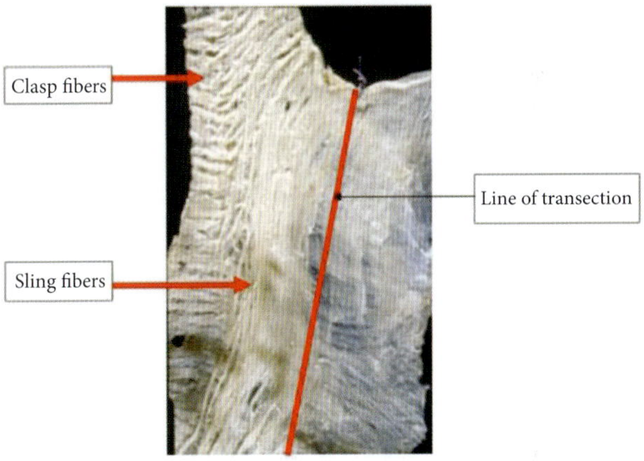

Figure 47-4 Cadaveric representation of LES showing clasp and sling fibers along with line of gastric transection. (Reproduced with permission from Braghetto I, Lanzarini E, Korn O, et al: Manometric changes of the lower esophageal sphincter after sleeve gastrectomy in obese patients. *Obes Surg*. 2010;20(3):357-362.)

repair of the hiatus remains recommended as per the Fourth International Consensus Summit on Sleeve Gastrectomy .

On the other hand, when GERD symptoms were evaluated pre- and postoperatively for patients undergoing LSG vs. RYGB, LSG was the strongest predictor for the development of postoperative GERD.[9]

3. **A.** Multiple surgical factors have been shown to potentially contribute to the development of worsened or de novo GERD following sleeve gastrectomy. Some of these factors are intrinsic to the sleeve operation itself, such as the decreased gastric compliance, increased intraluminal pressure with intact pylorus, and a lower LES pressure. Figures 47-3 and 47-4[10,11] demonstrate the disruption of LES sling and clasp

fibers due to the transection of the stomach, which can lead to the lower LES pressure and shortened intra-abdominal esophageal length.

Others factors such as a missed hiatal hernia, retained gastric fundus, or sleeve twisting are more preventable, and related to surgical technique.

Tables 47-1 and 47-2 summarize the many proposed mechanisms for increasing GERD following LSG, as well as the proposed mechanisms for which GERD may decrease.

Table 47-1 PROPOSED MECHANISMS FOR AN INCREASE IN PREVALENCE OF GERD SYMPTOMS AFTER LSG

Proposed mechanisms for increased GERD after LSG
Hypotension of the lower esophageal sphincter
Blunting of the angle of His
Decreased gastric compliance and volume (leading to increased gastric pressure)
Decreased gastric emptying
Decreased plasma ghrelin (dysmotility)
Gastric sleeve shape
Increase in hiatal hernia
Neofundus

Modified with permission from Laffin M, Chau J, Gill RS, Birch DW, Karmali S. Sleeve gastrectomy and gastroesophageal reflux disease. *J Obes*. 2013;2013:741097.

Table 47-2 PROPOSED MECHANISMS FOR A DECREASE IN PREVALENCE OF GERD SYMPTOMS AFTER LSG

Proposed mechanisms for decreased GERD after LSG
Accelerated gastric emptying
Decreased abdominal obesity
Increased long-term gastric compliance
Restoration of the angle of His
Decreased acid production
Gastric sleeve shape
Decreased wall tension

Modified with permission from Laffin M, Chau J, Gill RS, Birch DW, Karmali S. Sleeve gastrectomy and gastroesophageal reflux disease. *J Obes*. 2013;2013:741097.

The use of a smaller bougie <36-French in creation of the LSG may increase the risk of post sleeve reflux[12], presumably by causing further disruption to the LES mechanism, increasing intra-luminal pressure and further decreasing gastric compliance.

4. **A.** While the development of worsened or de novo GERD after LSG may be common, the majority of patients are able to be treated with lifestyle changes and medications alone. Some of these changes may include avoidance of overeating, ensuring separation of solids and liquids, and avoiding "trigger foods" such as acidic foods, coffee, or spices. If patients are eating appropriately then the addition of acid suppression medication such as H2 blockers or proton pump inhibitors (PPIs) is an appropriate first step in management. While some patients may be able to come off these medications as their weight loss and drop in intra-abdominal pressure continues, others will require ongoing medical therapy to control their symptoms.

   If lifestyle and medical therapy does not fully control symptoms, then the next steps would be to evaluate for an anatomic, and potentially reversible, cause for the reflux. This workup often begins with an upper gastrointestinal barium swallow and/or endoscopy to look for a retained fundus, a missed hiatal hernia, or an area of stricture. If these are normal, then further workup with manometry or pH monitoring may be indicated, especially if considering possible revision or conversion.

5. **B.** There are many revision procedure options for patients who have previously undergone LSG. Most of these revisions focus on failure of weight loss, rather than treatment of intractable GERD.

   The RYGB remains the "gold standard" for antireflux procedures in morbidly obese individuals, as well as the preferred revision surgery for patients who have developed worsened or de novo GERD following LSG. The bypass procedure not only decreases acid production by making a smaller gastric pouch, but also decreases the gastric pressure by creating a new gastric outlet and excluding the pylorus. The Roux-en-Y configuration also reduces the risk of bile reflux and its contributions to GERD symptoms. While the overall study size is low, a study by Landreneau et al.[13] showed that of the patients who underwent revision of sleeve gastrectomy to gastric bypass for refractory GERD, 75% of them had resolution of symptoms by 12 months postop.

The idea behind both DS-BPD is that in addition to the portion control achieved by the sleeve gastrectomy (see Figure 47-5), the addition of a significant intestinal bypass with relatively short common channel causes increased malabsorption. The newer SADI-S procedure is a modification of the DS-BPD with a single loop anastomosis, much like the one anastomosis gastric bypass or mini-gastric bypass (Figure 47-6). The SADI-S also results in a longer common channel than the DS, which is thought to decrease the overall risk of malnutrition. Both procedures maintain an intact sleeve gastrectomy, therefore there is no change in the increased intraluminal gastric pressure with intact pylorus or the decreased LES pressure felt to contribute to development of GERD symptoms.

A re-sleeve procedure has also been proposed as an option for patients who have had failure of primary weight loss or weight regain after sleeve gastrectomy, and for whom volumetric studies have shown dilation of the gastric sleeve.[14] While the resection of a retained fundus may be advantageous in some patients, the overall gastric pressure remains elevated and the LES pressure may in fact reduce due to further disruption of the LES clasp and sling fibers. Figure 47-7 suggests one algorithm for consideration of sleeve revision options based on presence or absence of pouch dilation or GERD.

Increasing the LES pressure has also been proposed as a mechanism to improve GERD following LSG. Novel approaches to this at the time of original sleeve have included concomitant fundoplication, although the data on this is quite lacking. However, for patients who develop worsened or de novo GERD following their SG, this is not an option. Magnetic LES augmentation via the LINX procedure as well as LES radiofrequency ablation via the STRETTA procedure have both been proposed methods to increase LES pressure and therefore decrease GERD symptoms. While both of these procedures have shown promise, they thus far seem to be reserved for patients who are unable or unwilling to proceed with the more invasive conversion to RYGB.

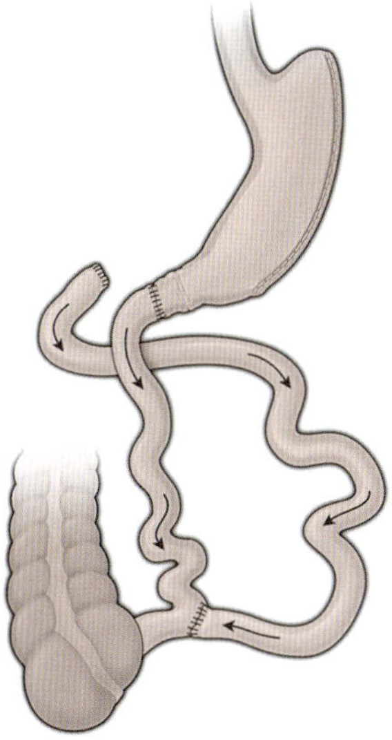

Figure 47-5 Duodenal switch (DS). (Reproduced with permission from Doherty GM. *CURRENT Diagnosis & Treatment Surgery, 15th ed.* New York, NY: McGraw Hill; 2020.)

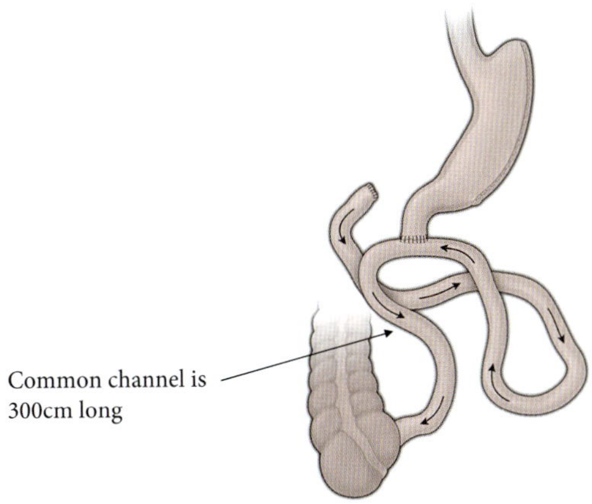

Figure 47-6 Single anastomosis duodeno-ileal (SADI). (Reproduced with permission from *Doherty GM: CURRENT Diagnosis & Treatment Surgery, 15th ed.* New York, NY: McGraw Hill; 2020.)

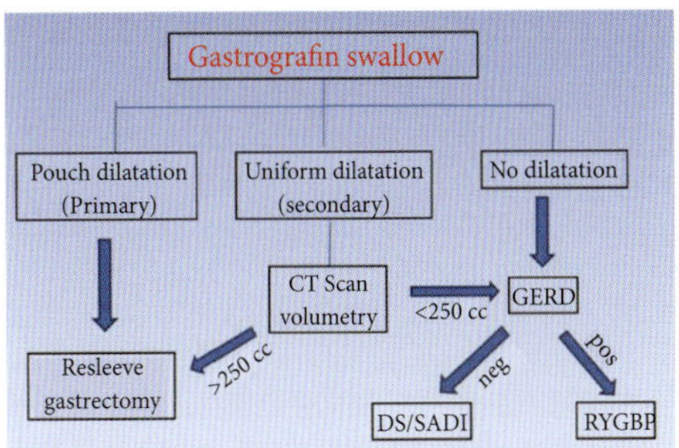

Figure 47-7 Bariatric algorithm of LSG failure. CT, computed tomography; GERD, gastroesophageal reflux disease; DS, duodenal switch; SADI, single-anastomosis duodenoileal bypass; LRYGB, laparoscopic Roux-en-Y gastric bypass. (Reproduced with permission from Nedelcu M, Noel P, Iannelli A, Gagner M. Revised sleeve gastrectomy (re-sleeve). *Surg Obes Relat Dis.* 2015;11(6):1282-1288.)

REFERENCES

1. ASMBS updated position statement on sleeve gastrectomy as a bariatric procedure. August 2017. https://asmbs.org/resources/updated-position-statement-on-sleeve-gastrectomy-as-a-bariatric-procedure
2. Patti MG, Schlottmann F. Gastroesophageal reflux after sleeve gastrectomy. *JAMA Surg*. 2018;153(12):1147-1148. doi:10.1001/jamasurg.2018.2437
3. Althuwaini S, Bamehriz F, Aldohayan A, et al. Prevalence and predictors of gastroesophageal reflux disease after laparoscopic sleeve gastrectomy. *Obes Surg*. 2018;28:916-922. doi:10.1007/s11695-017-2971-4
4. Janik M, Ibikunle C, Aryaie A. Safety of concurrent sleeve gastrectomy and hiatal hernia repair: a propensity score-matched analysis of the MSAQIP registry. *Surg Obes Relat Dis*. 2020;16:365-371.
5. Soricelli E, Iossa A, Casella G, et al. Sleeve gastrectomy and crural repair in obese patients with gastroesophageal reflux disease and/or hiatal hernia. *Surg Obes Relat Dis*. 2013;9(3):356-361.
6. Samaker K, McKenzie TJ, Tavakkoli A, et al. The effect of laparoscopic sleeve gastrectomy with concomitant hiatal hernia repair on gastroesophageal reflux disease in the morbidly obese. *Obes Surg*. 2016;26(1):61-66.
7. Snyder B, Wilson E, Wilson T, Mehta S, Bajwa K, Klein C. A randomized trial comparing reflux symptoms in sleeve gastrectomy patients with or without hiatal hernia repair. *Surg Obes Relat Dis*. 2016;12(9):1681-1688.
8. Dakour Aridi H, Asali M, Fouani T, et al. Gastroesophageal reflux disease after laparoscopic sleeve gastrectomy with concomitant hiatal hernia repair: an unresolved question. *Obes Surg*. 2017;27:2898-2904.
9. Navarini D, Madalosso CAS, Tognon AP, Fornari F, Barão FR, Gurski RR. Predictive factors of gastroesophageal reflux disease in bariatric surgery: a controlled trial comparing sleeve gastrectomy with gastric bypass. *Obes Surg*. 2020. doi:10.1007/s11695-019-04286-5.
10. Braghetto I, Lanzarini E, Korn O, et al. Manometric changes of the lower esophageal sphincter after sleeve gastrectomy in obese patients. *Obes Surg*. 2010;2(3):357-362.
11. Torquati A. Treatment for severe GERD after sleeve gastrectomy: conversion to gastric bypass or endoluminal radiofrequency. Duke University. 2015.
12. Alami R, Khatib D, Hejjani M, et al. A157 36F bougies have more complications and reflux than 40F in laparoscopic sleeve gastrectomy patients. *Surg Obes Relat Dis*. 2019;v15(10):S1-S268.
13. Landreneau JP, Strong AT, Rodriguez JH, et al. Conversion of sleeve gastrectomy to Roux-en-Y gastric bypass. *Obes Surg*. 2018;28(12):3843-3850.
14. Nedelcu M, Noel P, Iannelli A, Gagner M. Revised sleeve gastrectomy (re-sleeve). *Surg Obes Relat Dis*. 2015;11:1282-1288.

48

Marginal Ulcer and Gastrogastric Fistula

Xiao-Yue Han, MD, and Farah A. Husain MD

A 54-year-old woman with coronary artery disease (CAD), type 2 diabetes mellitus, hypersensitivity lung disease (HLD), asthma, tobacco use disorder, and obesity (body mass index [BMI] 45 kg/m^2) presents to your surgery clinic after completing a multidisciplinary bariatric surgery program. Her diabetes is well-controlled as is her asthma with daily use of her budesonide inhaler. She has significantly cut down on her smoking from 1-pack-per-day to only a few cigarettes daily, stating that she's been able to quit in the past but doesn't like the weight gain associated with smoking cessation.

She undergoes an uneventful laparoscopic Roux-en-Y gastric bypass (RYGB) after smoking cessation, but presents to the emergency department 9 months postoperatively with subacute gnawing epigastric pain with one episode of small-volume melena a few days ago now resolved. She is hemodynamically stable, afebrile, and nonperitoneal on exam.

1. **Which of her preoperative medical conditions places her at risk for a marginal ulcer after an RYGB?**
   A. CAD
   B. Type 2 diabetes mellitus
   C. Hyperlipidemia
   D. Asthma
   E. Age

2. **You order a computed tomography (CT) scan with intravenous (IV) and oral (PO) contrast to clarify the patient's anatomy and confirm your diagnosis. On the CT scan, you will most likely see:**
   A. A normal CT scan
   B. Enhancing mucosa at proximal Roux limb associated with fat stranding
   C. Intraabdominal free air over the liver
   D. Distention of the gastric remnant and the biliopancreatic limb

3. **What is the most appropriate treatment plan for this patient?**
   A. Discharge from the emergency department with Carafate, proton pump inhibitors (PPIs), smoking cessation, and expedited plan for endoscopy with return precautions discussed
   B. Admission for emergent inpatient upper endoscopy
   C. Admission for emergent surgery: Diagnostic laparoscopic possible laparotomy, possible Graham patch, and possible gastrojejunal revision
   D. Start misoprostol
   E. Clinic follow-up after 1 week of a liquid diet

4. **The patient presents 1 year later still intermittently smoking ("mostly when I'm stressed"). She has ongoing left upper quadrant pain, but no further evidence of bleeding. She describes increased pain in the left upper quadrant over the past 6 months, increased gastroesophageal reflux disease (GERD),**

and loss of satiety with weight regain (BMI 42). The next best step for this patient is:

A. Refer patient to a dietician for re-education on a post-bariatric diet
B. Refer patient for upper gastrointestinal (GI) series
C. Order CT scan with IV contrast
D. Refer patient to GI for further workup and management
E. Take patient to operating room for revision of her bariatric procedure

ANSWERS

1. **D.** Smoking, corticosteroid use (i.e. budesonide), and nonsteroidal anti-inflammatory drug (NSAID) use significantly increases risk of marginal ulcer after an RYGB.[1] The patient should be counseled on complete smoking cessation (at least 2 weeks preoperatively) and that her use of a corticosteroid inhaler places her at greater risk of possible marginal ulcer. Complete cessation of NSAIDs should also be counseled, particularly postoperatively. Rassmussen et al. evaluated preoperative *H. pylori* positive status, and found these patients had two times the risk of developing marginal ulcers after surgery, even when adequately treated.[2] Diabetes has been shown to be associated with increased risk of marginal ulcer in some case series, but not in prospective data series.[3]

2. **B.** Marginal ulcers after an RYGB are benign ulcerations occurring on the jejunal side of the gastrojejunostomy. Radiographically, they frequently result in edema at the gastrojejunal anastomosis causing gastric pouch distention and the area of ulceration is frequently in the proximal Roux limb. These ulcers appear as enhancement of the mucosa with hypoattenuation of edematous submucosa.[4] The patient's clinical exam is incongruent with perforated marginal ulcer and thus free air is less likely to be seen, although due to her body habitus, the physical exam is less reliable (C). Distention of the gastric remnant associated with dilation of the biliopancreatic limb has a broad differential of which marginal ulcer is an unlikely cause (D). While a normal CT scan (A) is possible in a patient with marginal ulcer, the patient most likely has radiographic abnormality. The clinical picture is not consistent with internal hernia or small-bowel obstruction but a CT scan can be helpful if there are concerns about other such pathology after an RYGB. Marginal ulcer may bleed or perforate causing cardiovascular and respiratory compromise, but most cause pain and PO intolerance due to fibrosis causing a stricture at the gastrojejunal anastomosis. A perforation may result in free air or a fluid collection but this patient does not appear ill enough to expect to see a fluid collection (E).

3. **A.** Most marginal ulcers can be managed nonoperatively with cessation of the offending agent (smoking, NSAIDs, steroids), Carafate, and PPI with timely upper endoscopy for diagnosis and management. Misoprostol can be added for refractory ulcers. The patient is hemodynamically stable with a subacute presentation enabling a window for outpatient-based therapy. If the patient had hemodynamic instability, stigmata of continued complicated marginal ulcer (i.e. continued GI bleeding) then admission for stabilization, workup, and treatment would be indicated.[1]

4. **B.** The patient most likely has complications from a gastrogastric fistula after previous marginal ulcer causing loss of bypass physiology and thereby weight gain. The best initial study to evaluate for presence of a gastrogastric fistula is an upper GI series looking for fistulous connection between the gastric pouch and remnant followed by endoscopic evaluation.[5] Once the diagnosis is confirmed, conservative therapies (i.e. PPI) should be initiated with consideration of endoscopic (i.e. fibrin ablation of the fistula) and surgical approaches for fistula treatment/closure.[6] Weight regain after an RYGB punctuated by a period of abdominal pain should raise suspicious for this infrequent but important complication. All patients with weight regain should reestablish care with a dietician, but in this case, that is not the only evaluation required. Smoking cessation will need to be addressed again to prevent further complications related to the original marginal ulcer.

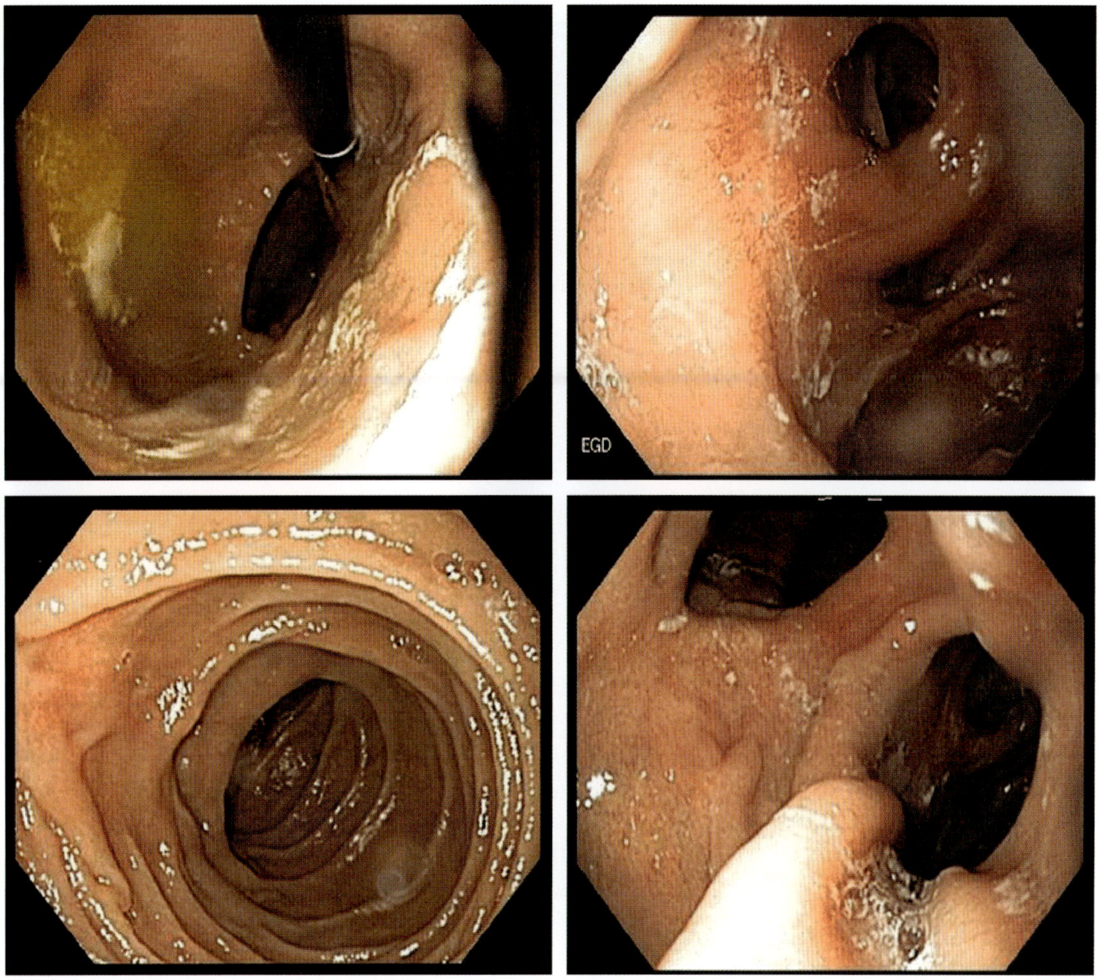

Figure 48-1 Gastrogastric fistula.

REFERENCES

1. Coblijn UK, Lagarde SM, de Castro SMM, et al. Symptomatic marginal ulcer disease after Roux-en-Y gastric bypass: incidence, risk factors and management. *Obes Surg*. 2015; 25(5):805-811.
2. Rasmussen JJ, Fuller W, Ali MR. Marginal ulceration after laparoscopic gastric bypass: an analysis of predisposing factors in 260 patients. *Surg Endo*. 2007;21(7):1090-1094.
3. Coblijn UK, Goucham AB, Lagarde SM, et al. Development of ulcer disease after Roux-en-Y gastric bypass, incidence, risk factors, and patient presentations: a systematic review. *Obes Surg*. 2014;24(2):299-309.
4. Adduci AJ, Phillips CH, Harvin H. Prospective diagnosis of marginal ulceration following Roux-en-Y gastric bypass with computed tomography. *Radiol Case Rep*. 2015;10(2):1063.
5. Pauli EM, Beshir H, Mathew A. Gastrogastric fistulae following gastric bypass surgery-clinical recognition and treatment. *Curr Gastro Rep*. 2014;16(9):405.
6. Gumbs AA, Duffy AJ, Bell RL. Management of gastrogastric fistula after laparoscopic Roux-en-Y gastric bypass. *Surg Obes Relat Dis*. 2006;2(2):117-121.

49

Malnutrition

Joel Brockmeyer, MD

VIGNETTE 1

A 35-year-old female with a body mass index (BMI) of 40 kg/m^2 and obstructive sleep apnea (OSA) presents for evaluation for bariatric surgery. She has completed her preoperative psychologic evaluation and nutrition education. Her preoperative labs have been completed.

1. What is the most likely cause of her preoperative anemia?

A. Vitamin B12 deficiency
B. Iron deficiency
C. Zinc deficiency
D. Protein deficiency

	Result	Reference Range
Hemoglobin	11.2 g/dL	(12–17.5 g/dL)
Hematocrit	33.4%	(35%–54%)
Mean corpuscular volume (MCV)	76.8 fL/cell	(80–96 fL/cell)
Mean corpuscular hemoglobin concentration (MCHC)	32.6 g/dL	(32–36 g/dL)
Vitamin B12 (cobalamin)	250 ng/mL	(200–900 ng/mL)
Folate	6 ng/mL	(2–20 ng/mL)
Zinc	85 μg/dL	(80–120 μg/dL)
Albumin	3.2 g/dL	(3.4–5.4 g/dL)
Serum Iron	40 μg/dL	(50–170 μg/dL)
Ferritin	15 μg/L	(20–335 μg/L)

2. Which of the listed surgeries would be least likely to worsen this type of anemia postoperatively?

A. Bilio-pancreatic diversion with duodenal switch (BPD/DS)
B. Roux-en-Y gastric bypass (RYGB) with long (200 cm) alimentary limb
C. Single anastomosis duodeno-ileal bypass with sleeve gastrectomy (SADI-S)
D. Sleeve gastrectomy (SG)

3. Which of the following supplementation needs is correct?

A. If she undergoes sleeve gastrectomy, 45 mg of elemental iron daily
B. If she undergoes BPD/DS, 20 mg of zinc daily
C. If she undergoes Roux-en-Y gastric bypass, 100 mg of elemental iron daily
D. If she undergoes sleeve gastrectomy, 350 μg of vitamin B12 orally daily

4. Which of the following improves the absorption of the latter?

A. Vitamin B6 for vitamin B12
B. Vitamin C for iron
C. Zinc for copper
D. Vitamin E for protein

ANSWERS

1. B. Preoperative laboratory analysis on the patient shows that she has microcytic anemia due to her decreased hemoglobin and hematocrit along with a low mean corpuscular volume (MCV). Iron deficiency is diagnosed by decreased serum iron and ferritin.[1] Iron is required for heme-containing molecules for oxygen transport, such as hemoglobin, and storage, such as myoglobin. It also contributes to electron transport and redox reactions via cytochromes. Deficiency leads to microcytic anemia, pallor, cheilosis (inflammation and cracking of the corners of the mouth), glossitis, hair loss, brittle fingernails, koilonychias (spoon nails), tissue hypoxia, exertional dyspnea, and heart enlargement.[2]

Vitamin B12 (cobalamin) is an essential coenzyme in DNA, RNA, and myelin synthesis. It is necessary for red blood cell synthesis and for the metabolism of amino acids and fatty acids. Deficiency is associated a macrocytic anemia, fatigue, pallor, shortness of breath, numbness and tingling of the extremities, abnormal gait, memory loss, and irreversible dementia.[3]

Zinc is a mineral that serves as an essential cofactor in a wide range of enzyme systems that are involved in protein synthesis, metalloenzymes, DNA replication, immune function, collagen formation, and cross linking. Zinc deficiency leads to hair loss, dermatitis, testicular atrophy, decreased appetite, depressed smell and taste acuity, depression, and diarrhea. In children, deficiency can lead to growth retardation and delayed sexual maturation. It leads to delayed wound healing.[2]

Protein or amino acids are used throughout the body and make up half of the dry weight of the cells of the body. They are required for tissue maintenance and growth and formation of hormones, enzymes, and nucleoproteins.[3] Severe protein malnutrition, or kwashiorkor, manifests as pedal edema, apathy, hepatic enlargement, skin atrophy and depigmentation, and decreased muscle mass.[2]

2. **D.** The microcytic anemia of the patient is likely due to iron deficiency. Iron is absorbed throughout the small intestine, but most efficiently in the duodenum. A slightly acidic environment is required for best absorption.[1] Iron deficiency is common in bariatric surgery patients preoperatively and can worsen after surgery. A systematic review found an incidence of 15.2% preoperatively and an incidence of iron-deficiency anemia at 1-year postop of 1.6% in patients who underwent SG and 16.7% in patients who underwent RYGB.[4] The range for patients undergoing RYGB is likely 15% to 50%.[5]

   Research on iron-deficiency following SADI-S and BPD/DS is sparse at this time. One study showed an incidence of iron-deficiency as high as 23% in BPD/DS patients at 28 months of follow-up. Other studies have shown a range of 8% to 50% following BPD/DS. Neither study clearly defined their iron supplementation protocol. Malabsorptive surgeries that bypass the duodenum and jejunum are likely to have higher rates of iron deficiency and its complications that can be treated with effective iron supplementation.[6]

3. **A.** The cause of this patient's anemia is iron deficiency. The American Society for Metabolic and Bariatric Surgeons (ASMBS) has released recommendations for postoperative nutritional supplementation.[5] For patients who undergo laparoscopic adjustable gastric banding (LAGB) and have no history of anemia, they should take 18 mg of elemental iron daily, likely from their multivitamin. For patients who are menstruating, have a history of iron deficiency, or have undergone RYGB, SG, or BPD/DS, they should take at least 45 to 60 mg of elemental iron daily. Iron absorption may be inhibited taken with calcium supplements, acid-reducing medications, and foods high in phytates or polyphenols, such as nuts and legumes. For patients with continued anemia, iron supplementation of 150 to 300 mg of elemental iron split 2 to 3 times per day should be given. If patients develop refractory iron deficiency despite oral supplementation, intravenous ferric gluconate or sucrose may be required.[7]

   Postoperative zinc supplementation varies based on the procedure. Patients who undergo BPD/DS should take 16 to 22 mg per day (200% of recommended daily allowance [RDA]). RYGB patients should take 8 to 22 mg per day (100%–200% of RDA). Patients who received SG or LAGB should take 8 to 11 mg per day (100% of RDA). It is likely that these levels can be found in a multivitamin.

   All patients who undergo bariatric surgery are recommended to receive vitamin B12 supplementation. The dose varies on the route of the supplementation. Orally by sublingual, liquid, or disintegrating tablet should be 350 to 500 μg daily. Intramuscular or subcutaneous dosing requires 1,000 μg monthly. New nasal spray formulations exist and the manufacturer's recommendations should be followed.

4. **B.** Vitamin C has been shown to significantly improve the absorption of iron.[7] Calcium, acid-reducing medications, and foods high in phytates and polyphenols will inhibit the absorption of iron.[5]

VIGNETTE 2

A 43-year-old female patient presents to your office with a history of a RYGB 14 years ago. She has not seen a bariatric surgeon or medical provider in 10 years. She was concerned because she is having difficulty maintaining weight and has had progressive weight loss over the past several years. Her preoperative weight was 106 kg, height 161.29 cm, and BMI 41 kg/m^2. Her ideal body weight is 58.6 kg. Her current weight is 46.27 kg and her BMI is 17.8 kg/m^2. Her percentage total body weight loss (%TBWL) is 56% and percentage excess weight loss (%EWL) is 125%.

The patient relates that she does not follow any prescribed diet. She was extremely satisfied with her weight loss for several years after her initial operation and had been in good health until she was laid off from her job "a while back." Her family has been unable to obtain insurance coverage due to financial hardship and, since that event, she has been unable to afford any protein supplements. Her husband accompanies her to the office today and notes that she has been somewhat forgetful and has had several falls at home. A limited dietary recall was performed, and it demonstrates a diet that is high in carbohydrates and starches. On exam, the patient is cachectic, has poor dentition, has patchy hair loss, and has poor short-term memory on recall. A brief neurological exam reveals discoordination of movement, nystagmus, and an unsteady gait in the office hallway.

1. **You decide to perform some lab work. When the results return, you are not surprised to find that her total protein levels and albumin levels are low. Based on her current symptoms, what common postbariatric surgery vitamin deficiency listed below *represents the most likely source* of her ataxia and short-term memory loss?**
   A. Selenium
   B. Thiamine
   C. Folate
   D. Vitamin D
   E. Vitamin C

2. **In an effort to boost her protein and calorie intake, the patient is scheduled to have an evaluation with your dietitian. During this evaluation, which of the tools listed below *would best determine* the optimal daily caloric intake for the patient?**
   A. Resting energy expenditure predictive equations
   B. Hamwi formula
   C. Nitrogen balance equation
   D. Lean tissue mass loss equation

3. **After 3 months, the patient has continued to lose weight. She has had several hospital admissions for a nonhealing sacral decubitus ulcer and her pre-albumin levels remain low despite attempts at maximizing oral feeding and protein supplementation. Which intervention is the *next best step* for long-term maintenance of her caloric and protein needs on the treatment algorithm until she is able to sustain herself with oral meals?**
   A. Total parenteral nutrition (TPN)
   B. Emergent reversal of her gastric bypass
   C. Remnant gastrostomy tube
   D. Nasojejunal feeds
   E. Roux limb lengthening procedure

4. **In a different scenario, assume that the patient has responded to the dietician recommendations, gained appropriate weight, and started taking her daily routine bariatric vitamins. The patient presents 6 months later, now with a BMI of 23 kg/m^2, and she is happier with her weight and appearance. Based on ASMBS guidelines, which of the following micronutrient *is the best example* of a lab value that should be followed on a routine basis in the absence of symptoms?**
   A. Vitamin A
   B. Vitamin E
   C. Vitamin K
   D. Vitamin B12
   E. Selenium

ANSWERS

1. **B.** Thiamine deficiency is one of the more well-known vitamin derangements following bariatric surgery. Thiamine is mainly absorbed in the proximal jejunum (Figure 49-1) and is involved in energy metabolism and ATP production, biosynthesis of nucleic acids, and antioxidant defense mechanisms.[8]

   Although the prevalence of thiamine deficiency in bariatric surgery patients is difficult to estimate, one study with a 2-year follow-up indicated an 18.3% prevalence rate after Roux-en-Y gastric bypass (RYGB).[9] It was once thought that restrictive operations would be less susceptible to micronutrient derangements; however, recent evidence suggests that patients undergoing the vertical sleeve gastrectomy (VSG) are also surprisingly at-risk, with a postoperative prevalence in one study of 25.7%.[10] Thiamine deficiency is known as beriberi and has several clinical manifestations.[11] Wet beriberi is associated with cardiac insufficiency and other cardiac manifestations, whereas dry beriberi is associated with neuritis and neuropathy.[12] Cerebral beriberi is known commonly as Wernicke-Korsakoff syndrome (WKS), which is characterized by nystagmus, ataxia, and mental status changes and can be an urgent medical issue. This patient is showing signs of WKS secondary to poor supplemental vitamin intake most likely due to her compromised socioeconomic condition. The combination of her clinical signs and symptoms indicates that her thiamine deficiency is severe, and she will require urgent administration of intravenous thiamine (500 mg IV over 30 minutes three times daily over 2 days).

For this patient with thiamine deficiency, the thiamine reserves must be replaced. As dehydration likely accompanies this diagnosis in cases of hyperemesis and food intolerance, resuscitation should be started with isotonic fluids and intravenous thiamine. The standard start for this patient would be the "banana bag." Each hospital and pharmacy may have different formulations, but a simple version includes 100 mg/L of thiamine, 1 mg/L of folate, 1 mg/L of magnesium, and a multivitamin formulation given in a liter of 0.9% normal saline. Because thiamine plays a role in carbohydrate metabolism, infusion of dextrose or carbohydrates would likely exacerbate the neurologic symptoms by depleting the last reserves of thiamine present.[13] After initial treatment with intravenous thiamine and a diagnosis is completed, her thiamine reserves should be repleted either orally or intravenously. The maximum amount of thiamine that may be absorbed in a healthy individual is 4.5 mg in a single oral dose. This amount may be reduced by 70% or more in patients with malnutrition or a bypassed

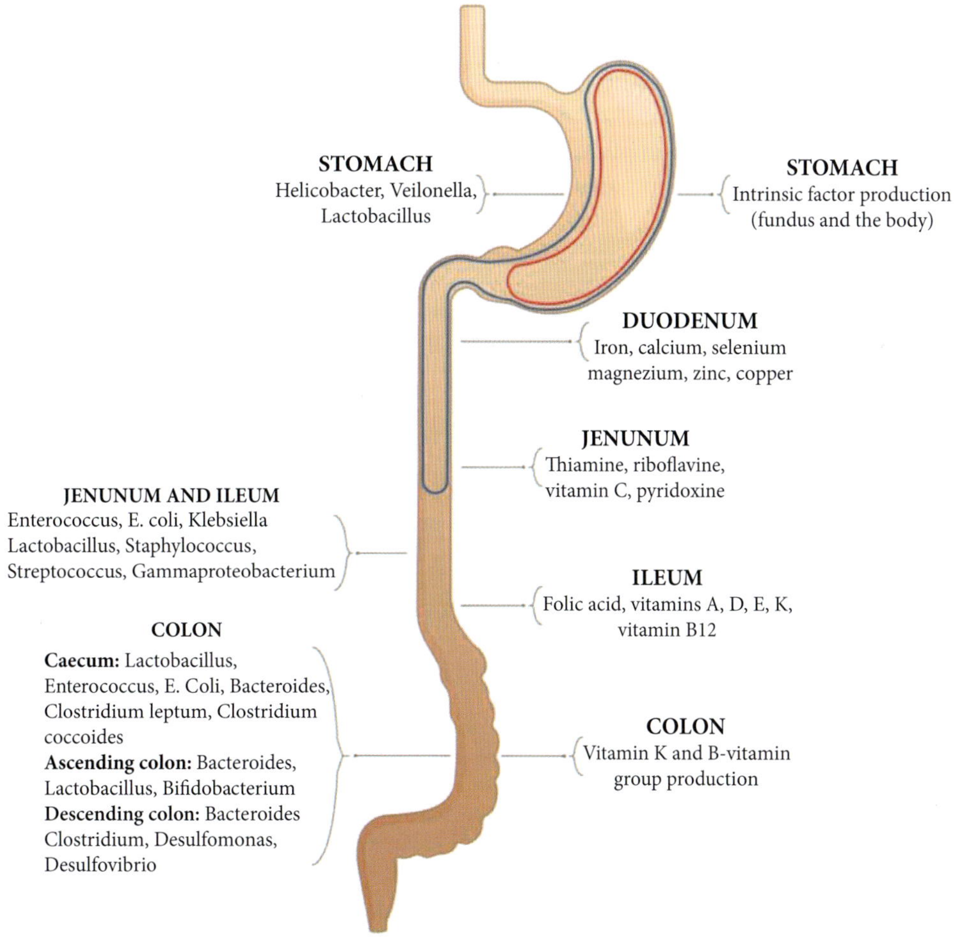

Figure 49-1 Site of micronutrient absorption within the gut and the location of gut microbiota. Red areas indicate areas excluded after VSG. Blue areas indicate those areas excluded after RYGB. (Reproduced with permission from Ciobârcă D, Cătoi AF, Copăescu C, et al: Bariatric Surgery in Obesity: Effects on Gut Microbiota and Micronutrient Status. *Nutrients*. 2020 16;12(1):235.)

duodenum. Intravenously, thiamine has a half-life of 96 minutes. Three times daily dosing of 120 to 500 mg intravenous thiamine is necessary to replenish deficiency.

Once that patient has had her thiamine deficiency corrected, she will need to be maintained on sufficient oral intake to prevent future deficiency. Postoperative thiamine supplementation for all patients who receive bariatric surgery should be at least 12 mg daily. Ideally, patients should receive 50 mg of thiamine from a multivitamin or B-complex supplement once or twice daily.[5] Excessive alcohol intake following bariatric surgery puts patients at increased for the development of thiamine deficiency.

The data on selenium deficiency in postoperative bariatric patients is very limited and should be followed up only if a patient displays unexplained anemia, fatigue, bone disease, chronic diarrhea, or heart failure.[14] Folate deficiency is a another micronutrient deficiency seen in bariatric surgery patients but is associated more with megaloblastic anemia, thrombocytopenia, glossitis, and elevated homocysteine levels rather than neurologic complications.[15] Vitamin D deficiency is also a common postsurgical micronutrient derangement that is associated with secondary hyperparathyroidism and osteomalacia. Although this patient more than likely has low levels of vitamin D, the vitamin D deficiency is not the source of her neurological dysfunction. Vitamin C deficiency may contribute to her poor dentition but vitamin C and has not been extensively studied in bariatric patients, although low serum concentrations of vitamin C have been reported in some RYGB patients.[16]

2. **A.** The gold standard for determination of a patient's resting energy expenditure (REE) is indirect calorimetry; however, this requires specialized equipment and resources that might not be available to all clinicians. There are a number of calculations that have been developed to estimate REE from indirect calorimetry. These tools yield an estimate of the daily caloric needs to maintain body weight and a variety of them are used in practice today. One of the more notable equations is the Harris–Benedict Equation. This was devised in 1918 and was in widespread use in clinical practice. It has recently fallen out of favor for other similar calculations that may have increased accuracy, such as the Mifflin–St. Jeor, the Ireton–Jones, and the Penn State equations.[17] Each REE equation is associated with modifiers or multipliers that account for activity or critical illness, and for this patient, an assessment of daily caloric needs would assist the dietitians to determine the best approach to improve the patient's nutritional status.

   The Hamwi formula is used to calculate ideal body weight (IBW). For women, the IBW is 45.4 kg for the first 152 cm in height and 2.3 kg for each 2.5 cm over 152 cm. For men, the IBW is 48 kg for the first 152 cm and 2.7 kg for each 2.5 cm over 152 cm. The nitrogen balance equation, or urinary urea nitrogen equation, is the total protein intake (protein)/6.25 – (gram of nitrogen excreted in urine + 4 grams). This represents a useful tool to estimate the protein caloric response during disease and therapy.[18] The lean tissue mass loss (LTM) equation estimates muscle and nonfat losses after a dietary intervention and can be used to estimate the overall nutrition status of a bariatric patient; however, this would be used to monitor a response to therapy rather than determining daily caloric intake.[19]

3. **C.** The best long-term strategy to improve overall calorie and micronutrient absorption in a postoperative RYGB patient is to access the remnant stomach for enteral feeds.[20] Although remnant enteral access devices are not without potential complications themselves, they represent the best approach to the highly absorptive area of the duodenum and proximal jejunum.[21] Remnant gastrostomy tubes can be maintained for a period of time measured in months and can assist with transition to oral feedings. When protein calorie oral intake has stabilized and the patient has transitioned out of a catabolic phase, the feeding access tube can be removed with a low risk of gastrocutaneous fistula formation. A laparoscopic jejunal feeding tube scan be utilized as well, but this procedure also carries a higher risk of complications without the added benefit of access to the proximal gut.[22]

   TPN, whether delivered peripherally or centrally, has the advantage of bypassing the gut in situations where gut-feeding is not feasible. Although the delivery of macro- and micronutrients can be closely monitored and adjusted, long-term delivery of nutrients by this method is associated with several serious complications, including catheter-related bloodstream infections, electrolyte disturbances, liver disease, and volume overload.[23] Reversal of this patient's gastric bypass in the setting of protein calorie malnutrition would be particularly hazardous due to poor healing of anastomoses and wounds. Nasojejunal feeding is a relatively good short-term feeding option, as long as feeding tubes are inserted safely under radiographic or endoscopic guidance; however, they are not a comfortable option for patients in need of long-term feeding access. Roux limb lengthening procedures would be contraindicated in this setting, because these procedures tend to decrease nutrient absorption and would lead to continued weight loss. Common channel lengthening procedures might be a viable option for this patient population depending on the degree of weight gain that is required to maintain a healthy weight.

4. **D.** Vitamin B12 is a water-soluble vitamin that plays an important role in neurologic function, red cell production, and DNA synthesis.[24] The absorption of vitamin B12 is facilitated by a carrier molecule produced in the stomach known as gastric intrinsic factor (IF) and the B12-IF complex is then absorbed in the jejunum (Figure 49-1). Medications and surgical procedures like the RYGB alter the production of gastric acid, required to free vitamin B12 from food sources and also inhibit the production of IF. The prevalence of vitamin B12 deficiency in RYGB is estimated to be near 20%, whereas in VSG patients, the rate is estimated to be between 4% and 20%.[25] ASMBS guidelines recommended screening of vitamin B12 levels at least annually in patients who have undergone RYGB, VSG, and BPD/DS.

Vitamin A is an important fat-soluble vitamin that plays a role in growth, development, and the production of retinal to maintain good vision. Although vitamin A deficiency is a concern for BPD/DS patients, it is rarely deficient in RYGB patients (8%–11%), unless it is in the setting of severe protein calorie malnutrition.[26] In this patient, now that she has returned to a normal BMI and is asymptomatic, vitamin A monitoring is not necessary. There is very little data on the absorption of fat-soluble vitamins E and K in bariatric surgery patients.[1] It is thought that deficiencies in these vitamins are relatively rare in weight loss surgery patients; therefore, routine annual monitoring of these vitamins is not necessary unless the patient is demonstrating signs and symptoms of deficiency. Selenium abnormalities, as stated before, are rare and bariatric patients do not require annual monitoring of this micronutrient.

VIGNETTE 3

A 35-year-old female underwent a BPD/DS and cholecystectomy 3 years ago. Her initial BMI was 60 kg/m^2 and is currently 33 kg/m^2. Her preoperative hypertension, hyperlipidemia, and type 2 diabetes mellitus have resolved. Most recent hemoglobin A1C is 5.9%. She has been taking a generic multivitamin twice daily. She was instructed to take a generic calcium supplement twice daily that is made of calcium carbonate 600 mg with 400 IU of vitamin D3. She suffered an ankle fracture while participating in a physical training class 2 weeks ago. She presents for her annual follow-up. She has completed her surveillance laboratory evaluation.

	Result	**Reference Range**
Hemoglobin	12.4 g/dL	(12–17.5 g/dL)
Hematocrit	36.1%	(35%–54%)
Mean corpuscular volume (MCV)	85.8 fL/cell	(80–96 fL/cell)
Mean corpuscular hemoglobin concentration (MCHC)	33.6 g/dL	(32–36 g/dL)
Vitamin B12 (cobalamin)	250 ng/mL	(200–900 ng/mL)
Calcium	7.8 mg/dL	(8.5–10.2 mg/dL)
25-OH Vitamin D	15 ng/mL	(25–40 ng/mL)
Folate	6 ng/mL	(2–20 ng/mL)
Albumin	2.8 g/dL	(3.4–5.4 g/dL)
Serum parathyroid hormone (PTH)	85 pg/mL	(<65 pg/mL)
Alkaline phosphatase	165 IU/L	(44–147 IU/L)
Serum Iron	56 μg/dL	(50–170 μg/dL)
Ferritin	23 μg/L	(20–335 μg/L)

1. Which of the following statements is correct?

A. Dietary 25-OH-vitamin D may be found in salmon, eggs, beef, pork, and dairy products.
B. 25-OH-vitamin D is hydroxylated in the liver to its active form, 1,25-OH-vitamin D.
C. Dietary vitamin D is absorbed in the proximal small intestine via active transport with protein absorption.
D. 1,25-OH-vitamin D is necessary for absorption of magnesium in the proximal small intestine.
E. Parathyroid hormone signals the liver to increase hydroxylation of vitamin D and increase vitamin D absorption.

2. Regarding her current disease process, which of the following statements is correct?

A. Preoperative deficiency of 25-OH-vitamin D is relatively rare amongst obese patients.
B. All female patients desiring bariatric surgery should undergo a routine dual-energy x-ray absorptiometry (DEXA) scan.
C. Primary hyperparathyroidism is common in both pre- and postoperative bariatric surgery patients.
D. All patients preparing for bariatric surgery should undergo laboratory analysis of 25-OH-vitamin D, PTH, and serum calcium.
E. The degree of bone turnover and loss of bone mineral density postoperatively is unrelated to procedure choice.

3. Regarding treatment and surveillance of her diagnosis, which of the following statements is true?

A. Calcium carbonate works well for all bariatric surgery patients, as long as vitamin D is added to the supplement.
B. Vitamin D supplementation for all bariatric surgery patients should be titrated to a level of at least 60 ng/mL.
C. Low vitamin D will resolve with standard suggested daily supplementation.
D. Patients who undergo bariatric surgery should receive a DEXA scan at 2 years after surgery.
E. Calcium supplementation after surgery is the same for a sleeve gastrectomy and RYGB.

4. Regarding her bariatric surgery, which of the following statements is correct?

A. Hypocalcemia following BPD/DS is less prevalent in patients with renal insufficiency.
B. The development of low vitamin D is rare following RYGB because the ileum is not bypassed allowing the fat-soluble vitamin to be absorbed normally.
C. The rate of vitamin D deficiency following RYGB is similar to that of SG due to a similar decrease in acid exposure in the alimentary tract.
D. Studies have shown no difference in the rate of hypocalcemia in patients who have undergone RYGB or SADI-S.
E. Multiple studies have shown that bariatric surgery increases the incidence of osteoporosis.

5. Deficiency of what other vitamin or mineral may also contribute to an increased risk of fracture?

A. Vitamin A
B. Vitamin E
C. Vitamin K
D. Copper
E. Zinc

ANSWERS

1. A. Vitamin D may come from two distinct sources. Most commonly, it comes from dietary sources. Foods rich in vitamin D include salmon, eggs, and dairy products. The vitamin D content of certain meats, such as poultry, pork, and beef, can be increased using vitamin D rich feeds for the animals. Vitamin D is absorbed in the diet in the jejunum and distal intestine (ileum) with fats. This absorption is decreased following cholecystectomy and in patients who consume excess polyunsaturated fats. Low serum magnesium and age also decrease absorption. An additional source of vitamin D (cholecalciferol) is via ultraviolet light exposure to the skin. 7-dehydrocholesterol can be converted in the skin via light in the UV-B spectrum. Cholecalciferol, either absorbed via the intestine or created in the skin, is converted to 25-OH-vitamin D (calcifediol) by the liver. The kidney then converts 25-OH-vitamin D to 1,25-OH-vitamin D, a process that is amplified in the presence of parathyroid hormone.[27] Calcium is absorbed through a complex process in the duodenum and upper jejunum via active and transcellular transport. It is absorbed throughout the small intestine via passive and paracellular transport. Active calcium transport is a multistep process that is stimulated by 1,25-OH-vitamin D. The paracellular pathway does not require vitamin D.[28]

2. **D.** Deficiency of vitamin D, defined as 25-OH-vitamin D levels less than 20 ng/mL, and insufficiency, defined as 25-OH-vitamin D levels between 21 and 29 ng/mL, are common in preoperative bariatric surgery patients with 60% to 84% of patients showing vitamin D deficiency.[29] Obesity has been protective of bone mass density in certain bones. Femur density has been shown to increase by 25% in some morbidly obese patients.[30]

Current recommendations from the ASMBS via a position statement are for female patients who are estrogen-deficient, in premenopausal females, and males who have conditions associated with bone loss or low bone mass to receive a preoperative DEXA scan. There is no recommendation for a routine preoperative DEXA scan in all female patients.[31]

Elevated PTH levels are present in up to 49% of obese patients, consistent with secondary hyperparathyroidism from low vitamin D blood levels.[31]

All patients preparing for bariatric surgery should be screened for preexisting conditions that may worsen following bariatric surgery. Laboratory analysis should include a complete blood count (CBC), kidney function and electrolyte panels, nutrition screening with 25-OH-vitamin D, and endocrine evaluation of the parathyroids, thyroid, and screening for diabetes.[7]

3. **D.** While calcium carbonate is inexpensive, calcium citrate is the preferred supplement in the setting of absence or reduction of gastric acid, such as after RGYB or BPD/DS.[31]

All patients who have had bariatric surgery should undergo at least annual measurement of albumin, calcium, 25-OH-vitamin D, and PTH. Twenty-four-hour urinary calcium excretion should be completed at 6 months post-operatively and then annually. Adjustments to vitamin D supplementation should be made to achieve a serum level of at least 30 ng/mL.[31]

Patients found to have vitamin D deficiency that fails to resolve shortly after beginning supplementation should be treated with 50,000 IU of vitamin D_2 or D_3 once a week for 8 weeks or daily 6,000 IU of vitamin D to achieve a goal 25-OH-vitamin D level of >30 ng/mL. Maintenance therapy then consists of daily 1,500 to 2,000 IU. In rare cases, ergocalciferol 100,000 IU intramuscular injection once a week can be used.[31]

Per the clinical practice guideline from the ASMBS, patients should receive a DEXA scan 2 years after surgery to verify their bone mineral density. This is recommended for the four surgeries reviewed: adjustable gastric band (AGB), SG, RYGB, and BPD/DS.[7] Routine surveillance or subsequent DEXA scan following this initial scan is not recommended.

Patients who undergo a BPD, BPD/DS, or RYGB should consume a daily multivitamin and additional calcium and vitamin D supplementation. These patients should consume at least 1,800 to 2,400 mg of calcium per day, split between two or three doses, and at least 3,000 IU of vitamin D per day. For patients who undergo a restrictive only surgery, such as AGB or SG, they should consume 1,200 to 1,500 mg of calcium per day, split between two or three doses. They should consume at least 3,000 IU of vitamin D per day, split between two or three doses, until they are nonobese. At that point, patients 19 to 70 years old should consume a minimum of 600 IU per day and patients older than 70 years old should consume 800 IU per day.[7]

4. **D.** The incidence of hypocalcemia following bariatric surgery increases in patients with concomitant renal insufficiency. One study on a cohort of BPD/DS patients showed that patients with renal insufficiency had an odds ratio of 16.8 (6.45–47.7) of developing albumin-corrected serum calcium levels of <7.5 mg/dL.[32]

Incidence of low vitamin D following malabsorptive procedures may be as high as 52%. Deficiencies in fat-soluble vitamins such as vitamin D in BPD/DS are high due to estimated fat malabsorption of about 72% after surgery.[33]

The rate of vitamin D deficiency in RYGB has been found to be higher in the majority of studies compared to SG patients with lower values of 25-OH-vitamin D on testing in RYGB patients. This is due to the malabsorptive effects of the RYGB via intestinal bypass on top of both surgeries having decreased gastric acid.[34]

As a newly accepted surgery, SADI-S has a paucity of data on its long-term outcomes. Currently, single institution, nonrandomized studies show that the surgery is similar to RYGB in terms of calcium absorption. Many studies fail to delineate the post-operative calcium and vitamin D supplementation.[35]

No studies thus far, including retrospective, prospective, and cross-sectional studies, have found any conclusive support for an increased incidence of osteoporosis or increased fracture risk after bariatric surgery.[31]

5. **C.** Vitamin K is well known as a cofactor in the coagulation cascade for factors II, VII, IX, and X. Vitamin K also serves to carboxylate osteocalcin. Carboxylated osteocalcin aids in the deposition of calcium in the bone matrix. It is absorbed throughout the small intestine and colon. Vitamin K deficiency has been showed to increase the risk of osteoporosis.[36] Vitamin K deficiency is rare following bariatric surgery and rarely leads to clotting disorders when present.

   Vitamin E deficiency is rare following bariatric surgery but manifests as hyporeflexia, gait disturbances, muscle weakness, and decreased proprioception. The patient can develop a hemolytic anemia and may have ophthalmoplegia or nystagmus.[5]

   Vitamin A deficiency is common in patients who have had a malabsorptive procedure. In BPD/DS patients, the incidence has been reported to be as high as 69% at 4-year follow-up. In RYGB patients, the incidence has been reported as high as 10% at 4 years. Deficiency manifests as night blindness and ocular xerosis (dry eye).[6]

   Mild zinc deficiency leads to rash and acne, change or absence of taste, and immune deficiency. Severe zinc deficiency manifests as alopecia, skin lesions (bullous pustular dermatitis and acrodermatitis enteropathica), diarrhea, anorexia, night blindness, and delayed wound healing.[5]

   Copper deficiency manifests as hypochromic anemia, neutropenia, or pancytopenia. Patients will also have hypopigmentation of the skin, hair, and nails. They will have hypercholesterolemia and can develop gait abnormalities. Deficiency symptoms are treated based on severity. For mild to moderate deficiency, patients should receive 3 to 8 mg per day of oral copper gluconate or sulfate until serum copper or ceruloplasmin labs have returned to normal. For patients with severe deficiency, they should receive 2 to 4 mg of intravenous copper per day until labs are normal.[5]

VIGNETTE 4

A 49-year-old male with an initial BMI of 51 kg/m^2 underwent a laparoscopic RYGB 4 weeks ago. His preoperative comorbidities include hypertension and type 2 diabetes mellitus. He tolerated his surgery well and was discharged on the morning of postoperative day 2. His blood sugars have remained normal over the last month. He tolerated his liquid diet for 2 weeks and has attempted to transition to a regular diet over the last 2 weeks. He reports drinking about 1 L of water per day and is consuming about 25 g of protein per day. He has not taken a multivitamin or other supplement since surgery.

1. Which statement concerning postoperative nutrition is correct?

A. Patients who underwent RYGB should consume 3 g of protein per kg of ideal body weight (IBW).
B. Following bariatric surgery, patients should slowly increase their water intake to an optimal goal of 2 L of water daily.
C. Vitamin E deficiency occurs in 1 out of 5 patients.
D. Patients with high albumin levels are at risk for developing vitamin A deficiency.
E. Patients who underwent SG should consume a solely liquid diet for the first 30 days after surgery to prevent staple line disruption and leak.

2. Regarding protein intake, which of the following statements is correct?

A. Protein malnutrition manifests itself most commonly following an SG because the decrease in gastric acid secretion leads to inhibition of protein intake.
B. A serum albumin of less than 3.0 g/dL would be consistent with severe protein malnutrition.
C. Severe protein malnutrition is associated with hepatosteatosis, exocrine pancreatic insufficiency, and edema.
D. Serum albumin level is the most accurate test for protein deficiency.
E. Severe protein malnutrition due to improper diet should be treated with total parenteral nutrition.

3. Three months after surgery, the patient notes that his hair is thinning. He has found several large clumps on his brush every morning. To prevent this known complication, he could have:

A. Supplemented biotin postoperatively
B. Supplemented selenium at 15 to 25 mg/day and zinc at 15 to 40 mg/day
C. Supplemented copper at 2 mg/day
D. Increased his over-the-counter multivitamin intake to three times a day
E. Increased his fat intake

4. Which of the following statements is correct?

A. This patient is only at risk for developing a microcytic anemia.

B. Folate deficiency is extremely rare in preoperative bariatric surgery patients and becomes common following bariatric surgery because it is absorbed in the duodenum.

C. Vitamin B12 is absorbed within the duodenum, so RYGB and BPD/DS put patients at higher risk for this deficiency.

D. Folate deficiency may manifest as edema and peripheral neuropathy that migrates proximally.

ANSWERS

1. B. Patients who undergo bariatric surgery, particularly malabsorptive surgeries, should consume 1.1 to 2.1 g/kg of protein based on IBW.[6] Protein is absorbed mostly in the jejunum to mid-ileum, therefore surgeries that bypass this portion of intestines place patients at higher risk for malnutrition. RYGB does not routinely bypass this region, so the most common cause of protein malnutrition in those patients is inadequate intake.[37] Patients who undergo BPD/DS will have portions of this intestine bypassed and should consume closer to 2 g/kg of IBW.[38]

Dehydration is a common cause for readmission in the early postoperative period for bariatric surgery patients. This is multifactorial but common across all bariatric surgeries. Patients should drink 30 mL of water every 15 minutes initially with a goal of about 1 L per day. This should increase to 2 L per day as the patients are able to tolerate more intake.[37]

Vitamin E is absorbed mostly in the jejunum as a fat-soluble vitamin and serves as an antioxidant helping protect cell membrane integrity, particularly muscle cells.[3] Deficiency is exceedingly rare. It is most common in BPD/DS patients and occurs in less than 4% of those patients. No reports of symptomatic bariatric surgery patients with vitamin E deficiency have been reported. Based on other patients, such as Crohn's disease patients, the likely presenting symptoms will be muscle weakness and ataxia.[6] Most over-the-counter multivitamins contain sufficient vitamin E to prevent deficiency. The ASMBS recommends at least 15 mg per day for all bariatric surgery patients.[5]

Vitamin A is a fat-soluble vitamin that is absorbed throughout the intestine. Provitamin A is converted to retinol in the intestines and absorbed. Patients with poor protein status, seen as low serum albumin, will have difficulty transporting and using vitamin A, leading to deficiency. Vitamin A is necessary for vision and maintenance of epithelial tissues. Vitamin A deficiency is a common complication following malabsorptive procedures. BPD/DS patients have an incidence of 69% of patients at 4-year follow-up.[39] In RYGB patients, the incidence is around 10% at 4-year follow-up.[6]

While a liquid diet is recommended for the first few days to 2 weeks after surgery, all bariatric surgery patients should progress to solid foods about 2 weeks after surgery.[6]

2. C. Protein malnutrition occurs least frequently with restrictive only bariatric surgeries, such as SG and AGB. The incidence associated with SG is less than 2%.[40] The incidence increases for patients with a malabsorptive surgery. As the length of common channel for absorption of nutrients decreases, incidence of protein malnutrition increases. For patients with proximal Roux limbs, the incidence is about 5%. It increases to 13% for more distal RYGB patients (Roux limb >150 cm).[41] For patients who have undergone BPD, protein malnutrition occurs in 3% to 18% of patients[42]; and for SADI-S, with a very short common channel, the incidence is 6% to 23%.[43]

Protein malnutrition can be recognized via evaluation of serum albumin (normal range 3.5–5.0 g/dL). A serum albumin of 3.0 to 3.5 g/dL is consistent with mild hypoalbuminemia, 2.5 to 3.0 g/dL is moderate, and <2.5 g/dL is severe.[42] Serum prealbumin is better short-term marker of protein deficiency because it has a shorter half-life of 1–2 days.[37]

Severe protein malnutrition may lead to secondary kwashiorkor. Kwashiorkor consists of several mechanisms that lead to organ dysfunction, particularly the liver and pancreas. Hepatosteatosis develops due to decreased hepatic synthesis of plasma beta-lipoproteins and intestinal epithelial barrier dysfunction leading to hepatic cell inflammation and death. Exocrine pancreatic insufficiency occurs due to the high rate of protein turnover. Edema occurs secondary to failure of hepatic inactivation of antidiuretic hormone and ferritin release from damaged hepatocytes that leads to further secretion of antidiuretic hormone and hyperaldosteronism. The hair becomes depigmented and brittle as well.[44]

Severe protein malnutrition may be treated with TPN, tube feeds, oral feeds, or a mixture of these. While no standardized treatment regimen exists for severe protein deficiency, multiple different techniques have been successful. These include high protein oral feeding, nasojejunal feedings, enteral feeding through a gastric feeding tube in the remnant stomach for RYGB patients, and TPN.[42]

3. **A.** Vitamin B6, also known as biotin, is an important cofactor in carboxylation reactions, such as gluconeogenesis, fatty acid, and propionate synthesis.[2] Symptomatic deficiency occurs rarely after bariatric surgery, particularly a malabsorptive procedure, but can occur. It can be prevented and treated by consuming 2,500 to 3,000 mcg of vitamin B6 daily.[37]

   Selenium is a mineral that works with enzymes to prevent cellular oxidation. It is not associated with hair loss.[3] Zinc is a mineral whose deficiency may contribute to hair loss. Zinc deficiency is common with bariatric surgeries, occurring in 70% of BPD/DS patients, 40% of RYGB patients, 19% of SG patients, and 34% of AGB patients. Consuming 15 to 40 mg of zinc in a multivitamin will prevent deficiency. Taking too much zinc after surgery may induce copper deficiency.[5]

   Inadequate protein intake is a risk factor for alopecia following bariatric surgery, particularly if the alopecia is not in a 3- to 6-month period after surgery. During that time period, the alopecia is likely secondary to the stress of surgery and low-calorie intake.[37]

   Copper deficiency is common in RYGB patients, occurring in up to 10%. In BPD/DS patients, the rate may be as high as 70%. This is due to bypassing the duodenum and proximal jejunum, where copper is absorbed.[5] Copper serves as cofactor for enzymes involved in hemoglobin synthesis and cell respiration. It is required for melanin pigment formation.[3] Deficiency will cause hypopigmentation of skin and hair, but it is not associated with hair loss. It can be prevented by taking 2 mg per day for BPD/DS and RYGB patients or 1 mg per day for SG and AGB patients.[5]

4. **A.** RYGB patients are at risk for developing vitamin B12 deficiency that will manifest as a macrocytic anemia. If present, vitamin B12 may be treated with either 1,000 μg of vitamin B12 orally or intramuscularly. Once resolved, preventive supplementation should be resumed.

   Folate deficiency is common in patients eating a Westernized diet with about 25% to 55% of patients being deficient in folate prior to bariatric surgery. This is likely due to low dietary intake of folate as it is absorbed throughout the entire small intestine.[6] Folate is necessary for DNA, RNA, and protein synthesis.[3] There is great variability in how folate is measured following bariatric surgery. The prevalence of folate deficiency after bariatric surgery is up to 65%.[5]

   Vitamin B12 (cobalamin) is absorbed in the distal ileum. Vitamin B12 in food is bound to protein. Gastric acid breaks the bond with the protein freeing the cobalamin. The free cobalamin then binds a protein called haptocorrin or transcobalamin I. Intrinsic factor is produced by gastric parietal cells and replaces the other proteins on cobalamin and binds it. The combined intrinsic factor and cobalamin are then absorbed by enterocytes in the distal ileum. About 1% to 5% of free vitamin B12 is absorbed in the small intestine. The incidence of vitamin B12 deficiency in RYGB patients is 12% to 33% and is likely higher in BPD/DS patients.[45] In SG patients, the rate of vitamin B12 deficiency ranges from 4% to 20%.[5]

   Folate deficiency is common following bariatric surgery. It may be prevented by taking 400 to 800 μg of folate orally from a multivitamin. Women of childbearing age should increase their intake to 800 to 1,000 μg per day. Deficiency will manifest fatigue and weakness. Examination will reveal changes in the pigmentation or ulceration of the skin, nails, or oral mucosa.[3] Deficiency is treated with 1,000 μg of folate orally daily until normal levels are achieved. Taking more than 1 mg of folate per day may mask vitamin B12 deficiency.[5] Thiamine deficiency may manifest with edema and peripheral neuropathy that migrates proximally.

REFERENCES

1. Fernandez-Bañares F, Monzón H, Forne M. A short review of malabsorption and anemia. *World J Gastroenterol.* 2009;15(37):4644-4652.
2. Carson J, Al-Mousawi A, Rodriguez NA, et al. Metabolism in Surgical Patients. In: Townsend C, Beauchamp RD, Evers BM, Mattox K, eds. *Sabiston Textbook of Surgery.* 20th ed. Philadelphia: Elsevier; 2017: 103-105.
3. Lutz CA, Pryztulski KR. *Nutrition and Diet Therapy.* 5th ed. Philadelphia: F.A. Davis Co.; 2011:92-142.
4. Enani G, Bilgic E, Lebedeva E, et al. The incidence of iron deficiency anemia post-Roux-en-Y gastric bypass and sleeve gastrectomy: a systematic review. *Surg Endosc.* 2019 Sep 4; epub ahead of print.
5. Parrott J, Frank L, Rabena R, et al. American Society for Metabolic and Bariatric Surgery integrated health

nutritional guidelines for the surgical weight loss patient 2016 update: micronutrients. *Surg Obes Relat Dis.* 2017;13(5):727-741.
6. Handzlik-Orlik G, Holecki M, Orlik B, et al. Nutrition management of the post-bariatric surgery patient. *Nutr Clin Pract.* 2015;30(3):383-392.
7. Mechanick JI, Youdim A, Jones DB, et al. Clinical practice guidelines for perioperative nutritional, metabolic, and nonsurgical support of the bariatric surgery patients-2013 update. *Surg Obes Relat Dis.* 2013;9(2):159-191.
8. Ciobârcă D, Cătoi AF, Copăescu C, Miere D, Crişan G. Bariatric surgery in obesity: effects on gut microbiota and micronutrient status. *Nutrients.* 2020;12(1):235–227. doi:10.3390/nu12010235
9. Clements RH, Katasani VG, Palepu R, et al. Incidence of vitamin deficiency after laparoscopic Roux-en-Y gastric bypass in a university hospital setting. *Am Surg.* 2006;72(12):1196–1204.
10. Tang L, Alsulaim HA, Canner JK, Prokopowicz GP, Steele KE. Prevalence and predictors of postoperative thiamine deficiency after vertical sleeve gastrectomy. *SOARD.* 2018;14(7):943-950. doi:10.1016/j.soard.2018.03.024
11. Oudman E, Wijnia JW, Dam M, Biter LU, Postma A. Preventing Wernicke encephalopathy after bariatric surgery. *Obes Surg.* 2018:1–9. doi:10.1007/s11695-018-3262-4
12. Stroh C, Meyer F, Manger T. Beriberi, a severe complication after metabolic surgery - review of the literature. *Obes Facts.* 2014;7(4):246-252. doi:10.1159/000366012
13. Iannelli A, Addeo P, Novellas S, et al. Wernicke's encephalopathy after laparoscopic Roux-en-Y gastric bypass: a misdiagnosed complication. *Obes Surg.* 2010;20(11):1594-1596.
14. Zadeh MH, Farsani GM, Zamaninour N. Selenium status after Roux-en-Y gastric bypass: interventions and recommendations. *Obes Surg.* 2019:1–6. doi:10.1007/s11695-019-04148-0
15. Shankar P. Boylan M, Sriram K. Micronutrient deficiencies after bariatric surgery. *Nutrition.* 2010;26(11–12): 1031-1037. doi:10.1016/j.nut.2009.12.003
16. Netto BD, Moreira EA, Patiño JS, Benincá JP, Jordão AA, Fröde TS. Influence of Roux-en-Y gastric bypass surgery on vitamin C, myeloperoxidase, and oral clinical manifestations: a 2-year follow-up study. *Nutr Clin Pract.* 2012;27(1):114–121. doi:10.1177/0884533611431462
17. Zusman O, Theilla M, Cohen J, Kagan I, Bendavid I, Singer P. Resting energy expenditure, calorie and protein consumption in critically ill patients: a retrospective cohort study. *Crit Care.* 2016;20(1):367. doi:10.1186/s13054-016-1538-4
18. Mackenzie TA, Clark NG, Bistrian BR, Flatt JP, Hallowell EM, Blackburn GL. A simple method for estimating nitrogen balance in hospitalized patients: a review and supporting data for a previously proposed technique. *J Am Coll Nutr.* 1985;4(5):575–581. doi:10.1080/07315724.1985.10720100
19. Moizé V, Andreu A, Rodríguez L, et al. Protein intake and lean tissue mass retention following bariatric surgery. *Clin Nutr.* 2013;32(4):550–555. doi:10.1016/j.clnu.2012.11.007
20. Mogensen KM. Nutritional support therapy for the bariatric surgery patient. *Weight Management Matters.* 2010 (Winter): 8-16.
21. Strong AT, Fayazzadeh H, Sharma G, El-Hayek K, Kroh M, Rodriguez J. Feeding the gut after revisional bariatric surgery: the fate of 126 enteral access tubes. *Surg Obes Relat Dis.* 2018;14(7):986–991. doi:10.1016/j.soard.2018.03.008
22. Young MT, Troung H, Gebhart A, Shih A, Nguyen NT. Outcomes of laparoscopic feeding jejunostomy tube placement in 299 patients. *Surg Endosc.* 2016;30(1): 126–131. doi:10.1007/s00464-015-4171-4
23. Mirtallo J, Canada T, Johnson D, et al. Safe practices for parenteral nutrition [published correction appears in JPEN J Parenter Enteral Nutr. 2006; 30(2): 177]. *JPEN J Parenter Enteral Nutr.* 2004;28(6):S39–S70. doi:10.1177/0148607104028006s39
24. Langan RC, Goodbred AJ. Vitamin B12 deficiency: recognition and management. *Am Fam Physician.* 2017;96(6):384-389.
25. Parrott J, Frank L, Rabena R, Craggs-Dino L, Isom KA, Greiman L. American Society for Metabolic and Bariatric Surgery Integrated Health Nutritional Guidelines for the Surgical Weight Loss Patient 2016 Update_ micronutrients. *SOARD.* 2017;13(5):1-15. doi:10.1016/j.soard.2016.12.018
26. Stein J, Stier C, Raab H, Weiner R. Review article: the nutritional and pharmacological consequences of obesity surgery. *Aliment Pharmacol Ther.* 2014;40(6):582–609. doi:10.1111/apt.12872
27. Simoliunas E, Rinkunaite I, Bukelskiene Z, et al. Bioavailability of different vitamin D oral supplements in laboratory animal model. *Medicina.* 2019;55(265).
28. Balsa JA, Botella-Carretero JI, Peromingo R, et al. Role of calcium malabsorption in the development of secondary hyperparathyroidism after biliopancreatic diversion. *J Endocrinol Invest.* 2008;31(10):845-850.
29. Carlin AM, Rao DS, Meslemani AM, et al. Prevalence of vitamin D depletion among morbidly obese patients seeking gastric bypass surgery. *Surg Obes Relat Dis.* 2006;2:98-103.
30. Beck TJ, Petit MA, Wu G, et al. Does obesity really make the femur stronger? BMD, geometry, and fracture incidence in the women's health initiative-observational study. *J Bone Miner Res.* 2009;24:1369-1379.
31. Kim J, Brethauer S. Metabolic bone changes after bariatric surgery. *Surg Obes Relat Dis.* 2015;11(2):406-411.
32. Shah M, Sharma A, Wermers RA, et al. Hypocalcemia after bariatric surgery: prevalence and associated risk factors. *Obes Surg.* 2017;27:2905-2911.
33. Furtado MM. Identification, assessment, and treatment of vitamin and mineral deficiencies after bariatric surgery. In: Still C, Sarwer DB, Blankenship J, eds. *The ASMBS Textbook of Bariatric Surgery.* Volume 2. New York: Springer; 2014:111-117.
34. Chaktoura M, Rahme M, Fuleihan GE. Vitamin D metabolism in bariatric surgery. *Endocrinol Metab Clin N Am.* 2017;46:947-982.

35. Lee WJ, Lee KT, Kasama K, et al. Laparoscopic single-anastomosis duodenal-jejunal bypass with sleeve gastrectomy (SADJB-SG): short-term result and comparison with gastric bypass. *Obes Surg*. 2014;24(1): 109-113.
36. Wen L, Chen J, Duan L, et al. Vitamin K-dependent proteins involved in bone and cardiovascular health. *Mol Med Rep*. 2018;18(1):3-15.
37. LeBrun CM. Managing common nutrition problems after bariatric surgery. In: Still C, Sarwer DB, Blankenship J, eds. *The ASMBS Textbook of Bariatric Surgery*. Volume 2. New York: Springer; 2014:119-127.
38. Litchford MD. Macronutrient recommendations: protein, carbohydrate, and fat. In: Still C, Sarwer DB, Blankenship J, eds. *The ASMBS Textbook of Bariatric Surgery*. Volume 2. New York: Springer; 2014:101-110.
39. Slater GH, Ren CJ, Siegel N, et al. Serum fat-soluble vitamin deficiency and abnormal calcium metabolism after malabsorptive bariatric surgery. *J Gastrointest Surg*. 2004 Jan;8(1):48-55.
40. Verger EO, Aron-Wisnewsky J, Dao MC, et al. Micronutrient and protein deficiencies after gastric bypass and sleeve gastrectomy: a 1-year follow-up. *Obes Surg*. 2016;26(4):785-796.
41. Stein J, Stier C, Raab H, et al. The nutritional and pharmacological consequences of obesity surgery. *Aliment Pharmacol Ther*. 2014;40(6):582-609.
42. Kuin C, den Ouden F, Brandts H, et al. Treatment of severe protein malnutrition after bariatric surgery. *Obes Surg*. 2019;29(10):3095-3102.
43. Shoar S, Poliakin L, Rubenstein R, et al. A single anastomosis duodeno-ileal switch (SADIS): a systematic review of efficacy and safety. *Obes Surg*. 2018;28(1):104-113.
44. William JH, Tapper EB, Yee EU, et al. Secondary Kwashiorkor: a rare complication of gastric bypass surgery. *Am J Med*. 2015;128(5): e1-e2.
45. Majumder S, Soriano J, Cruz AL, et al. Vitamin B12 deficiency in patients undergoing bariatric surgery: preventive strategies and key recommendations. *Surg Obes Relat Dis*. 2013;9(6):1013-1019.

50

Venous Thromboembolic Events (DVT, PE, Splenic Vein Thrombosis)

Christopher Yheulon, MD

A 49-year-old female with a body mass index (BMI) of 43 kg/m^2 with no weight-related comorbidities undergoes an uncomplicated laparoscopic sleeve gastrectomy (operative time 90 minutes).

1. **Which of the following is a risk factor for venous thrombo-embolism (VTE) in bariatric surgery?**
    A. Increasing BMI class II obesity
    B. Conversion to open from robot-assisted surgery
    C. Revisional bariatric surgery
    D. Operative time of 2 hours
    E. Family history of VTE

2. **Which strategy has the highest risk of VTE occurrence after bariatric surgery?**
    A. Standard-dose unfractionated heparin
    B. Adjusted-dose unfractionated heparin
    C. Low-molecular-weight heparin
    D. Vena cava filters
    E. Lower extremity compression

3. **Two weeks after discharge, the patient presents to the emergency room with fatigue, nausea, low-grade fever (38°C), and moderate central abdominal pain. A computed tomography (CT) scan with oral and intravenous contrast shows no evidence of leak. However, there is a nonobstructive portal vein thrombosis (PVT). The bowel appears otherwise heathy. What is the next step in management?**
    A. Aspirin
    B. Thrombolytic therapy
    C. Admission and systemic anticoagulation
    D. Diagnostic laparoscopy
    E. Portal venous thrombectomy

4. **Which of the following is a proposed mechanism for portal venous thrombosis after sleeve gastrectomy?**
    A. Prolonged liver retraction
    B. Ligation/division of the left gastroepiploic artery with energy devices
    C. Injury to the splenic vein
    D. Increased portal vein flow
    E. Increased intraluminal pressure from intraoperative leak test

5. **After initial observation, the patient's pain worsens with associated tachycardia. Repeat CT scan shows progression of the thrombosis along with bowel wall edema. The patient is taken for diagnostic laparoscopy which reveals a large (50 cm segment) necrotic-appearing bowel. The case is converted to an exploratory laparotomy and a bowel resection is performed. Which of the following is an important adjunct for this patient's care?**
    A. Vena cava filter
    B. Leave the bowel in discontinuity, plan for second look operation
    C. Administration of activated protein C

D. Feeding jejunostomy
E. Venting gastrostomy

ANSWERS

1. **C.** Bariatric surgery patients are moderate-high risk for VTE. Risk factors include increasing age, male sex, increasing BMI (>50kg/m^2), personal history of VTE, smoking, open surgery, revisional surgery, and operative time greater than 3 hours.[1]

2. **D.** Many different societies provide recommendations for prophylaxis of VTE in bariatric surgery patients. However, there is no consensus regarding the exact therapy, timing, or duration. Unfractionated heparin has shown to be effective in reducing VTE in bariatric surgery patients in both standard and adjusted doses. However, adjusted doses may be associated with increased rates of bleeding. There is no direct comparison of low-molecular-weight heparin and unfractionated heparin in bariatric surgery patients and meta-analyses have demonstrated similar outcomes between the two medications. A Michigan study shows that Lovenox before and after is better than heparin. Although there is no data regarding compression therapy in bariatric surgery patients, it has shown a reduction of 65% in other sets of patients. Given that compression therapy is cheap and safe, it is recommended in all bariatric surgery patients. Early ambulation (within 2–4 hours after the operation) is also thought to reduce the incidence of VTE.

   Meta-analyses have demonstrated that vena cava filters do not decrease the rate of pulmonary emboli, but actually increase the rates of VTE and mortality. These should only be used on a very select basis such as patients with a very recent acute VTE within 3 to 4 weeks of surgery. As the overwhelming majority of bariatric procedures are elective, it may be best to delay those procedures to a time when a vena cava filter is not necessary.[1,2,4]

3. **C.** Porto-mesenteric venous thrombosis has an incidence of 0.3% to 1.0% after sleeve gastrectomy, although it can also be identified after other bariatric surgeries. Although considered a harbinger for impending bowel ischemia/infarction, >90% of cases can be treated effectively with 3 to 6 months of systemic anticoagulation. More aggressive therapies are reserved for bowel ischemia/infarction. There is no evidence supporting the use of aspirin in these patients.[3,5]

4. **E.** Proposed mechanisms of PVT after sleeve gastrectomy/bariatric surgery include prolonged liver retraction, decreased blood flow from increased intra-abdominal pressure due to pneumoperitoneum, and ligation/division of both the right gastroepiploic artery and short gastric vessels with energy devices. Endoscopic sclerotherapy is a described cause of portal vein thrombosis, but performance of an endoscopic intra-abdominal leak test is not. While an injury or retraction on the splenic vein may cause portal vein thrombosis, it is unlikely to be injured during an SG.[3,5]

5. **B.** A patient who worsens clinically with PVT should be taken to the operating room. Although surgeons can begin with diagnostic laparoscopy, conversion to laparotomy should be performed if bowel ischemia/infarction is noted. A second-look procedure should be planned to evaluate the extent of ischemia/infarction prior to reestablishing continuity. Drotrecogin alfa (activated protein C) is no longer manufactured and there is no routine role for vena cava filters in these patients. Nutrition should be established parenterally until the extent of ischemia is determined. In addition, many of these patients will develop a postoperative ileus. We advocate against venting gastrostomy in post-sleeve patients, although this could be considered in the remnant stomach of a gastric bypass patient. Also of note, immunofluorescence imaging with the use of a near-infrared camera or light can help identify ischemic bowel but there is no evidence that it accurately predicts the extent of resection that is needed.[3,5]

REFERENCES

1. ASMBS updated position statement on prophylactic measures to reduce the risk of venous thromboembolism in bariatric surgery patients. *Surg Obes Relat Dis.* 2013;9(4): 493-497.
2. Bartlett MA, Mauck KF, Daniels PR. Prevention of venous thromboembolism in patients undergoing bariatric surgery. *Vasc Health Risk Manage.* 2015;11:461-477.
3. Belnap L, Rodgers GM, Cottam D, Zaveri H, Drury C, Surve A. Portal vein thrombosis after laparoscopic sleeve gastrectomy: presentation and management. *Surg Obes Relat Dis.* 2016;12(10):1787-1794.

4. Brotman DJ, Shihab HM, Prakasa KR, et al. Pharmacologic and mechanical strategies for preventing venous thromboembolism after bariatric surgery: a systematic review and meta-analysis. *JAMA Surg*. 2013;148(7):675-686.

5. Tan SBM, Greenslade J, Martin D, Talbot M, Loi K, Hopkins G. Portomesenteric vein thrombosis in sleeve gastrectomy: a 10-year review. *Surg Obes Relat Dis*. 2018;14(3):271-275.

51

Nausea, Vomiting, and Diarrhea after Bariatric Surgery

Jesse R. Conner, MD, and Laura E. Fischer, MD, MS

SCENARIO 1

A 36-year-old female with a body mass index (BMI) of 43 kg/m^2 and a medical history of hypertension and obstructive sleep apnea undergoes a Roux-en-Y gastric bypass. Her postoperative course is uncomplicated and she is discharged home on postoperative day 2 on a full liquid diet. Upon return to clinic after advancing to solid foods, she complains of postprandial abdominal pain, nausea, fatigue, and diarrhea. After careful questioning, you determine that her symptoms are associated with carbohydrate-rich meals.

Which answer is the most correct regarding appropriate management of this patient's symptoms?

A. Supplements that increase the viscosity of food (e.g. pectin) are the mainstay of treatment.
B. Octreotide should be the first-line treatment.
C. This self-limiting condition can be treated with reassurance alone.
D. A majority of patients will respond to dietary modification.
E. Surgical intervention has no role.

ANSWER

D. This patient is exhibiting symptoms of dumping syndrome. Treatment approaches for dumping syndrome include dietary modification, pharmacological intervention, and, rarely, surgical intervention.[1]

Early dumping syndrome is thought to be caused by the rapid delivery of hyperosmolar, carbohydrate-rich food to the small intestine causing fluid shifts from the intravascular space to the intestinal lumen.[8,9] These fluid shifts, as well as the release of various gastrointestinal hormones, can cause abdominal bloating, fatigue, nausea, vomiting, and diarrhea. Symptoms typically occur within 30 minutes of eating. In some studies, up to one-third of postbariatric patients experience symptoms of dumping at some point in their postoperative course.[2,3]

Late dumping syndrome, or hyperinsulinemic hypoglycemia, is thought to be related to increased insulin secretion combined with improved insulin sensitivity after bariatric surgery.[5,8,9] Late dumping typically doesn't appear until at least 1 year after surgery and often occurs 2 to 3 hours after eating. Late dumping is associated with more severe symptoms such as diaphoresis, palpitations, severe fatigue, syncope, neuroglycopenia, coma, and even death.[2] Severe hyperinsulinemic hypoglycemia is thought to be rare, occurring in only a small percentage of postbariatric patients.[4,6,7]

Dietary modification should be the initial management approach, because a majority of patients will respond.[6,8] Dietary modification consists of limiting the diet to small portions of low-carbohydrate, high-fiber, and protein-rich food.[3] Patients should be instructed to delay fluid intake until at least 30 min after meals and alcohol should be avoided.

For patients that do not have relief from dietary modification, medical management can assist with symptom management.[6,8,9] Acarbose is an antidiabetic medication that slows the rate of carbohydrate digestion and influx into the bloodstream. Somatostatin analogues can also be considered.

Somatostatin analogues delay gastric emptying, delay transit through the small intestine, and inhibit the release of gastrointestinal hormones. Dietary supplementation such as pectin have been thought to increase viscosity of food and slow the rate of gastric emptying. There are several small studies suggesting that dietary supplementation slows gastric emptying, and improves glucose tolerance and vasomotor symptoms; however, tolerance can be poor because some patients can experience bloating and gas as well as concern for choking hazard and bowel obstruction with the increased viscosity.

Surgical intervention is poorly studied with variable outcomes.[8] For refractory hyperinsulinemic hypoglycemia, small studies with reversal of Roux-en-Y gastric bypass have shown improvement in postprandial hypoglycemia.[1] Several case reports have shown good symptomatic relief with continuous feeds through gastrostomy tubes into the remnant stomach. Results of surgical intervention have been variable and should be a last resort on a select few patients.

SCENARIO 2

1. A 46-year-old male with a past medical history of smoking, type 2 diabetes mellitus, and morbid obesity, now 1-year status post–Roux-en-Y gastric bypass, presents to your office with complaints of postprandial epigastric pain, nausea, and vomiting. Upper endoscopy is significant for a nonbleeding marginal ulcer.

Which statement regarding margin ulcers is correct?

A. Gastric pouch size has no relation to incidence of marginal ulcer.
B. Prophylactic proton pump inhibiters (PPIs) have not been shown to decrease the incidence of marginal ulcers.
C. The most common indication for operative treatment of marginal ulcers is bleeding.
D. Age is a significant risk factor for the formation of marginal ulcers.
E. Diagnosis of marginal ulcers requires subsequent endoscopic surveillance.

ANSWER

E. Marginal ulcers are a frequent complication after bariatric surgery with an incidence ranging from 1% to 16%.[10] Risk factors for marginal ulcers include a history of diabetes mellitus, smoking or other nicotine use, nonsteroidal anti-inflammatory drug (NSAID) use, and gastric pouch size.[10,13] The most common presentation is upper abdominal or epigastric pain, often with eating, followed by nausea, vomiting, and dysphagia.[15] Patients can exhibit anemia on complete blood count if their marginal ulcer bleeds.

Studies have shown that prophylactic PPIs significantly decrease the incidence of marginal ulcers and should be continued at least 60 to 90 days postoperatively.[12,14] Patients should be strongly encouraged to quit smoking or using other forms of nicotine prior to surgery. Patients should also be educated on avoiding all NSAIDs after surgery.

Initial management of marginal ulcers consists of medical therapy with high-dose PPIs in addition to modification of risk factors. Most ulcers will respond to medical management; however, approximately 10% will be refractory requiring operative intervention.[10]

Refractory marginal ulcers place the patient at risk for bleeding, perforation, stricture, and gastrogastric fistula formation; therefore resolution should be confirmed with endoscopic surveillance. Indications for operative intervention include perforation, uncontrolled bleeding, gastrogastric fistula formation, or medically refractory disease causing symptoms that interfere with daily life.[14] Surgical options include revision of the gastrojejunostomy, gastrectomy with esophagojejunostomy, and laparoscopic truncal vagotomy.[11]

2. The patient has resolution of his marginal ulcer approximately 6 weeks after initiating medical management with high-dose PPIs. Six months later, he develops nausea, vomiting, and dysphagia to solid foods consistent with an anastomotic stricture.

Which statement is correct regarding anastomotic strictures?

A. There is no difference in anastomotic stricture rate between 21-mm and 25-mm circular staplers.
B. Anastomotic stricture aids in weight loss after Roux-en-Y gastric bypass.
C. The majority of strictures will resolve with one balloon dilation.
D. Anastomotic stricture is a rare complication after Roux-en-Y gastric bypass occurring in 1% to 5% of patients.

ANSWER

C. Gastrojejunal anastomotic stricture after Roux-en-Y gastric bypass is a common complication occurring in 7% to 25% of patients.[16,18] Several case series and retrospective studies have shown a significantly higher stricture rate when using a 21-mm versus 25-mm circular stapler to create the gastrojejunal anastomosis.[19,20] Anastomotic strictures have not been shown to aid in weight loss.[20] Many patients are unable to tolerate solid foods and tend to revert to a high-carbohydrate diet, leading to weight regain after surgery. The majority of anastomotic strictures are amendable to pneumatic balloon dilation with 80% resolving after one dilation.[20] However, some strictures may require additional dilations.[17,18] It is rare to require surgical revision of the anastomosis with the most common indication being perforation after dilation.[17,19] The patient should be counseled to modify risk factors for marginal ulceration, such as avoiding nicotine products and NSAID usage.

SCENARIO 3

A 36-year-old female undergoes a distal Roux-en-Y gastric bypass with a 250-cm alimentary limb and a 40-cm biliopancreatic limb. She presents to your office 2 months postoperatively complaining of chronic, greasy, loose stools that occur primarily after meals. She has had excellent weight loss, but notes some mild lower extremity swelling and persistent fatigue.

Which is true regarding this patient's symptoms?

A. Symptoms are likely secondary to the length of the alimentary limb.
B. Symptoms are likely secondary to the length of the biliopancreatic limb.
C. Exocrine pancreatic insufficiency is extremely common and should be treated with oral supplementation of pancreatic enzymes.
D. Bile acid malabsorption is the likely cause and trial of octreotide should be given.

ANSWER

A. Diarrhea can occur after any bariatric procedure and there are multiple possible causes.[21] Common causes of diarrhea include lactose intolerance and carbohydrate malabsorption.

Short bowel syndrome occurs in about 4% of bariatric patients and is more common in distal gastric Roux-en-Y gastric bypass and biliopancreatic diversion with duodenal switch (BPD-DS).[21,22,25,26] Although appropriate limbs lengths are controversial, a common channel length of less than 100 cm puts the patient at high risk for malabsorption and severe protein calorie malnutrition.[21,25] Initial treatment includes dietary modification, such as increasing protein intake. Surgical options include placing a feeding gastrostomy or jejunostomy, lengthening the common channel, or restoring normal gastrointestinal anatomy.[23]

Exocrine pancreatic insufficiency can occur after gastric bypass or BPD-DS and leads to subsequent malabsorption of fat-soluble vitamins (A, D, E, and K).[21,22,25] There are several mechanisms by which this occurs including: (1) less mixing time of food with chyme, and (2) an increased breakdown of pancreatic enzyme within the biliopancreatic limb in the absence of nutrients. Exocrine pancreatic insufficiency usually manifests as greasy and loose stools that are worse after fatty meals.[24] Patients with these symptoms should be given a trial of pancreatic enzymes, and if they do not have improvement, other causes should be considered.

Patients undergoing bariatric surgery are also at increased risk of bile acid malabsorption, which can cause chronic diarrhea; however, this is less common.[21] The mechanism of bile acid malabsorption is not completely understood. It is thought to be associated with reduced intestinal transit time as well as the prevalence of small intestine bacterial overgrowth, which can alter the absorption of bile acids within the ileum. Treatment of bile acid malabsorption is with cholestyramine, a bile acid binder.[21]

REFERENCES

1. Campos GM, Ziemelis M, Paparodis R, Ahmed M, Davis DM. Laparoscopic reversal of Roux-en-Y gastric bypass: technique and utility for treatment of endocrine complications. *Surg Obes Relat Dis*. 2014;10(1):36-43.
2. Halperin F, Patti ME, Skow M, Bajwa M, Goldfine AB. Continuous glucose monitoring evaluation of glycemic excursions after gastric bypass. *J Obes*. 2011;2011:869536.
3. Kellogg TA, Bantle JP, Leslie DB, et al. Postgastric bypass hyperinsulinemic hypoglycemia syndrome: characterization and response to a modified diet. *Surg Obes Relat Dis*. 2008;4:492-499.
4. Marsk R, Jonas E, Rasmussen F, Naslund E. Nationwide cohort study of post-gastric bypass hypoglycaemia

including 5,040 patients undergoing surgery for obesity in 1986-2006 in Sweden. *Diabetologia.* 2010;53:2307-2311.
5. Meier JJ, Butler AE, Galasso R, Butler PC. Hyperinsulinemic hypoglycemia after gastric bypass surgery is not accompanied by islet hyperplasia or increased beta-cell turnover. *Diabetes Care.* 2006;29(7):1554-1559.
6. Patti ME, Goldfine AB. Hypoglycaemia following gastric bypass surgery–diabetes remission in the extreme? *Diabetologia.* 2010;53:2276-2279.
7. Sarwar H, Chapman WH III, Pender JR, et al. Hypoglycemia after Roux-en-Y gastric bypass: the BOLD experience. *Obes Surg.* 2014;24:1120-1124.
8. van Beek AP, Emous M, Laville M, Tack J. Dumping syndrome after esophageal, gastric or bariatric surgery: pathophysiology, diagnosis, and management. *Obes Rev.* 2017;18:68-85.
9. Vavricka SR, Greuter T. Gastroparesis and dumping syndrome: current concepts and management. *J Clin Med.* 2019;8(8):E1127.
10. Azagury D, Dayyeh BA, Greenwalt I, Thompson C. Marginal ulceration after Roux-en-Y gastric bypass surgery: characteristics, risk factors, treatment, and outcomes. *Endoscopy.* 2011;43(11):950-954.
11. Chau E, Youn H, Ren-Fielding CJ, Fielding GA, Schwack BF, Kurian MS. Surgical management and outcomes of patients with marginal ulcer after Roux-en-Y gastric bypass. *Surg Obes Relat Dis.* 2015;11(5):1071-1075.
12. Coblijn UK, Lagarde SM, de Castro SM, Kuiken SD, van Tets WF, van Wagensveld BA. The influence of prophylactic proton pump inhibitor treatment on the development of symptomatic marginal ulceration in Roux-en-Y gastric bypass patients: a historic cohort study. *Surg Obes Relat Dis.* 2016;12(2):246-252.
13. Dittrich L, Schwenninger MV, Dittrich K, Pratschke J, Aigner F, Raakow J. Marginal ulcer after laparoscopic Roux-en-Y gastric bypass: analysis of the amount of daily and lifetime smoking smoking on postoperative risk. *Surg Obes Relat Dis.* 2020;16(3):389-396.
14. Kang X, Zurita-Macias L, Hong D, Cadeddu M, Anvari M, Gmora S. A comparison of 30-day versus 90-day proton pump inhibitor therapy in prevention of marginal ulcers after laparoscopic Roux-en-Y gastric bypass. *Surg Obes Relat Dis.* 2016;12(5):1003-1007.
15. Moon RC, Teixeira AF, Goldbach M, Jawad MA. Management and treatment outcomes of marginal ulcers after Roux-en-Y gastric bypass at a single high volume bariatric center. *Surg Obes Relat Dis.* 2014;10(2):229-234.
16. Alasfar F, Sabnis AA, Liu RC, Chand B. Stricture rate after laparoscopic Roux-en-Y gastric bypass with a 21-mm circular stapler: the Cleveland Clinic experience. *Med Princ Pract.* 2009;18(5):364-367.
17. Almby K, Edholm D. Anastomotic strictures after Roux-en-Y gastric bypass: a cohort study from the Scandinavian obesity surgery registry. *Obes Surg.* 2019;29(1): 172-177.
18. Carrodeguas L, Szomstein S, Zundel N, Lomenzo E, Rosenthal R. Gastrojejunal anastomotic strictures following laparoscopic Roux-en-Y gastric bypass surgery: analysis of 1291 patients. *Surg Obes Relat Dis.* 2006;2(2): 92-97.
19. Markar SR, Penna M, Venkat-Ramen V, Karthikesalingam A, Hashemi M. Influence of circular stapler diameter on postoperative stenosis after laparoscopic gastrojejunal anastomosis in morbid obesity. *Surg Obes Relat Dis.* 2012;8(2):230-235.
20. Nguyen NT, Stevens CM, Wolfe BM. Incidence and outcome of anastomotic stricture after laparoscopic gastric bypass. *J Gastrointest Surg.* 2003;7(8):997-1003.
21. Borbély YM, Osterwalder A, Kröll D, Nett PC, Inglin RA. Diarrhea after bariatric procedures: diagnosis and therapy. *World J Gastroenterol.* 2017;23(26):4689-4700.
22. Borbély Y, Plebani A, Kröll D, Ghisla S, Nett PC. Exocrine pancreatic insufficiency after Roux-en-Y gastric bypass. *Surg Obes Relat Dis.* 2016;12(4):790-794.
23. Horsley B, Cottam D, Cottam A, et al. Bowel reconstruction to treat chronic diarrhea and hypoproteinemia following single anastomosis duodenal-ileal bypass with sleeve gastrectomy: a single-site experience. *Obes Surg.* 2019;29(8):2387-2391.
24. Keller J, Layer P. Human pancreatic exocrine response to nutrients in health and disease. *Gut.* 2005;54(suppl 6): 1-28.
25. Lupoli R, Lembo E, Saldalamacchia G, Avola CK, Angrisani L, Capaldo B. Bariatric surgery and long-term nutritional issues. *World J Diabetes.* 2017;8(11):464-474.
26. van der Burgh Y, Boerboom A, de Boer H, Witteman B, Berends F, Hazebroek E. Weight loss and malnutrition after conversion of the primary Roux-en-Y gastric bypass to distal gastric bypass in patients with morbid obesity. *Surg Obes Relat Dis.* 2020;16(3):381-388.

52

Gallstones and Accessing the CBD

Nikdokht Rashidian, MD, PhD, Mohammad Abu Hilal, MD, PhD, and Adnan Alseidi, MD, EdM

A 32-year-old man with a body mass index (BMI) of 41 kg/m^2 is referred to a tertiary center for management of obesity disorders. After a thorough clinical assessment, he is found to be a good candidate for a Roux-en-Y gastric bypass (RYGB). He has no history of biliary colic or other gallstone-related symptoms. In the preoperative abdominal ultrasound examination, his gallbladder has a normal shape, 2-mm wall thickness, and contains multiple 8- to 10-mm stones. The liver has a normal appearance and there is no evidence of biliary duct dilatation. Liver function tests are in the normal range.

1. **Concerning the management of his gallstones in this setting, which of the following is true?**
   A. RYGB and subsequent laparoscopic cholecystectomy in 3 to 6 months has the lowest complication rate.
   B. RYGB with a concomitant cholecystectomy increases risk of perioperative complications.
   C. The risk of symptomatic biliary disease will decrease after RYGB.
   D. For symptomatic gallstones, cholecystectomy and subsequent RYGB is indicated (two-stage operation).
   E. Concomitant RYGB and cholecystectomy is indicated for asymptomatic gallstones.

2. **The patient has undergone an uneventful RYGB. Two years after this surgery, he presents with abdominal pain, nausea, vomiting, and mild jaundice. He has no fever and the clinical examination is normal. His BMI is 29 kg/m^2 with desirable nutritional status. The ultrasound examination reveals multiple stones in the gallbladder without signs of cholecystitis. The intrahepatic biliary ducts are mildly dilated, the common bile duct (CBD) is 10 mm, and there is no clear evidence of stone or ampullary lesions. Laboratory tests show a mild elevation in bilirubin and alkaline phosphatase levels, along with a normal level of inflammatory parameters, transaminase, and amylase. What would be the next step?**
   A. Preoperative endoscopic ultrasound (EUS)
   B. Endoscopic retrograde cholangiopancreatography (ERCP)
   C. Percutaneous trans-hepatic cholangiography
   D. Laparoscopic cholecystectomy and intraoperative cholangiography
   E. Magnetic resonance cholangiopancreatography (MRCP)

3. **The patient is scheduled for a minimally invasive surgery. An intraoperative cholangiogram reveals two stones in a distal part of the CBD and passage of the contrast agent into the duodenum. A laparoscopic attempt and choledococoscopy fail to retrieve the stones through the cystic duct. What would be the best approach?**
   A. Conversion to open and performing choledochoduodenostomy
   B. Completing the cholecystectomy, draining the CBD, and planning postoperative ERCP
   C. Laparoscopic Roux-en-Y hepaticojejunostomy

D. Laparoscopic cholecystectomy and CBD exploration
E. Retrograde ERCP with sphincterotomy via biliopancreatic limb

ANSWERS

1. **B.** After rapid weight loss, emptying of the gallbladder is significantly compromised. Altered anatomy following RYGB results in decreasing the secretion of cholecystokinin. Therefore, the gallbladder becomes distended, and the risk of biliary sludge and stone formation increases.[1] Despite increasing the rate of stone formation, the incidence of biliary complications after bariatric procedures is still low. Thus, concomitant prophylactic cholecystectomy at the time of bariatric operations is generally not recommended. Performing both procedures at the same time increases the operation time and perioperative complications significantly.[2,3] When cholecystectomy is not indicated, a careful follow-up with attention to biliary complications is recommended. Performing post-bariatric cholecystectomy is reported to be associated with higher risk of complications and reoperation. The reason for the increased postoperative complication is probably because post-bariatric indications for cholecystectomy are commonly due to acute cholecystitis and biliary complications.[2] The administration of ursodeoxycholic acid during the period of rapid weight loss may prevent gallstone formation.[3]

   In the case of symptomatic gallstone disease, however, a concurrent cholecystectomy and bariatric surgery is justified. It has been reported that concomitant operations for symptomatic gallstones did not affect the mortality rate and the risk of major complications.[4]

2. **D.** A dilated CBD on ultrasound and a mildly elevated bilirubin level (>1.7 mg/dL) are strong predictors of choledocholithiasis. In patients at high probability of a CBD stone, due to frequent need for an intervention, additional biliary imaging may not be required. Preoperative MRCP is useful when clinical data is suggestive of a passed stone.[5] In this patient, however, the level of bilirubin and alkaline phosphatase is still elevated; therefore, the diagnosis of passed stone is clinically less likely. Further assessment of bile ducts in these patients is typically performed either by preoperative ERCP or operative cholangiography and CBD exploration. At least a couple meta-analyses, one Cochrane review, and few randomized studies have shown that there is no advantage to either approach in terms of any patient-linked outcome (morbidity or mortality) or patient safety; although the single step surgical approach is cost-effective and reduces the length of hospital stay.[6-10] Furthermore, following bariatric procedures in which the duodenum is bypassed, classic access through ERCP to the biliary tree is not feasible. Considering the local expertise and available technology, intraoperative cholangiography and direct surgical approach to the biliary tree seems to be the best option for this patient. Flushing or removing the stones via cystic ducts, intravenous administration of glucagon, and choledocoscopy may result in safe and uncomplicated treatment of the choledocholithiasis.[11]

3. **D.** Laparoscopic choledochotomy and direct CBD exploration is a good choice when the duct measures more than 7 mm at the operative cholangiogram and the surgical expertise is available.[12] In experienced hands, the success rates of laparoscopic CBD exploration is more than 90%.[13] The decision to add a drainage procedure (choledochoduodenostomy or hepaticojejunostomy) could be considered for complicated CBD stones with available duct diameter > 10 to 12 mm.[14] Different alternative approaches have been described for CBD access after RYGB. Approaching to the CBD through the remnant stomach has been reported by several studies to be a safe and reliable technique with a success rate of more than 90%. In this procedure, a surgeon can laparoscopically open the remnant stomach and give access to the endoscopist to enter from a port to the stomach. It requires advanced endoscopic and minimally invasive techniques as well as adequate team work between the surgeon and the endoscopist.[15-17] The technique of retrograde ERCP after RYGB has a success rate of 33% to 70%, depending on the experience of the center and the availability of advanced endoscopic techniques. It is especially more difficult in the case of a long limb gastrojejunostomy.[15]

REFERENCES

1. Bastouly M, Arasaki CH, Ferreira JB, Zanoto A, Borges FG, Del Grande JC. Early changes in postprandial gallbladder emptying in morbidly obese patients undergoing Roux-en-Y gastric bypass: correlation with the

occurrence of biliary sludge and gallstones. *Obes Surg.* 2009;19(1):22-28.
2. Tustumi F, Bernardo WM, Santo MA, Cecconello I. Cholecystectomy in patients submitted to bariatric procedure: a systematic review and meta-analysis. *Obes Surg.* 2018;28(10):3312-3320.
3. Leyva-Alvizo A, Arredondo-Saldaña G, Leal-Isla-Flores V, et al. Systematic review of management of gallbladder disease in patients undergoing minimally invasive bariatric surgery. *Surg Obes Relat Dis.* 2020;16(1):158-164.
4. Wood SG, Kumar SB, Dewey E, Lin MY, Carter JT. Safety of concomitant cholecystectomy with laparoscopic sleeve gastrectomy and gastric bypass: a MBSAQIP analysis. *Surg Obes Relat Dis.* 2019;15(6):864-870.
5. ASGE Standards of Practice Committee, Maple JT, Ben-Menachem T, et al. The role of endoscopy in the evaluation of suspected choledocholithiasis. *Gastrointest Endosc.* 2010;71(1):1-9.
6. Rogers SJ, Cello JP, Horn JK, et al. Prospective randomized trial of LC+LCBDE vs ERCP/S+LC for common bile duct stone disease. *Arch Surg.* 2010;145(1):28-33. doi:10.1001/archsurg.2009.226.
7. Liu JG, Wang YJ, Shu GM, Lou C, Zhang J, Du Z. Laparoscopic versus endoscopic management of choledocholithiasis in patients undergoing laparoscopic cholecystectomy: a meta-analysis. *J Laparoendosc Adv Surg Tech A.* 2014;24:287-294.
8. Nagaraja V, Eslick GD, Cox MR. Systematic review and meta-analysis of minimally invasive techniques for the management of cholecysto-choledocholithiasis. *J Hepatobiliary Pancreat Sci.* 2014;21:896-901.
9. Bansal VK, Misra MC, Garg P, Prabhu M. A prospective randomized trial comparing two-stage versus single-stage management of patients with gallstone disease and common bile duct stones. *Surg Endosc.* 2010;24:1986-1989.
10. Dasari BV, Tan CJ, Gurusamy KS, et al. Surgical versus endoscopic treatment of bile duct stones. *Cochrane Database Syst Rev.* 2013;2013(12):CD003327.
11. Brockmeyer JR, Grover BT, Kallies KJ, Kothari SN. Management of biliary symptoms after bariatric surgery. *Am J Surg.* 2015;210(6):1010-1017.
12. Nathanson LK, O'Rourke NA, Martin IJ, et al. Postoperative ERCP versus laparoscopic choledochotomy for clearance of selected bile duct calculi: a randomized trial. *Ann Surg.* 2005;242(2):188-192.
13. Bansal VK, Misra MC, Rajan K, et al. Single-stage laparoscopic common bile duct exploration and cholecystectomy versus two-stage endoscopic stone extraction followed by laparoscopic cholecystectomy for patients with concomitant gallbladder stones and common bile duct stones: a randomized controlled trial. *Surg Endosc.* 2014;28 (3):875-885.
14. Senthilnathan P, Sharma D, Sabnis SC, et al. Laparoscopic choledochoduodenostomy as a reliable rescue procedure for complicated bile duct stones. *Surg Endosc.* 2018;32 (4):1828-1833.
15. Somasekar K, Chan DSY, Sreekumar NS, Anwer S. Choledocholithiasis after bariatric surgery-more than a stone's throw to reach? *J Gastrointest Surg.* 2018;22(3):529-537.
16. Borel F, Branche J, Baud G, Gérard R, Pattou F, Caiazzo R. Management of acute gallstone cholangitis after Roux-en-Y gastric bypass with laparoscopic transgastric endoscopic retrograde cholangiopancreatography. *Obes Surg.* 2019;29(2):747-748.
17. Bures C, Seika P, Veltzke-Schliecker W, Adler A, Kröll D, Zorron R. Intragastric single-port surgery (IGS) accesses the gastric remnant and allows ERCP for common bile duct stones after RYGB: a simple solution for a difficult problem. *Surg Obes Relat Dis.* 2019;15(8):1326-1331.

53

SBO/Intussusception after Gastric Bypass Surgery

Andrea Moon, MD, and Chan W. Park, MD

A 45-year-old woman with diabetes, gastroesophageal reflux disease, obstructive sleep apnea, hypertension, and a body mass index (BMI) of 43 kg/m^2 is seen in consultation for bariatric surgery. She is interested in both sleeve gastrectomy and gastric bypass procedures. However, she has a cousin who underwent gastric bypass 7 years prior who recently required a reoperation for a "bowel obstruction." As such, she is very concerned about her risk of developing small bowel obstruction (SBO) after gastric bypass surgery.

1. What is an appropriate response regarding the risk of SBO after surgery?

A. SBO is a relatively rare complication after gastric bypass with rates less than 1%.
B. Isolated biliopancreatic limb bowel obstruction is a benign type of obstruction that can be managed without surgical intervention.
C. Intussusception is the most common cause of SBO after gastric bypass.
D. SBOs have a reported incidence of 1.5% to 16%.
E. Internal hernias are the least common cause of SBO after gastric bypass.

2. What is the impact of the following surgical techniques with regards to developing SBO?

A. A retrocolic Roux limb reduces the risk of SBO caused by internal hernias.
B. Closing mesenteric defects may reduce the risk of adhesions.
C. Closing mesenteric defects will decrease her risk of developing an internal hernia but may increase the risk of adhesions.
D. Closing mesenteric defects will have no impact on her risk of developing SBO.
E. Closing mesenteric defects will increase her risk of developing intussusception.

The above patient undergoes uncomplicated laparoscopic Roux-en-Y gastric bypass (RYGB). On postoperative day 2, she continues to have a difficult time with oral intake and complains of abdominal pain localized to the left upper quadrant. Her vital signs are pulse of 94, blood pressure of 135/90, respiratory rate of 12, temperature of 37.2°C, and oxygen saturation of 99% on room air. Her abdominal exam reveals mild distention and generalized discomfort, but without evidence of peritonitis. Her labs are significant for white blood cell count of 12, hemoglobin/hematocrit of 8.9/20 respectively, and platelet count of 198. An abdominal x-ray demonstrates what appears to be a dilated gastric remnant with dilated loops of small bowel, but without evidence of free air. Computed tomography (CT) abdomen/pelvis is obtained (Fig. 53-1).

3. What is your initial diagnosis?

A. Obstruction of the Roux limb before the jejunojejunal (JJ) anastomosis
B. JJ anastomotic leak
C. Obstruction at the JJ anastomosis
D. Ileus
E. Obstruction of the biliopancreatic limb only

4. How should one manage this patient?

A. Bowel rest
B. Blood transfusion and discontinuation of any anticoagulants
C. Esophagogastroduodenoscopy (EGD) and percutaneous endoscopic gastrostomy (PEG) tube placement
D. Diagnostic laparoscopy with possible EGD
E. Exploratory laparotomy

5. With regards to internal hernia after gastric bypass surgery, what key finding has the best positive predictive value?

A. Dilated small bowel loops
B. Dilated remnant stomach
C. JJ anastomosis on the right side of the abdomen
D. Swirling pattern of small bowel mesentery
E. Target sign

ANSWERS

1. **D.** The patient should be counseled that SBO is a known complication after gastric bypass surgery, and should be educated on a low threshold to return to the hospital and seek out a bariatric surgeon particularly early in their postoperative course. While some patients may respond to medical management, there should a low threshold for surgical exploration in post–gastric bypass surgery patients suspected of having an internal hernia and/or SBO resulting in dilation of the biliopancreatic limb/gastric remnant because these "closed loop" types of obstructions will not be decompressed with nasogastric tube placement and they can result in catastrophic outcomes. SBOs have a variety of etiologies to include internal hernia, incisional hernias, adhesions, anastomotic narrowing, intraluminal hematoma, and intussusception, among others. Studies estimate the overall prevalence of SBO after gastric bypass anywhere from 1.5% to 16%.[1] Early SBO after RYGB occur within 30 days of surgery and are reported in 0.5% to 5.2% of cases.[2] Intussusception is a rare and uncommon cause of intestinal obstruction after RYGB with reported prevalence of 0.07% up to 1.2% depending on the study.[3] Most intussusceptions will involve the JJ anastomosis. When this is determined to be the cause of the obstruction, then revision of the anastomosis is recommended.

2. **C.** While there is no single agreed upon technique that definitively minimizes the risk of SBO after gastric bypass, there are several techniques than aim to mitigate those risks. Routine closure of the mesenteric defect is performed by many bariatric surgeons in order to prevent internal herniation. A 2016 multicenter randomized controlled trial published in *The Lancet* including 2507 patients reported a reduced cumulative incidence of reoperation for SBO secondary to internal hernia (HR, 0.56; 95% CI, 0.41–0.76; $P = 0.0002$) for the study period of 3 years. However, the incidence of re-operative early SBO was higher in the closure versus nonclosure group (1.27% vs. 0.24%), and this was most commonly due to kinking at the JJ anastomosis or early adhesions. Despite the increased risk of early obstruction, there is a reduction in overall incidence of obstruction (particularly internal hernias) over time by closing the mesenteric defects.[4] The antecolic orientation of the Roux limb eliminates the need for creation of a mesocolic window, and reduces the number of potential anatomic locations for internal hernia—the JJ mesenteric defect and the Peterson's space (between the Roux limb mesentery and transverse mesocolon).

   Acute angulation (or "kinking") caused by adhesive disease is a well-described early complication of laparoscopic RYGB. It is particularly associated with closure of the JJ mesenteric defect.[5] Methods to attempt to reduce the incidence of kinking of the JJ defect include the antiobstruction stitch,[6] a wide division of the mesentery under the blind limb, and double-stapling of the anastomosis. In a 2018 retrospective cohort study of 1327 patients, the authors compared a "unidirectional jejunojejunostomy" with a single staple load to a "bidirectional jejunojejunostomy" with two staple loads. The authors reported 11/626 obstructions by kinking in the unidirectional group and 0/701 in the bidirectional group.[4]

3. **C.** Figure 53-1 shows two CT images[2] of early SBO after laparoscopic RYGB due to a jejunojejunostomy obstruction. The key findings in these images are the dilated Roux limb proximal to the JJ (image A) and the abrupt caliber change at the JJ (image B). The small bowel is decompressed past the JJ anastomosis, which can be found easily by the staple line. The JJ anastomosis obstruction must block travel down the common channel because there was distention into the gastric remnant on plain film meaning the biliopancreatic limb and gastric remnant are also distended by the obstruction at the JJ anastomosis. A blockage of only the biliopancreatic limb may be more difficult to determine because contrast would not enter this limb nor would any refluxant be able to distend that limb or the gastric remnant.

   While an anastomotic leak and bleeding are always on the differential in the early postoperative period, it is much less likely in this patient with imaging that reveals dilated small bowel with abrupt caliber change at the JJ. An ileus would show diffusely dilated loops of bowel without an abrupt caliber change.

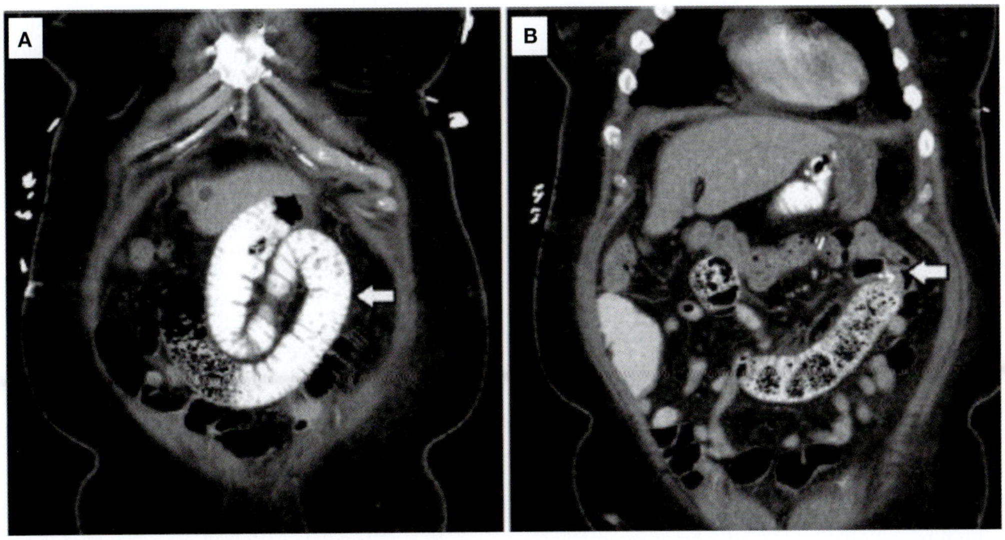

Figure 53-1 CT abdomen/pelvis. (Reproduced with permission from Khoraki J, Mazzini GS, Shah AS, et al: Early small bowel obstruction after laparoscopic gastric bypass: a surgical emergency. *Surg Obes Relat Dis*. 2018;14(8):1118-1125.)

4. **D.** This patient has SBO at the level of the JJ anastomosis, most likely from an internal anastomotic bleed resulting in an obstructing intralumenal blood clot. Laparoscopic exploration and opening of the JJ anastomosis could allow the evacuation of the obstructing blood clot and allow the surgeon to control the intralumenal bleeding source. Opening the stapled blind end of the biliopancreatic limb could eliminate the need to completely re-do the JJ anastomosis and/or reduce the risk of JJ anastomotic complications such as stricture, leak, and so on.

   This complication is potentially life-threatening if left untreated and requires urgent diagnosis and treatment. If the biliopancreatic limb and remnant stomach becomes dilated resulting in a "closed-loop" obstruction, a gastric staple line disruption or perforation could occur. If the Roux limb becomes overly dilated, the patient could be at high risk for anastomotic disruption, and aspiration pneumonitis resulting in acute respiratory distress. The patient should be promptly taken to the operating room for early surgical intervention, but close coordination with the anesthesia team is necessary to limit the possibility of aspiration during induction.

   A PEG will not be possible in a post–gastric bypass patient. Placement of a decompressive gastrostomy tube into the remnant stomach may be possible and relieve some tension in the remnant stomach/biliopancreatic limb, but it will not address the underlying cause of the JJ obstruction. EGD is an important adjunct that should always be considered in gastric bypass patients in order to adequately evaluate the intraluminal status of the anastomoses, and it may be helpful in decompressing the dilated Roux limb. However, care must be taken when insufflating an already dilated and obstructed Roux limb. Diagnostic laparoscopy with laparoscopic repair/revisions are commonly successful and most patients do not require exploratory laparotomy. While exploratory laparotomy should be pursued if absolutely necessary, a large open incision in a morbidly obese patient could add significant and unnecessary morbidity and increase wound related complications postoperatively.

5. **D.** CT scan of the abdomen with a "mesenteric swirl" is a very concerning radiologic finding for internal hernia after a gastric bypass that must be correlated clinically. This finding along with the presence of dilated small bowel as is seen in any SBO, a "beaking" appearance of the superior mesenteric vein, the presence of small bowel behind the superior mesenteric artery, the presence of the JJ anastomosis on the right side of the abdomen, and a "mushroom" appearance of small bowel, among others, are all suggestive of an internal hernia on CT imaging. In several studies that reviewed CT interpretations in post–gastric bypass surgery patients presenting with symptoms of SBO, the finding of a "mesenteric swirl" had the highest sensitivity (86%–89%) and specificity (85%–90%) as well

as the highest predictive value for internal hernia.[7–9] The presence of dilated small bowel on a plain film is a nonspecific finding that is suggestive of an ileus or a bowel obstruction, but the presence of a dilated gastric remnant must be acted upon with urgency because this suggests a closed loop obstruction that could lead to gastric perforation if left untreated. A barium swallow can be helpful diagnosing a gastrojejunal leak or obstruction, but a CT scan is much more helpful when evaluating for a possible internal hernia. A target sign seen on CT scan is indicative of an intussusception and should be a reason for exploration either laparoscopically or via laparotomy.

REFERENCES

1. Clapp B. Small bowel obstruction after laparoscopic gastric bypass with nonclosure of mesenteric defects. *JSLS.* 2015;19(1):e2014.00257.
2. Khoraki J, Mazzini GS, Shah AS, Del Prado PAR, Wolfe LG, Campos GM. Early small bowel obstruction after laparoscopic gastric bypass: a surgical emergency. *Surg Obes Relat Dis.* 2018;14(8):1118-1125.
3. Facchiano E, Soricelli E, Leuratti L, et al. Intussusception after Roux-en-Y gastric bypass: laparoscopic management. *Obes Surg.* 2018;28:2145-2147.
4. Stenberg E, Szabo E, Agren G, et al. Closure of mesenteric defects in laparoscopic gastric bypass: a multicentre, randomised, parallel, open-label trial. *Lancet.* 2016;387:1397-1404.
5. Aghajani E, Jacobsen HJ, Nergaard BJ, Hedenbro JL, Leifson BG, Gislason H. Internal hernia after gastric bypass: a new and simplified technique for laparoscopic primary closure of the mesenteric defects. *J Gastrointest Surg.* 2012;16:641-645.
6. Munier P, Alratrout H, Siciliano I, Keller P. Bidirectional jejunojejunal anastomosis prevents early small bowel obstruction due to the kinking after closure of the mesenteric defect in the laparoscopic Roux-en-Y gastric bypass. *Obes Surg.* 2018;28(7):1838-1844.
7. Dilauro M, McInnes M, Schidea N, et al. Internal hernia after laparoscopic Roux-en-Y gastric bypass: optimal CT signs for diagnosis and clinical decision making. *Radiology.* 2017;282(3):752-760.
8. Sunnapwar A, Sandrasegaran K, Menias C, et al. Taxonomy and imaging spectrum of small bowel obstruction after Roux-en-Y gastric bypass surgery. *AJR.* 2010;194:120-128.
9. Karila-Cohen P, Cuccioli F, Tammaro P, et al. Contribution of computed tomographic imaging to the management of acute abdominal pain after gastric bypass: correlation between radiological and surgical findings. *Obes Surg.* 2017;27:1961-1972.

54

Roux Stasis Syndrome

Anne P. Ehlers, MD, MPH and Laura M. Mazer, MD

A 45-year-old woman presents to your office 3 years after her laparoscopic Roux-en-Y gastric bypass (RYGB). She reports symptoms of abdominal pain, distention, and postprandial bloating. She also reports frequent nausea, nonbilious emesis, and significant weight loss. Upper gastrointestinal (GI) series demonstrates no delay of contrast from the pouch through the Roux limb. Scintigraphy demonstrates delayed emptying of solid food. Based on her symptoms and imaging, you suspect that she has Roux stasis syndrome.

1. **An esophagogastroduodenoscopy is most likely to show which of the following?**
   A. Dilated gastric pouch containing residual food
   B. Narrowing of the gastrojejunal anastomosis
   C. Ulceration of the gastrojejunal anastomosis
   D. Excessive length of the afferent (blind) limb
   E. No abnormality

2. **Which of the following is the most likely underlying cause of this patient's symptoms?**
   A. Bacterial overgrowth in the small intestine
   B. Disruption of the autonomic nervous system
   C. Mechanical obstruction at the gastrojejunal anastomosis
   D. Mechanical obstruction at the jejunojejunal anastomosis
   E. Neuropathy from malnutrition

3. **Treatment of her condition may include:**
   A. Dilation of gastrojejunal anastomosis
   B. Surgical revision of jejunojejunal anastomosis
   C. Prokinetic agents
   D. Antibiotics
   E. High-carbohydrate diet

4. **Which of the following factors is associated with development of Roux stasis syndrome?**
   A. Female sex
   B. Irritable bowel syndrome
   C. Achalasia
   D. Chronic opioid use
   E. Gastric resection and Roux-en-Y reconstruction for peptic ulcer disease

ANSWERS

1. **A.** Roux stasis syndrome is a complication of Roux-en-Y reconstruction, both in bariatric surgery and other operations requiring this anatomy. It refers to a complex of symptoms including early satiety, nausea, nonbilious emesis, and postprandial abdominal pain. The most common endoscopic finding in Roux stasis syndrome is a dilated gastric pouch containing residual food. Other findings can include mucosal irritation and a dilated Roux limb. Other diagnostic studies that can be considered in the evaluation of Roux stasis syndrome include upper GI series, computed tomography scan, or scintigraphy. As in this patient, Roux syndrome is not associated with any evidence of mechanical obstruction on imaging, and there is usually no delay for emptying of liquids. Emptying of solid food is typically delayed, as demonstrated by the scintigraphy in this patient.[1]

2. **B.** The primary disorder is disruption of the autonomic nervous system in the small intestine.[2,3] One hypothesis to explain these symptoms is that the Roux limb is disrupted from the primary pacing center located on the duodenum[4] and ultimately acts as a functional obstruction for the patient.[2] A second hypothesis is that there are disruptions to the normal pacesetting mechanisms that occur due to creation of the gastric pouch.[5]

   Some evidence also suggests that ectopic pacemakers present in the Roux limb lead to retrograde peristalsis, further contributing to the symptoms. Delayed gastric emptying may also contribute.[4] More recent studies suggest that the primary problem exists in the stomach due to delayed gastric emptying. The most common symptoms include nausea, vomiting, and abdominal pain worse after eating. Imaging findings do not demonstrate any evidence of obstruction. While bacterial overgrowth can occur as a result of Roux stasis syndrome, it is not the underlying cause.[1] There are many neurologic symptoms that can occur from malnutrition to include deficiencies in thiamine, vitamin B12, calcium, copper, iron, and vitamin A, but none of them seem to cause GI dysfunction.

3. **C.** Because the underlying problem is neurological in nature, the therapies are aimed at symptom control (i.e. switching to a liquid diet) and therapies that aim to improve intestinal motility, such as prokinetic agents and gastric or intestinal pacemakers.[4] Surgical revision of the gastric pouch can be considered as a last resort. One suggested surgical option is subtotal gastrectomy given the concern for abnormal gastric emptying. However, patients who have already undergone a Roux-en-Y gastric bypass have functionally undergone a subtotal gastrectomy. In these scenarios, reversal of the bypass has been reported with some success.[6] Narrowing of the gastrojejunal anastomosis has not been proposed as a contributor to the development of Roux syndrome and thus is not suggested as a potential treatment option.[1] Antibiotics may be used as an adjunct if the patient has also developed small intestine bacterial overgrowth (SIBO). Patients with SIBO may present with diarrhea, bloating, anemia, or malabsorption. A diagnosis of SIBO can be made either by culturing fluid from the small bowel (obtained through endoscopy) or using a hydrogen and methane breath test.[7] Antibiotics should be initiated in confirmed cases. However, given the limitations of the current testing modalities, antibiotics are also sometimes prescribed in patients who exhibit signs and symptoms of SIBO. An improvement in symptoms following initiation of antibiotics may help to confirm the diagnosis.[8]

4. **E.** Roux stasis syndrome is thought to result from delayed gastric emptying, or disruption of the autonomic nervous system due to transection of the jejunum. While there are some technical factors that may be related to development of this syndrome (e.g. size of gastric pouch, length of Roux limb), none of the listed factors have been cited as being contributory. In Roux-en-Y reconstructions done for peptic ulcer disease, likely a vagotomy would be done to help control acid secretion, and consequently, these patients are at risk for Roux stasis syndrome. Up to 30% of patients who have Roux-en-Y anatomy after gastrectomy suffer from Roux stasis syndrome.[4] In an RYGB done for obesity, this is a rare complication.

REFERENCES

1. Zinner MJ, Ashley SW, Maingot R, et al. Chapter 29. In: Zinner MJ, Ashley SW, Hines OJ, eds. *Maingot's Abdominal Operations*. 13th ed. McGraw Hill; 2018.
2. Mathias JR, Fernandez A, Sninsky CA, et al. Nausea, vomiting, and abdominal pain after Roux-en-Y anastomosis: motility of the jejunal limb. *Gastroenterology*. 1985;88:101-107.
3. Daram SR, Tang SJ, Vick K, et al. Novel application of GI electrical stimulation in Roux stasis syndrome (with video). *Gastrointest Endosc*. 2011;74:683-686.
4. Tu BN, Kelly KA. Motility disorders after Roux-en-Y gastrojejunostomy. *Obes Surg*. 1994;4:219-226.
5. Noh SM. Improvement of the Roux limb function using a new type of "uncut Roux" limb. In: *Am J Surg*. 2000;180:37-40.
6. Simper SC, Erzinger JM, McKinlay RD, et al. Laparoscopic reversal of gastric bypass with sleeve gastrectomy for treatment of recurrent retrograde intussusception and Roux stasis syndrome. *Surg Obes Relat Dis*. 2010;6:684-688.
7. Dolan RD, Baker J, Harer K, et al. Small intestinal bacterial overgrowth: Clinical presentation in patients with Roux-en-Y gastric bypass. *Obes Surg*. 2021;31:564-569.
8. Achufusi TGO, Sharma A, Zamora EA, et al. Small intestinal bacterial overgrowth: Comprehensive review of diagnosis, prevention, and treatment methods. *Cureus*. 2020;12:e8860.

55

Weight Regain after Bariatric Surgery

Geoffrey S. Chow, MD

A 39-year-old female with a history of a Roux-en-Y gastric bypass 3 years ago is referred for surgical evaluation after regaining 2.3 kg over the last year. She currently has a body mass index (BMI) of 26.4 kg/m^2. Preoperatively, the patient had diabetes mellitus, hypertension, and obstructive sleep apnea, and has not needed any treatment for these since her prior surgery. Vitals are normal and physical exam does not have any acute concerns. The patient has not had any follow-up since 6 months after her bariatric operation.

1. Regarding the 5-year weight outcomes after bariatric surgery, which of the following is correct?

A. Less than 5% of patients will encounter any weight regain.
B. Significant weight gain is expected for the majority of patients.
C. Up to 50% of patients may regain a small amount of weight in the first 5 years after surgery.
D. The majority of weight regain occurs within the first 1 year after surgery.

2. Regarding the 1-year outcomes after bariatric surgery, which of the following is correct?

A. Patients who have less than 50% excess weight loss should undergo revision surgery.
B. Less than expected initial weight loss followed by weight gain may be due to a technical issue.
C. Weight regain is common between 6 and 12 months after surgery.
D. Weight loss does not follow a standard trend during this time frame.

3. Which of these factors is most often associated with weight regain in long-term follow-up after a gastric bypass?

A. Gastrogastric fistula
B. New onset adjustment disorder
C. Lack of follow-up with a multidisciplinary bariatric program
D. Increased consumption of high calorie foods

4. Which of the following is correct regarding revisional surgery for weight regain after a primary bariatric operation?

A. Revision rates for weight regain and refractory complications are highest after gastric banding.
B. Ten percent of all patients will require revisional surgery for weight regain.
C. Leak rates after revision are the same as with primary bariatric surgery.
D. Risk of post-operative complications are decreased compared to primary bariatric surgery.

ANSWERS

1. C. The majority of patients undergoing bariatric surgery will have a nadir weight between 12 and 18 months after the index operation. Patients who do not have adequate weight loss during this time should prompt multidisciplinary evaluation to see whether there are dietary-, psychosocial-, medical-, or surgery-related factors that have caused the patient to not lose an expected amount of weight in the postoperative period.[1,2] In follow-up to 5 years, a small amount of weight regain is often observed in up to 50% of patients.[3,4] Patients should receive regular multidisciplinary evaluation during this time to ensure that they are following the recommend dietary and postsurgical care.[5,6]

2. **B.** Almost all patients will experience weight loss during the first year after bariatric surgery. Weight regain during this time frame is unusual and should prompt review of records to ensure that the patient has been compliant with postoperative recommendations and has not developed any medical problems, or psychological concerns. Further, they should be evaluated to see if they are compliant with the prescribed postsurgical nutritional plan.[1] Patients who do not experience initial weight loss or begin to have weight regain during the first year should also have an evaluation of their surgical anatomy to see if there are any anatomic factors contributing to their results.[2] This work up can incorporate upper endoscopy, upper gastrointestinal contrast study, and computed tomography with oral and intravenous contrast. Up to 50% of patients in this group with inadequate weight loss in the first year may have an anatomic issue as a source of failure. These can include retained fundus, retained antrum, large pouch size, too large of a gastro-jejunal anastomosis, gastro-gastric fistula, and too short of a roux or biliopancreatic limb.[1] Most patients will follow a trend where weight decreases over the first 12 months after surgery, and the highest amount of excess weight loss will occur at 12 to 18 months after surgery.[3–5]

3. **D.** Poor dietary compliance and incorporation of unhealthy dietary habits are the most common cause of weight regain after bariatric surgery. Patients who adopt regular snaking or grazing on food throughout the day may inadvertently increase caloric intake with the result of weight regain over a longer period of time. The regular intake of high-calorie liquids or snack foods that dissolve in the mouth may also put patients at risk of weight gain after initial weight loss after bariatric surgery. Lifelong follow-up with a comprehensive program that includes dietary care, surgical follow-up, and psychosocial support every 3 months for the first year, every 6 months for the second year, and then annually after that time frame is associated with maintenance of weight loss and less weight regain after bariatric surgery.[6] Gastrogastric fistulas are found in 1% to 6% of patients after bariatric surgery and may often present with abdominal pain, and are also associated with anastomotic leakage and marginal ulcers.[1]

4. **A.** Revisional surgery can benefit patients who have ongoing challenges with morbid obesity and weight regain after a primary bariatric operation. Inadequate weight loss and rates of weight regain that require reoperation are higher after gastric banding than other operations.[1] Out of all patients who undergo bariatric surgery, less than 5% will require revisional surgery for weight regain. The postoperative complication rates after revisional surgery are higher than primary bariatric surgery, including the leak rate.[7] In patients with weight regain after sleeve gastrectomy, a repeat sleeve may be of benefit if there is evidence of a dilated sleeve, excess fundus, or a large retained antrum. Conversion to Roux-en-Y gastric bypass or duodenal switch is based on the patient's weight, comorbidities, and long-term goals. However, weight loss after a revision is less predictable than after a primary procedure.[7]

REFERENCES

1. Karmali S, Brar B, Shi X, et al. Weight recidivism post-bariatric surgery: a systematic review. *Obes Surg*. 2013;23(11): 922-1933.
2. Brethauer S, Kothari S, Sudan R, et al. Systematic review on reoperative bariatric surgery American Society for Metabolic and Bariatric Surgery Revision Task Force. *Surg Obes Relat Dis*. 2014;10:952-972.
3. Lauti M, Kularatna M, Hill AG, et al. Weight regain following sleeve gastrectomy—a systematic review. *Obes Surg*. 2016;26:1326-1334.
4. Magro D, Geloneze B, Delfini R, et al. Long-term weight regain after gastric bypass: a 5-year prospective study. *Obes Surg*. 2008;18:648-651.
5. Carlsson L, Jacobson P, Peltonen M, et al. Life expectancy after bariatric surgery in the Swedish Obese Subjects Study. *N Engl J Med*. 2020;383:1535-1543.
6. Kushner F, Webb K. Medical approach to a patient with postoperative weight regain. In: Still C, Sarwer D, Blankenship J, eds. *The ASMBS Textbook of Bariatric Surgery*. Philadelphia, PA: Springer; 2014: 205-216.
7. Qui J, Lundberg PW, Birriel TJ, et al. Revisional bariatric surgery for weight regain and refractory complications in a single MBSAQIP accredited center: what are we dealing with? *Obes Surg*. 2018;28:2789-2795.

56

Psychiatric Complications of Bariatric Surgery

Henry Lin, MD

During your bariatric educational session, several of your prospective patients express concern about reports of increased mental health complications after bariatric surgery. One particular woman expressed that she thought that postoperatively she would be more attractive, better able to deal with her anxiety, and decrease her likelihood of another admission for severe depression.

1. How does bariatric surgery change the risk of depression?

A. Increases recurrent depression
B. Does not change rates of depression
C. Decreases probability of depression
D. Is unrelated
E. Can only decrease depression if preoperative mental health treatment is initiated

2. During postoperative bariatric care, which statement about mental health trends is false? Increased psychiatric emergency room visits:

A. Increased psychiatric emergency room visits
B. Decreased hospital admissions rate for psychiatric reasons
C. Increased need for outpatient mental health visits
D. Likelihood of mental health emergencies is related to history of preoperative depression, anxiety, or bipolar disorder.
E. Uncontrolled schizophrenia usually helps in the interpretation of a patient's postoperative abdominal symptoms.

3. Suicide rates postbariatric surgery are

A. Not known
B. Increased
C. Decreased
D. Unaffected
E. Do not require a discussion in low-risk low patients

4. Substance abuse trends after bariatric surgery include

A. Decreased tobacco use
B. Increased cocaine use
C. Decreased opioid addiction
D. Increased alcohol use
E. Decreased cannabinoid use

5. What relationships change after bariatric surgery?

A. Marriage rates improve during the weight loss.
B. Roux-en-Y gastric bypass (RYGB) improves marriages more so than laparoscopic adjustable gastric banding.
C. The less the weight loss, the more negative the effect on relationships.
D. Single patients are more likely to develop relationships postoperatively.
E. Divorces decrease postoperatively.

ANSWERS

1. C. There are several psychologic changes that occur after bariatric surgery, both beneficial and detrimental. Overall, bariatric surgery decreases the probability of depression. Behavioral psychotherapy and behavioral-motivational nutritional education decrease the risk of postoperative depression. Furthermore, patients who develop postoperative depression do not lose as much weight. Although preoperative mental health treatment is important in ensuring patients receive appropriate cognitive behavioral therapy, but postoperative initiation of mental health counseling improves follow-up with psychological therapy and thus decreases risk of depression.[1]

2. **E.** Increased hospital admission for psychiatric reasons occurs after bariatric surgery by an incidence rate ratio (IRR) of 3.0. Postoperatively, there is also increased psychiatric emergencies (IRR 3.0) and increased outpatient mental health visits (IRR 2.3). The likelihood of mental health emergencies is higher in patients with a history of preoperative severe depression, anxiety, bipolar disorder, psychosis, or schizophrenia.[2]

3. **A.** Suicide rates post–bariatric surgery are controversial and the true rate is unknown. Multiple studies, including meta-analyses, show conflicting results. Some studies suggest suicide rates increase after 2 years but not all studies support this conclusion. The risk of mental health complications is higher after bariatric surgery, therefore mental health screening at postop appointments and early referral to a mental health provider is important.[3,4]

4. **D.** Alcohol use increases (hazard ratio 1.7). Likelihood of alcohol use postoperatively increases with risk factors of youth (odds ratio [OR] 1.3), male gender (OR 2.1), history of preoperative smoking (OR 2.6), regular alcohol consumption (OR 6.4), recreational drug use (OR 2.4), lower "belonging" interpersonal support (OR 1.1), and gastric bypass surgery (OR 2.1). After bariatric surgery, the following substance uses are increased: tobacco, stimulants other than cocaine, and cannabinoids. Narcotic addictions are also increased.[5]

5. **D.** A patient who is single preoperatively is more likely to develop a new relationship postoperatively by an adjusted hazard ratio (aHR) of 2.03. Divorces and separations increase after bariatric surgery (aHR 1.28). RYGB compared to other bariatric surgeries increases divorce rates (aHR 1.41); but it also improves marriage rates in patients who were unmarried preoperatively (aHR 1.35). The higher the weight loss postoperatively, the more likely the patient will have a relationship status change.[6]

REFERENCES

1. Sogg S, Lauretti J, West-Smith L, et al. ASMBS guidelines/statements recommendations for the presurgical psychosocial evaluation of bariatric surgery patients. *Surg Obes Relat Dis*. 2016:731-749.
2. Kovacs Z, Valentin J, Nielsen R, et al. Risk of psychiatric disorders, self-harm behaviour and service use associated with bariatric surgery. *Acta Psychiatrica Scandinavica*. 2016:135:10.
3. Kalarchian MA, Marcus M, Levine M, et al. Optimizing long-term weight control after bariatric surgery: a pilot study. *Surg Obes Relat Dis*. 2012:710-716.
4. Leahey TM, Bond D, Irwin S, et al. When is the best time to deliver behavioral intervention to bariatric surgery patients: before or after surgery? *Surg Obes Relat Dis*. 2009:99-103.
5. Bruze G, Holmin T, Peltonen M, et al. Associations of bariatric surgery with changes in interpersonal relationship status: results from 2 Swedish cohort studies. *JAMA Surg*. 2018:153(7):654-661.
6. Yen YC, Huang C, Tai C, et al. Psychiatric aspects of bariatric surgery. *Curr Opin: Psychiat Med Behavior Sci*. 2014;27(5):374-379.

57

Post-Bariatric Hypoglycemia

Christopher Mulla, MD, MS

A 46-year-old woman with a body mass index (BMI) of 40 kg/m^2 and progressive weight gain along with hypertension, hyperlipidemia, osteoarthritis, and obstructive sleep apnea (OSA) has scheduled a visit for discussion and preevaluation for surgical management of her obesity- and weight-related comorbidities. She recently heard from a friend that she should not pursue any form of bariatric surgery because her "blood sugar will always be too low and she'll be passing out."

1. How would you describe the occurrence of post-bariatric hypoglycemia (PBH) syndrome?

A. PBH develops in 50% of patients who undergo Roux-en-Y gastric bypass (RYGB).
B. PBH does not develop in patients who undergo sleeve gastrectomy (SG).
C. PBH occurs in up to 30% of patients after RYGB and SG.
D. PBH develops only develops in patients with a history of diabetes prior to bariatric surgery.

2. This same patient completed perioperative screening that reveals she had failed to lose weight in commercial programs in the past. She had previously been prescribed metformin but stopped it due to feeling shaky and sweaty, especially when exercising. She decided to proceed with laparoscopic RYGB, which was uncomplicated. However, she returns to your clinic 2 months postoperatively after several emergency room visits for episodes of sweating, confusion, palpitations, and hunger combined with fingerstick glucose readings <50 mg/dL that occur between 2 and 3 hours after meals. Symptoms improve after consuming 15 to 25 g of glucose. Which of the following characteristics of this patient's symptoms are atypical for PBH?

A. Episodes beginning 2 months postoperatively
B. Symptoms occurring 2 to 3 hours after meals
C. Unsuccessful weight loss prior to surgery
D. Preoperative treatment with metformin

In your follow-up clinic, a 54-year-old man who is 3 years postop from RGYB returns after a recent visit to the emergency room. He recently had an episode of confusion and agitation at a local supermarket. Emergency medical services responded to a call and found him lethargic and sweaty with a fingerstick glucose of 42 mg/dL. He was given intravenous fluids and intramuscular glucagon, and had gradual improvement in cognition and symptoms. At the emergency room, his workup was negative for CVA, cardiac arrhythmia, or other electrolyte abnormalities and he was discharged home.

3. What is the next most appropriate step in evaluation?

A. Place a referral for him to see neurology
B. Confirm Whipple's Triad
C. Refer for a 72-hour inpatient fast
D. Rule out pheochromocytoma

4. The patient had been keeping a diary of similar episodes that occur every few days. Approximately 2 to 3 hours after meals, he has documented several fingerstick glucose levels less than 60 mg/dL. What is the next best step in management?

A. Mixed-meal tolerance test
B. Venous glucose, insulin, c-peptide, pro-insulin after an overnight fast

C. Urine metanephrines
D. Computed tomography (CT) scan of the pancreas

5. This same patient had a normal morning cortisol ruling out adrenal insufficiency. His workup also ruled out fasting hypoglycemia. He was given a mixed-meal tolerance test to evaluate his response. Three hours after initiating his mixed meal test, his glucose dropped to 47 mg/dL accompanied by sweating, dizziness, and palpitations. How would you treat this patient?

A. Give reassurance and allow the patient to feel better on his own.
B. Provide an intravenous infusion of dextrose.
C. Provide 15 to 20 g of oral carbohydrate mixed with protein and fat (glucose tablets or glucose gel, as well as a whole wheat cracker and natural peanut butter).
D. Referral for partial pancreatectomy.

6. Subsequently, when his glucose was 47 mg/dL his concurrent insulin was found to be elevated to 19 μU/mL (reference range 3–25 μU/mL) and c-peptide was 3.1 (reference range 1–4 ng/mL). What is the appropriate counseling approach for diet modification to reduce the frequency and severity of episodes of hypoglycemia in PBH?

A. Increase high-glycemic index carbohydrates and limit low-glycemic index carbohydrates and consume beverages during meals.
B. High protein, low fat, high-glycemic index carbohydrate diet.
C. Increase low-glycemic index carbohydrates and limit high-glycemic index carbohydrates and limit beverages during meals.
D. Avoid complex carbohydrates and consume beverages during meals.

7. One and a half months later, the patient returns to clinic following your recommended dietary changes. He initially experienced fewer episodes of hypoglycemia with neuroglycopenia; however, they have persisted. What is the recommended next step?

A. Metformin
B. Calcium channel blocker
C. Octreotide
D. Acarbose

8. Eight months later, the patient returns to your clinic in desperation. He has worked closely with endocrinology and nutrition colleagues and despite diet adherence, acarbose, diazoxide, and octreotide, he has frequent debilitating episodes of postprandial hypoglycemia. Which of the following is considered an option for treatment at this point?

A. Gastric remnant feeding tube
B. Distal or partial pancreatectomy
C. Conversion to a one anastomosis gastric bypass
D. Gastric pouch restriction

ANSWERS

1. C. PBH has been identified and reported in patients with a history of both RYGB as well as a SG.[1] Due to several factors, including difficulties in establishing the diagnosis, low awareness among patients and clinicians, and challenges in testing at the time of a hypoglycemic episode, the diagnosis is often missed or delayed. Nevertheless, the prevalence ranges from 0.1% to 1% of post-bariatric surgery patients who were hospitalized for severe hypoglycemia in one series, to 38% of patients who reported symptoms of PBH by survey or provocative meal testing[1-3] (see Table 57-1).

Unfortunately, the natural history and preoperative risk factors for developing PBH are still not understood. Survey data from Lee et al. suggested that lower preoperative hemoglobin A1c and BMI as

Table 57-1 PREVALENCE OF PBH

Method of Ascertainment	Prevalence of PBH after RYGB
Hospitalization	0.1%–1%
Clinical recognition	0.4%–7.6%
Severe hypoglycemia requiring assistance (self-report)	11.60%
Symptoms (survey)	33%–38%, or 0.1%
Diagnostic testing	**Prevalence of PBH after RYGB**
MMTT glucose below 55 mg/dL	22%–29%
CGMS sensor glucose below 55 mg/dL	75%

Modified with permission from Goldfine AB, Patti ME. How common is hypoglycemia after gastric bypass? Obesity (*Silver Spring*). 2016;24(6):1210-1211.

well as greater weight loss by 6 months were associated with an increased incidence of hypoglycemia.[4] Another study found that lower fasting glucose, lower preoperative BMI, and higher insulin sensitivity and beta-cell responsiveness to glucose were associated with a higher incidence of PBH.[5] Although, together, these data as well as other studies using provocative mixed-meal tolerance testing[6] have still not clearly identified a cohort at risk for developing PBH.

When a patient with a history of bariatric surgery describes vague symptoms that could be related to hypoglycemia or another clinical phenomenon appropriate screening should be conducted. PBH is should be evaluated in patients who are at least 6 months out from bariatric surgery along with other causes of hypoglycemia or other conditions (see Figure 57-1).[7]

2. **A.** This patient describes episodes that satisfy Whipple's Triad[9] for hypoglycemia, namely (1) symptomatic hypoglycemia, (2) blood glucose level <50mg/dL, and (3) resolution of symptoms with glucose ingestion. The pattern of hypoglycemic episodes is typical for PBH: occurring 1 to 3 hours after meals (see Figure 57-2). However, the onset of these episodes is uncharacteristic of PBH because they occurred soon after surgery and it is possible that the patient also had similar episodes prior to surgery. PBH typically arises between 1 and 3 years following bariatric surgery and is considered a late complication.[8] This raises the possibility for another etiology of hypoglycemia such as an insulinoma that was unmasked by her bariatric surgery and subsequent dietary restriction. Insulinomas have been uncovered following bariatric surgery, and can be characterized by both fasting and postprandial symptoms that can occur at any time after surgery including immediately after surgery.[10] Unsuccessful weight loss attempts prior to surgery are common but not exclusive to patients with preoperative hypoglycemia syndromes and would not be unusual for PBH. Preoperative diabetes or hyperglycemia requiring metformin or other therapies have been reported in patients with PBH.[1]

3. **B.** This patient's symptoms are classic for post-bariatric hypoglycemia. It is important to confirm

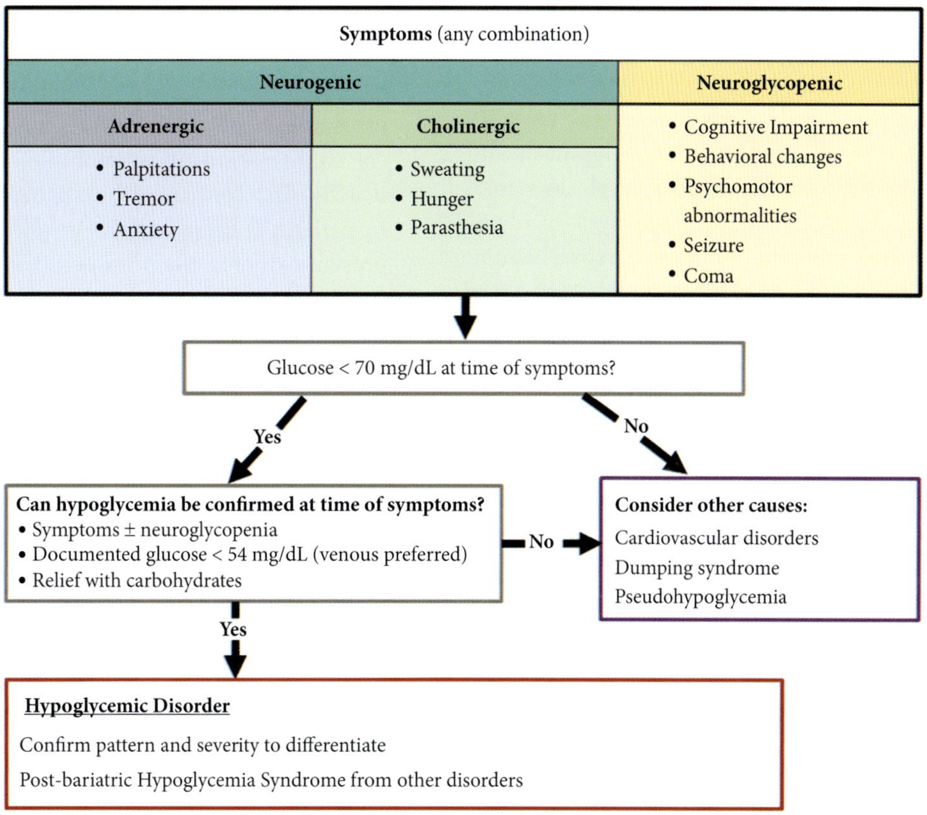

Figure 57-1 Evaluation of symptoms for hypoglycemia.

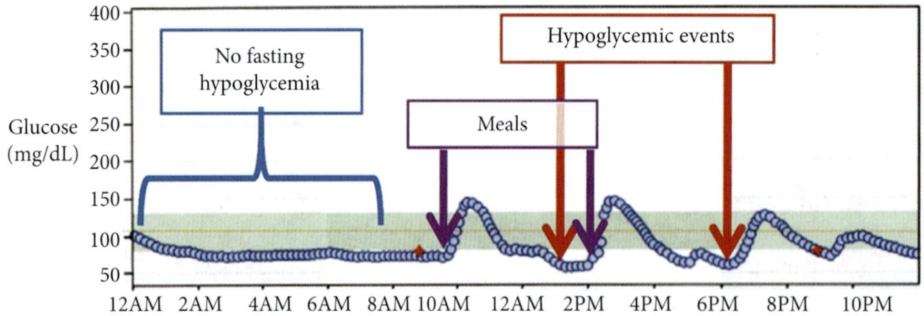

Figure 57-2 Typical pattern of hypoglycemia in untreated post-bariatric hypoglycemia syndrome. (Reproduced with permission from Suhl E, Anderson-Haynes SE, Mulla C, et al: Medical nutrition therapy for post-bariatric hypoglycemia: practical insights. *Surg Obes Relat Dis.* 2017;13(5):888-896.)

Whipple's Triad for hypoglycemia. Does this patient have PBH or an insulinoma? An endocrinologist would be an appropriate specialist rather than a neurologist to evaluate metabolic disturbances following bariatric surgery. A 72-hour fast is an appropriate evaluation for a patient who describe episodes of fasting hypoglycemia, suggested by fingerstick glucose, continuous glucose monitoring tracings, or confirmed by venous blood draw. These described episodes would be atypical for other pathology such as a pheochromocytoma but could be investigated if hypoglycemia has been ruled out.

4. **A.** This patient has documented several episodes where he developed symptoms following meals and has had some fingerstick glucose levels less than 60 mg/dL. The gold standard for analysis of hypoglycemia is measurement of plasma glucose, insulin, c-peptide, pro-insulin, and sulfonylurea screen at the time of one of these symptomatic episodes.[11] Ruling out fasting hypoglycemia is an important step in analysis and is relatively easy to perform. However, this is often not feasible for the patient or the clinician. Therefore, a combination of approaches is often utilized when attempting to evaluate for PBH. Having the patient keep a diary with meals eaten, exercise performed, and symptoms along with fingerstick glucose or blinded continuous glucose monitoring (CGM) data can be very illustrative to identify the patterns and triggers for glycemic excursions. This can then be supported by provocative testing. However, oral glucose tolerance testing is not an appropriate test for reactive hypoglycemia,[12] especially in patients with a history of bariatric surgery. Oral glucose challenges are not well tolerated and usually lead to dumping syndrome. In addition, 25% of healthy subjects can develop nadir glucose levels <55 mg/dL following oral glucose tolerance testing, rendering this test unable to distinguish between healthy and abnormal.[13] However mixed-meal tolerance testing with a combination of protein, carbohydrate, and fat have been used to stimulate postprandial hypoglycemia in patients suspected of having PBH.[14,15] Provocative testing should be performed in a supervised clinical setting to ensure ability to assist and treat patients if they develop severe hypoglycemia.

   Because this patient has not had his hypoglycemia diagnosed or ruled out, a workup for pheochromocytoma with 24-hour urine metanephrines is not indicated. A CT scan of the abdomen to rule out an insulinoma could be done but only after biochemical confirmation of autonomous insulin secretion, usually first confirmed by an overnight fast or an in-patient 72-hour fast. An insulinoma would likely present earlier in the postoperative course.

5. **C.** Hypoglycemia will not likely resolve on its own without intervention so reassurance and observation would not be appropriate. Hypoglycemia should initially be treated with rapid acting oral glucose, in the form of glucose tablets, hard candies, or glucose gels. We recommend utilizing the "rule of 15" for treating symptomatic glucose levels less than 70 mg/dL, which entails 15 g of glucose and then wait 15 minutes to check glucose and confirm correction. Glucose levels less than 50 mg/dL usually require 30 or more grams of glucose to correct to above 80 mg/dL. The advantage of glucose gels is that they can be held in between the cheek and gum for faster absorption through the buccal mucosa.[16]

   Intravenous dextrose infusion can be utilized for severe hypoglycemia, especially in patients who cannot tolerate or reliably swallow due to altered mental status, but would not be first line except in hospitalized patients with established intravenous access. Other immediate treatments could include mini-dose glucagon that has demonstrated to be effective in restoring normal glucose in episodes of PBH; glucagon-pump systems for automated detection of hypoglycemia are in development.[18,19]

Partial pancreatectomy is not recommended for first-line or even refractory PBH due to findings that it has not been effective in fully resolving hypoglycemia and would not be helpful for an acute episode of hypoglycemia.[17] Reversing the RYGB to normal anatomy may be indicated in the most severe cases but that is a complicated procedure with a high risk of morbidity, so it is not recommended as a first- or second-line treatment.

6. **C.** First-line therapy for PBH is medical nutrition therapy. Other strategies to avoid severe and frequent episodes of hypoglycemia can be combined; however, some patients will respond well to diet intervention alone.[1,16,20] In addition to medical nutrition therapy, a personal continuous glucose monitor (CGM) has been demonstrated to be a very effective tool for patients to observe the impact on different foods and activities on their glucose and identify patterns to their hypoglycemic episodes. In addition, CGM therapy can alert patients when their glucose is dropping to avoid severe episodes before driving, operating machinery, or walking near stairs. Providing a CGM for patients is often limited by insurance coverage and high out of pocket expenses when there is no insurance coverage.

The cornerstone for dietary management of PBH is to reduce the postprandial glucose spikes, which in turn leads to reduced production of insulin and other incretin hormones thought to be responsible for postprandial hypoglycemia. Several reports[16] and one study by Kandel and colleagues[21] demonstrated that reducing high-glycemic index carbohydrates and favoring low-glycemic index carbohydrates can prevent episodes of postprandial hypoglycemia. Addition of slow absorbing corn starch in addition to low glycemic-index carbohydrates has also demonstrated some benefit for nocturnal hypoglycemia in PBH.[22]

Hypoglycemia is often a component of dumping syndrome. Part of the strategy to avoid dumping syndrome is to avoid consuming liquids with meals to attenuate the rapid delivery of nutrients including glucose to the intestine.[23] Suhl and colleagues have recommended that beverages be spaced apart from meals by 30 to 60 minutes.[16] Other dietary recommendations for PBH are summarized in Table 57-2.

Table 57-2 SUMMARY OF DIETARY RECOMMENDATIONS FOR PBH

1.Control portions of carbohydrates.
- 30 grams/meal, 15 grams/snack.

2. Choose low-glycemic carbohydrates.
- Steel-cut oats (regular, not quick-cook or instant)
- Oat bran cereal
- Beans/legumes (e.g., garbanzo, navy, kidney, lime, pinto, black-eyed and pea bens, edamame (soybeans), lentils
- Bean products (e.g., hummus, tofu)
- Pearled barley, cooked al dente
- Yams
- Some fruits (e.g., grapefruit, apples, pears, berries, apricots, peaches)
- Some pasta (whole wheat), cooked al dente
- Some whole grain breads (e.g., oat bran & whole wheat Pita/Lavash/Tortillas)
- Some whole grain crackers

3. Avoid high-glycemic carbohydrates.
- Refined breakfast cereals (including cream of rice, instant oatmeal)
- Regular pasta
- Most starchy vegetables (e.g., white potatoes,corn,winter (orange) squash)
- White rice, rice cakes
- Popcorn, pretzels, chips
- Some fruits (e.g., ripe bananas, pineapple, mango, watermelon, grapes)
- All fruit juices and sweetened drinks (e.g., sodas, sweetened iced tea)
- Bread, rolls, bagels, muffins, and crackers made with refined flour
- Sweets (e.g, candy, cake, cookies, ice cream, syrup)

4. Emphasize optimal protein intake.

5. Space meals/snacks 3–4 hours apart.

6. Avoid consuming liquids wih meals.

7. Include (heart-healthy) fats in each meal or snack
- 15 grams/meal, 5grams/snack

8. Avoid alcohol.

9. Avoid caffeine.

10. Maintain post-bariatric vitamin and mineral intake.

Data from Suhl E, Anderson-Haynes SE, Mulla C, et al: Medical nutrition therapy for post-bariatric hypoglycemia: practical insights. *Surg Obes Relat Dis.* 2017;13(5):888-896.

Imaging the pancreas is only appropriate if the clinical history and biochemical testing, which usually involves prolonged observed fasting, suggests autonomous insulin production in the fasting state.[10,24]

7. **D.** The most safe and inexpensive medication for patients with PBH who continue to have hypoglycemia despite adherence to a PBH diet is acarbose. Acarbose is an alpha-glucosidase inhibitor that works in the gut and small intestine to slow carbohydrate digestion and therefore delay absorption of glucose. It is recommended to start with 25 mg given before the first bite of a meal and can be titrated up to 100 mg before all meals and snacks containing carbohydrates. The most common side effect is bloating and gas, which is a common reason why it is not well tolerated. However, in patients who can tolerate the gastrointestinal side effects, it has been demonstrated to reduce both early dumping syndrome and the frequency and severity of hypoglycemia in PBH.[25,26]

8. **B.** After medical therapies for preventing and treating PBH have been exhausted including medical nutrition therapy, acarbose, somatostatin analogues including octreotide, diazoxide, and calcium channel blockers, further surgical management may be required. As previously discussed, partial pancreatectomy is no longer recommended for surgical management of post-bariatric hypoglycemia due to incomplete response and high morbidity associated with the procedure.

   One surgical therapy is gastrostomy tube (G-tube) placement into the gastric remnant pouch for patients who have had RYGB. This tube can allow passage of nutrients into the excluded remnant stomach that will enter the bypassed duodenum and proximal small intestine and thereby reduce stimulation of insulin and other incretin hormones.[27–29] However, although this approach has been successful in some patients, it is limited by impacts on quality of life caused by insurance coverage, discomfort during feeds, presence of a feeding tube, and challenges in finding optimal supplies and formulas.

   Revision and restriction of gastric outlet to further slow the absorption of food into the small intestine has been demonstrated to provide benefit in one series of patients.[30] Another approach has been reversal of gastric bypass, which has been successful in eliminating PBH episodes in some[27,29] but not all patients.[31]

   It should be noted that promising experimental approaches are in development, including automated glucagon-pump,[18,19] GLP-1 receptor antagonism,[32] and insulin receptor blockade.[33] Clinicians should continue to monitor for signs of PBH in their patients and monitor for new approaches to reduce its burden on affected patients.

REFERENCES

1. Lee CJ, Clark JM, Schweitzer M, et al. Prevalence of and risk factors for hypoglycemic symptoms after gastric bypass and sleeve gastrectomy. *Obesity (Silver Spring)*. 2015;23(5):1079-1084.
2. Brix JM, Kopp HP, Hollerl F, Schernthaner GH, Ludvik B, Schernthaner G. Frequency of hypoglycaemia after different bariatric surgical procedures. *Obes Facts*. 2019;12(4):397-406.
3. Goldfine AB, Patti ME. How common is hypoglycemia after gastric bypass? *Obesity (Silver Spring)*. 2016;24(6): 1210-1211.
4. Lee CJ, Wood GC, Lazo M, et al. Risk of post-gastric bypass surgery hypoglycemia in nondiabetic individuals: A single center experience. *Obesity (Silver Spring)*. 2016;24(6): 1342-1348.
5. Nannipieri M, Belligoli A, Guarino D, et al. Risk factors for spontaneously self-reported postprandial hypoglycemia after bariatric surgery. *J Clin Endocrinol Metab*. 2016;101(10):3600-3607.
6. Raverdy V, Baud G, Pigeyre M, et al. Incidence and predictive factors of postprandial hyperinsulinemic hypoglycemia after Roux-en-Y gastric bypass: a five year longitudinal study. *Ann Surg*. 2016;264(5):878-885.
7. Chalew SA, McLaughlin JV, Mersey JH, Adams AJ, Cornblath M, Kowarski AA. The use of the plasma epinephrine response in the diagnosis of idiopathic postprandial syndrome. *JAMA*. 1984;251(5):612-615.
8. Salehi M, Vella A, McLaughlin T, Patti ME. Hypoglycemia after gastric bypass surgery: current concepts and controversies. *J Clin Endocrinol Metab*. 2018;103(8):2815-2826.
9. Whipple AO. The surgical therapy of hyperinsulinism. *J International de Chirurgie*. 1938;3:237-276.
10. Mulla CM, Storino A, Yee EU, et al. Insulinoma after bariatric surgery: diagnostic dilemma and therapeutic approaches. *Obes Surg*. 2016;26(4):874-881.
11. Service FJ. Diagnostic approach to adults with hypoglycemic disorders. *Endocrinol Metabol Clin N Am*. 1999;28(3): 519-532.
12. Cryer PE, Axelrod L, Grossman AB, et al. Evaluation and management of adult hypoglycemic disorders: an Endocrine Society Clinical Practice Guideline. *J Clin Endocrinol Metab*. 2009;94(3):709-728.
13. Charles MA, Hofeldt F, Shackelford A, et al. Comparison of oral glucose tolerance tests and mixed meals in patients with apparent idiopathic postabsorptive hypoglycemia: absence of hypoglycemia after meals. *Diabetes*. 1981;30(6):465-470.

14. Salehi M, Gastaldelli A, D'Alessio DA. Altered islet function and insulin clearance cause hyperinsulinemia in gastric bypass patients with symptoms of postprandial hypoglycemia. *J Clin Endocrinol Metab*. 2014;99(6):2008-2017.
15. Shah M, Law JH, Micheletto F, et al. Contribution of endogenous glucagon-like peptide 1 to glucose metabolism after Roux-en-Y gastric bypass. *Diabetes*. 2014;63(2):483-493.
16. Suhl E, Anderson-Haynes SE, Mulla C, Patti ME. Medical nutrition therapy for post-bariatric hypoglycemia: practical insights. *Surg Obes Relat Dis*. 2017;13(5):888-896.
17. Vanderveen KA, Grant CS, Thompson GB, et al. Outcomes and quality of life after partial pancreatectomy for noninsulinoma pancreatogenous hypoglycemia from diffuse islet cell disease. *Surgery*. 2010;148(6):1237-1245; discussion 1245-1246.
18. Mulla CM, Zavitsanou S, Laguna Sanz AJ, et al. A randomized, placebo-controlled double-blind trial of a closed-loop glucagon system for postbariatric hypoglycemia. *J Clin Endocrinol Metab*. 2020;105(4).
19. Laguna Sanz AJ, Mulla CM, Fowler KM, et al. Design and clinical evaluation of a novel low-glucose prediction algorithm with mini-dose stable glucagon delivery in post-bariatric hypoglycemia. *Diabetes Technol Ther*. 2018;20(2):127-139.
20. Michaels AD, Hunter Mehaffey J, Brenton French W, Schirmer BD, Kirby JL, Hallowell PT. Hypoglycemia following bariatric surgery: our 31-year experience. *Obes Surg*. 2017;27(12):3118-3123.
21. Kandel D, Bojsen-Moller KN, Svane MS, et al. Mechanisms of action of a carbohydrate-reduced, high-protein diet in reducing the risk of postprandial hypoglycemia after Roux-en-Y gastric bypass surgery. *Am J Clin Nutr*. 2019;110(2):296-304.
22. Lembo E, Lupoli R, Ciciola P, et al. Implementation of low glycemic index diet together with cornstarch in post-gastric bypass hypoglycemia: two case reports. *Nutrients*. 2018;10(6).
23. van Beek AP, Emous M, Laville M, Tack J. Dumping syndrome after esophageal, gastric or bariatric surgery: pathophysiology, diagnosis, and management. *Obes Rev*. 2017;18(1):68-85.
24. Placzkowski KA, Vella A, Thompson GB, et al. Secular trends in the presentation and management of functioning insulinoma at the Mayo Clinic, 1987-2007. *J Clin Endocrinol Metab*. 2009;94(4):1069-1073.
25. Cadegiani FA, Silva OS. Acarbose promotes remission of both early and late dumping syndromes in post-bariatric patients. *Diabetes Metab Syndr Obes*. 2016;9:443-446.
26. Scarpellini E, Arts J, Karamanolis G, et al. International consensus on the diagnosis and management of dumping syndrome. *Nat Rev Endocrinol*. 2020.
27. Davis DB, Khoraki J, Ziemelis M, Sirinvaravong S, Han JY, Campos GM. Roux en Y gastric bypass hypoglycemia resolves with gastric feeding or reversal: Confirming a non-pancreatic etiology. *Mol Metab*. 2018;9:15-27.
28. Craig C, Lamendola C, Holst J, Deacon C, McLaughlin T. The use of gastrostomy tube for the long-term remission of hyperinsulinemic hypoglycemia after Roux-en-y gastric bypass: a case report. *AACE Clin Case Rep*. 2015;1:e84-e87.
29. Qvigstad E, Gulseth HL, Risstad H, et al. A novel technique of Roux-en-Y gastric bypass reversal for postprandial hyperinsulinemic hypoglycaemia: a case report. *Int J Surg Case Rep*. 2016;21:91-94.
30. Leitman IM, Virk CS, Avgerinos DV, et al. Early results of trans-oral endoscopic plication and revision of the gastric pouch and stoma following Roux-en-Y gastric bypass surgery. *JSLS*. 2010;14(2):217-220.
31. Lee CJ, Brown T, Magnuson TH, Egan JM, Carlson O, Elahi D. Hormonal response to a mixed-meal challenge after reversal of gastric bypass for hypoglycemia. *J Clin Endocrinol Metab*. 2013;98(7):E1208-1212.
32. Craig CM, Liu LF, Deacon CF, Holst JJ, McLaughlin TL. Critical role for GLP-1 in symptomatic post-bariatric hypoglycaemia. *Diabetologia*. 2017;60(3):531-540.
33. Johnson KW, Gordon A, Neale AC, et al. Single administration of xoma 358, an insulin receptor attenuator, improves post-meal and nighttime hypoglycemia profiles in post gastric bypass hypoglycemia (PGBH) patients. *Endocrine Rev*. 2019;38(Supplement):i1-i1431.

58

Mortality Following Bariatric Surgery

Colston Edgerton, MD, and Ali Tavakkoli, MD

A 63-year-old female with a body mass index (BMI) of 55 kg/m^2 and medical comorbidities of insulin-dependent diabetes mellitus, hypertension controlled with two medications, and obstructive sleep apnea presents for consideration of bariatric surgery. She is interested to learn more about the common bariatric procedures offered and would like to know about her risks in undergoing surgery. She had a relative who died following complications from a nonbariatric surgery and is specifically interested in the mortality risk.

1. What is the patient's risk of perioperative mortality after Roux-en-Y gastric bypass (RYGB)?

A. The risk is similar in both the open and laparoscopic approach.
B. It is 5-times higher than that of laparoscopic sleeve gastrectomy (LSG).
C. It is higher than common laparoscopic procedures such as a cholecystectomy and appendectomy.
D. Counseling of risk should include individual patient risk factors.

2. Which of her following characteristics will increase her risk of mortality following bariatric surgery?

A. BMI >50
B. Age >60
C. White race
D. Female sex

3. Which of the following comorbidities increase her risk of mortality?

A. Hypertension
B. Independent functional status
C. Family history of deep vein thrombosis (DVT)/pulmonary embolism (PE)
D. Hypothyroidism

4. Which of the following is true regarding the cause of perioperative mortality after bariatric surgery?

A. Bariatric center volume has strong influence on mortality.
B. Perioperative mortality is more likely associated with bleeding than leaks.
C. The majority of perioperative deaths following bariatric surgery are related to a technical complication from surgery rather than systemic complications.
D. Most perioperative deaths occur following hospital discharge from the index procedure.

5. To what extent would bariatric surgery decrease her risk of dying compared to if she decides to forego surgery?

A. Randomized, prospective data demonstrates increased life expectancy in patients undergoing bariatric surgery.
B. Her all-cause mortality is decreased following surgery.
C. If she had surgery earlier in her life, the more effective the surgery will have on her all-cause mortality.
D. Her risk of dying from cancer will be increased after bariatric surgery.

ANSWERS

1. D. Mortality following RYGB has decreased with the adoption of laparoscopic techniques.[1–6]

A meta-analysis including 361 studies with 85,048 patients from 1995 to 2004 found a 30-day mortality rate for open gastric bypass to be 0.41% (95% CI, 0.24–0.58) compared to 0.16% (95% CI, 0.09–0.23) for laparoscopic gastric bypass.[7] A systematic review of 4,030 patients that analyzed 30-day mortality following bariatric surgeries included studies through the year 2016, with most within 10 years of publication. The all-cause 30-day mortality rate was 0.27% and was higher for open (0.31%; 95% CI, 0.03%–0.97%) than for laparoscopic surgeries (0.16%; 95% CI, 0.03%–0.36%).[8]

Data from the American College of Surgeons National Surgical Quality Improvement Program (NSQIP) database also showed no difference in 30 day mortality between patients undergoing LSG and RYGB.[9,10] However, more recent data from the 2015 Metabolic and Bariatric Surgery Accreditation and Quality Improvement Program (MBSAQIP) registry showed a slightly higher mortality rate in LSG compared to RYGB (0.1% vs. 0.2% respectively, P <0.001).[11,12] These findings in the modern laparoscopic era of bariatric surgery are similar to reported 30-day mortality following other common laparoscopic procedures such as cholecystectomy (0.15%) and laparoscopic appendectomy (0.21%).[13,14]

Mortality following bariatric surgery can be stratified according to patient risk factors. A risk calculator was developed from the MBSAQIP database comprising 775,000 operations from 925 centers in 2013 to 2018. For 30-day outcomes, the calculator uses 20 patient predictors, such as age, American Society of Anesthesiologists Physical Status classification, and preoperative BMI to predict the likelihood that patients will experience any of nine different outcomes within the first 30 days after an operation, including death.[15] A patient's risk of mortality should be based on their individual risk factors.

2. **A.** Studies have shown an increased mortality rate in superobese patients with some specifying a BMI >50 as a cutoff after which this difference can be appreciated.[2,3,5,7,16–18]

There are mixed data regarding the influence of age on mortality following bariatric surgery. Many studies have shown an acceptable mortality rate in patients >60 years old across all types of bariatric surgery.[2,7,19–24] Data from the NSQIP database from 2011 to 2015 showed an increase risk in 30-day mortality following LSG in patients >60 years old, but not after RYGB.[24] However, a contemporaneous review of 21,571 LSG patients in the German Bariatric Surgery Registry found that while there was higher morbidity, there was no difference in mortality among older patients.[25] The safety of LSG in older patients has likewise been published in single institutional reviews.[26–28] On the contrary, data from 2015 in the MBSAQIP registry showed higher 30-day mortality in patients in the highest two quintiles of patient age.[29]

While there is variable prevalence of medical comorbidities and rates of obesity in different racial groups,[30] there is no reliable evidence that in controlling for these factors, race alone influences mortality following bariatric surgery.[2,3]

Data across all types of bariatric surgery has shown an increased mortality rate in males.[1,3,5,7,16] A retrospective review including over 11,800 patients undergoing LSG from 2005 to 2013 showed an overall 30-day mortality within the study period to be 0.25%, with twice the rate of mortality in males (0.4%) compared to females (0.2%) patients (P=0.022). Although not able to prove causality, there was noted to be statistically significant differences in bleeding (1.7% vs. 1.1%, P = 0.012) and sepsis (0.9% and 0.5%, P = 0.009). There were no differences between males and females for cardiac (0.6 vs. 0.4, P = 0.69), pulmonary (1.3 vs. 1.1, P = 0.244), or VTE (0.1 vs. 0.1) complications. Such data suggests but does not prove that increased intra-abdominal visceral adiposity in males male lead to a higher rate of technical failures and a higher risk of perioperative mortality in LSG.[26]

3. **A.** Patients who meet the criteria for metabolic syndrome have been shown to have a 3.2-fold increase risk of mortality.[31] Other studies have demonstrated a higher mortality in patients with the comorbidities that make up metabolic syndrome such as hypertension and diabetes mellitus.[1,3,5,16,18]

Functional status has been shown to be an independent predictor of mortality following bariatric surgery.[2,18] Khan et al. reviewed 30-day mortality following bariatric surgery in 44,408 patients from the NSQIP database. The majority (54%) of procedures were laparoscopic RYGB followed by laparoscopic adjustable gastric banding (33%) and open RYGB (7%). The cumulative 30-day perioperative mortality rate was 0.14%. The single greatest independent predictor of mortality with an odds ratio of

27.6% was functional status of total dependency before surgery. Risk stratification showed an exponential increase in mortality as the number of comorbid conditions increased: 0 to 1 comorbidities (0.03 %), 2 to 3 comorbidities (0.16 %), and 4 comorbidities or more (7.4 %).[3]

Patients with a prior diagnosis of DVT/PE have also been found to have a higher rate of perioperative mortality on multivariate analysis, which has led its inclusion as an element in bariatric mortality risk calculators.[2,15–17] A family history of VTE has not been proven to increase the mortality risk.

While studies have investigated the effect of bariatric surgery on thyroid homeostasis and the influence of thyroid pathologies on postoperative weight loss, there is no evidence that thyroid hormone imbalances increase postoperative mortality.[32–35]

4. **D.** Fortunately, a challenge of studying mortality after bariatric surgery is its low incidence. Many institutional series are not powered to detect a significant difference between causes, and larger national database sampling may not offer specifics for the cause of death. Initially, it had been shown that the adoption of minimally invasive techniques and the accreditation of high-volume bariatric centers of excellence have resulted in a decrease in perioperative mortality.[4,5,36–38] However, mortality between accredited and nonaccredited hospitals is the same if the centers use the recommended pathways and guidelines of a center of excellence.

A review of prospectively collected data from four centers for 4,431 patients undergoing open and laparoscopic RYGB demonstrated a 30-day mortality rate of 0.7% that was caused by PE in 30% of cases, cardiac events in 27%, and anastomotic leak in 21%.[17] A retrospective review of The Italian Society of Obesity Surgery national registry was performed from 1996 to 2006 and included 13,871 patients. Perioperative mortality was defined as death within 60 days of surgery and was found to be 0.25% overall. Specific causes were identified as PE/DVT (38.2%), cardiac events (17.6%), anastomotic leak (17.6%), and respiratory failure (11.8%). Overall, 29.4% were attributable to technical surgical complications. When examined by procedure type, there was a 0.8% mortality rate for biliopancreatic diversion (BPD), 0.54% for RYGB (open and laparoscopic), 0.15% vertical banded gastroplasty, and 0.1% adjustable gastric banding, although these differences were not noted to be statistically significant. There was a significant difference in the contribution of open versus laparoscopic surgery to mortality, including systemic complications such as DVT/PE.[4]

The Longitudinal Assessment of Bariatric Surgery (LABS) database analyzed 30-day mortality in 6,118 patients from March 2005 to April 2009. The leading causes of death were found to be abdominal sepsis (33%), cardiac events (28%), and DVT/PE (17%), with most occurring after hospital discharge.[39] Similarly, data from the Scandinavian Obesity Surgery Registry from 2008 to 2017 classified perioperative mortality as that occurring within 90 days after surgery, and found the average time after surgery for mortality due to a technical factor to be 17.1 days, and that from nontechnical factors including PE, cardiac, and stroke to be 53.6 days.[40]

5. **B.** Mortality rates are increased in obese subjects.[41–44] Estimates include 5 to 20 years of life lost due to obesity depending on demographic and age cohorts.[45] Not surprisingly, with the known health benefits of weight loss, modification of medical comorbidities, and attenuation of metabolic syndrome, bariatric surgery is increasingly being proven to be a powerful tool to combat obesity-related mortality. Many of the studies examining this question were done in patients undergoing RYGB or gastric banding.

Although there are no long-term results from randomized studies, multiple studies have shown improved life expectancy after surgery. In the Swedish Obese Subjects (SOS) study, Sjöström et al. studied 2010 patients who underwent bariatric surgery and 2,037 matched controls, which included 265 patients undergoing RYGB, 1,369 VBG, and 376 adjustable or nonadjustable gastric banding. After a mean follow up of 10.9 years, the unadjusted overall hazard ratio for mortality was 0.76 in the surgery group (95% CI, 0.59–0.99), as compared with the control group, and the hazard ratio adjusted for sex, age, and risk factors was 0.71 ($P = 0.01$).[46]

Several large population-based retrospective series have similarly demonstrated decreased all-cause mortality with median follow up ranging from 4.3 to 9 years following all types of bariatric surgery compared to matched controls. Several specifically identify decreased mortality related to cardiovascular causes or complications from diabetes.[47–51]

The only cause of death that has been shown to be higher in bariatric surgery cohorts is that from accidents or suicide.[47,51,52] Because of this, one review found that when analyzed by age group, the only cohort that did not experience a reduction in mortality was in those <35 years old. This was driven largely by the finding that the hazard ratio for mortality from external causes in women <35 years old was 3.08 (95% CI, 1.4–6.7). External deaths were defined as unintentional or undetermined injuries or poisonings and intentional injury or poisonings (e.g. suicide, homicide, assault, or legal intervention).[53]

A single institution study followed the patients who had been evaluated for an initial bariatric surgery consultation between 1997 and 2006, and compared 908 patients who later underwent surgery to 112 patients who did not. RYGB was performed almost exclusively. After 9 years of follow-up and adjusting for age, gender, and body mass index, patients who had undergone surgery had an 82% reduction in mortality (HR 0.18; 95% CI, 0.09–0.35).[54]

A recent review analyzed 8 studies ranging from 1984 to 2014, which involved 23,647 operated patients compared to 89,628 nonoperated obese controls. All studies showed a decrease in long-term mortality following bariatric surgery. The pooled effect estimate showed a reduction in mortality of 41% (HR 0.59; 95% CI, 0.52–0.67). Operated patients had a hazard ratio of 0.42 (95% CI, 0.25–0.72) for mortality due to cardiovascular events, and 0.47 (95% CI, 0.3–0.63) for cancer-related mortality.[8]

Bariatric surgery has been shown to decrease cancer-related mortality.[8,47,51,55] While one study showed a decreased incidence of hormone-related cancers for all bariatric surgeries and an increase in colorectal cancer incidence following RYGB,[55] other studies have demonstrated lower incidence of colorectal cancer in all types of bariatric surgery including RYGB.[56,57] Data from the SOS study demonstrated a decreased the incidence of cancer in female but not male bariatric surgery patients.[58] A meta-analysis found a decreased cancer risk following bariatric surgery (OR 0.56; 95% CI, 0.48–0.66), in terms of both incidence (HR 0.56; 95% CI, 0.46–0.68) and mortality (HR 0.56; 95% CI, 0.41–0.75). In subgroup analysis, bariatric surgery was significantly associated with decreased breast and endometrial cancer risk, but not associated with other cancer subtypes.[59]

REFERENCES

1. Nguyen NT, Nguyen B, Smith B, Reavis KM, Elliott C, Hohmann S. Proposal for a bariatric mortality risk classification system for patients undergoing bariatric surgery. *Surg Obes Relat Dis*. 2013;9(2):239-246.
2. Consortium LAoBS. Perioperative safety in the longitudinal assessment of bariatric surgery. *N Eng J Med*. 2009;361(5):445-454.
3. Khan MA, Grinberg R, Johnson S, Afthinos JN, Gibbs KE. Perioperative risk factors for 30-day mortality after bariatric surgery: is functional status important? *Surg Endosc*. 2013;27(5):1772-1777.
4. Morino M, Toppino M, Forestieri P, Angrisani L, Allaix ME, Scopinaro N. Mortality after bariatric surgery: analysis of 13,871 morbidly obese patients from a national registry. *Ann Surg*. 2007;246(6):1002-1009.
5. Lazzati A, Audureau E, Hemery F, et al. Reduction in early mortality outcomes after bariatric surgery in France between 2007 and 2012: a nationwide study of 133,000 obese patients. *Surgery*. 2016;159(2):467-474.
6. Hutter MM, Randall S, Khuri SF, Henderson WG, Abbott WM, Warshaw AL. Laparoscopic versus open gastric bypass for morbid obesity: a multicenter, prospective, risk-adjusted analysis from the National Surgical Quality Improvement Program. *Ann Surg*. 2006;243(5):657.
7. Buchwald H, Estok R, Fahrbach K, Banel D, Sledge I. Trends in mortality in bariatric surgery: a systematic review and meta-analysis. *Surgery*. 2007;142(4):621-635.
8. Cardoso L, Rodrigues D, Gomes L, Carrilho F. Short- and long-term mortality after bariatric surgery: a systematic review and meta-analysis. *Diabet Obes Metabol*. 2017;19(9):1223-1232.
9. Spaniolas K, Trus TL, Adrales GL, Quigley MT, Pories WJ, Laycock WS. Early morbidity and mortality of laparoscopic sleeve gastrectomy and gastric bypass in the elderly: a NSQIP analysis. *Surg Obes Relat Dis*. 2014;10(4):584-588.
10. Young MT, Gebhart A, Phelan MJ, Nguyen NT. Use and outcomes of laparoscopic sleeve gastrectomy vs laparoscopic gastric bypass: analysis of the American College of Surgeons NSQIP. *J Am Coll Surg*. 2015;220(5):880-885.
11. Kumar SB, Hamilton BC, Wood SG, Rogers SJ, Carter JT, Lin MY. Is laparoscopic sleeve gastrectomy safer than laparoscopic gastric bypass? A comparison of 30-day complications using the MBSAQIP data registry. *Surg Obes Relat Dis*. 2018;14(3):264-269.
12. El Chaar M, Lundberg P, Stoltzfus J. Thirty-day outcomes of sleeve gastrectomy versus Roux-en-Y gastric bypass: first report based on Metabolic and Bariatric Surgery Accreditation and Quality Improvement Program database. *Surg Obes Relat Dis*. 2018;14(5):545-551.
13. Sandblom G, Videhult P, Crona Guterstam Y, Svenner A, Sadr-Azodi O. Mortality after a cholecystectomy: a population-based study. *HPB*. 2015;(3):239-243.
14. Kotaluoto S, Ukkonen M, Pauniaho S-L, Helminen M, Sand J, Rantanen T. Mortality related to appendectomy;a population based analysis over two decades in Finland. *World J Surg*. 2017;41(1):64-69.

15. Bariatric Surgical Risk/Benefit Calculator. https://riskcalculator.facs.org/bariatric/patientoutcomes.jsp. 2019. Accessed March 15, 2020.
16. DeMaria EJ, Portenier D, Wolfe L. Obesity surgery mortality risk score: proposal for a clinically useful score to predict mortality risk in patients undergoing gastric bypass. *Surg Obes Relat Dis*. 2007;3(2):134-140.
17. DeMaria EJ, Murr M, Byrne TK, et al. Validation of the obesity surgery mortality risk score in a multicenter study proves it stratifies mortality risk in patients undergoing gastric bypass for morbid obesity. *Ann Surg*. 2007;246(4):578-584.
18. Gupta PK, Franck C, Miller WJ, Gupta H, Forse RA. Development and validation of a bariatric surgery morbidity risk calculator using the prospective, multicenter NSQIP dataset. *J Am Coll Surg*. 2011;212(3):301-309.
19. O'Keefe KL, Kemmeter PR, Kemmeter KD. Bariatric surgery outcomes in patients aged 65 years and older at an American Society for Metabolic and Bariatric Surgery Center of Excellence. *Obes Surg*. 2010;20(9):1199-1205.
20. Abbas M, Cumella L, Zhang Y, et al. Outcomes of laparoscopic sleeve gastrectomy and Roux-en-Y gastric bypass in patients older than 60. *Obes Surg*. 2015;25(12):2251-2256.
21. Varela JE, Wilson SE, Nguyen NT. Outcomes of bariatric surgery in the elderly. *Am Surg*. 2006;72(10):865-869.
22. Sugerman HJ, DeMaria EJ, Kellum JM, Sugerman EL, Meador JG, Wolfe LG. Effects of bariatric surgery in older patients. *Ann Surg*. 2004;240(2):243.
23. Sosa J, Pombo H, Pallavicini H, Ruiz-Rodriguez M. Laparoscopic gastric bypass beyond age 60. *Obes Surg*. 2004;14(10):1398-1401.
24. Koh CY, Inaba CS, Sujatha-Bhaskar S, Nguyen NT. Outcomes of laparoscopic bariatric surgery in the elderly population. *Am Surg*. 2018;84(10):1600-1603.
25. Hajer AA, Wolff S, Benedix F, et al. Trends in Early Morbidity and Mortality after Sleeve Gastrectomy in Patients over 60 Years. *Obes Surg*. 2018;28(7):1831-1837.
26. Stroh C, Köckerling F, Volker L, et al. Results of more than 11,800 sleeve gastrectomies. *Ann Surg*. 2016;263(5):949-955.
27. Danan M, Nedelcu A, Noel P, Zulian V, Carandina S, Nedelcu M. Operative morbidity of laparoscopic sleeve gastrectomy in subjects older than age 65. *Surg Obes Relat Dis*. 2019;15(1):8-11.
28. Garofalo F, Denis R, Pescarus R, Atlas H, Bacon SL, Garneau P. Long-term outcome after laparoscopic sleeve gastrectomy in patients over 65 years old: a retrospective analysis. *Surg Obes Relat Dis*. 2017;13(1):1-6.
29. Haskins IN, Ju T, Whitlock AE, et al. Older age confers a higher risk of 30-day morbidity and mortality following laparoscopic bariatric surgery: an analysis of the metabolic and bariatric surgery quality improvement program. *Obes Surg*. 2018;28(9):2745-2752.
30. Ward ZJ, Bleich SN, Cradock AL, et al. Projected US State-Level Prevalence of Adult Obesity and Severe Obesity. *N Engl J Med*. 2019;381(25):2440-2450.
31. Lak KL, Helm MC, Kindel TL, Gould JC. Metabolic syndrome is a significant predictor of postoperative morbidity and mortality following bariatric surgery. *J Gastrointest Surg*. 2019;23(4):739-744.
32. Gokosmanoglu F, Aksoy E, Onmez A, Ergenç H, Topkaya S. Thyroid homeostasis after bariatric surgery in obese cases. *Obes Surg*. 2020;30(1):274-278.
33. Neves JS, Oliveira SC, Souteiro P, et al. Effect of weight loss after bariatric surgery on thyroid-stimulating hormone levels in patients with morbid obesity and normal thyroid function. *Obes Surg*. 2018;28(1):97-103.
34. Zendel A, Abu-Ghanem Y, Dux J, Mor E, Zippel D, Goitein D. The impact of bariatric surgery on thyroid function and medication use in patients with hypothyroidism. *Obes Surg*. 2017;27(8):2000-2004.
35. Rudnicki Y, Slavin M, Keidar A, et al. The effect of bariatric surgery on hypothyroidism: sleeve gastrectomy versus gastric bypass. *Surg Obes Relat Dis*. 2018;14(9):1297-1303.
36. Davis S, Babidge W, Kiermeier A, Aitken R, Maddern G. Perioperative mortality following bariatric surgery in Australia. *Obes Surg*. 2018;28(5):1329-1334.
37. Podnos YD, Jimenez JC, Wilson SE, Stevens CM, Nguyen NT. Complications after laparoscopic gastric bypass: a review of 3464 cases. *Arch Surg*. 2003;138(9):957-961.
38. Flum DR, Salem L, Elrod JAB, Dellinger EP, Cheadle A, Chan L. Early mortality among Medicare beneficiaries undergoing bariatric surgical procedures. *JAMA*. 2005;294(15):1903-1908.
39. Smith MD, Patterson E, Wahed AS, et al. Thirty-day mortality after bariatric surgery: independently adjudicated causes of death in the longitudinal assessment of bariatric surgery. *Obes Surg*. 2011;21(11):1687-1692.
40. Sundbom M, Näslund E, Vidarsson B, Thorell A, Ottoson J. Low overall mortality during 10 years of bariatric surgery: nationwide study on 63,469 procedures from the Scandinavian Obesity Registry. *Surg Obes Relat Dis*. 2020;16(1):65-70.
41. Preston SH, Vierboom YC, Stokes A. The role of obesity in exceptionally slow US mortality improvement. *Proc National Academy of Sciences*. 2018;115(5):957-961.
42. Flegal KM, Graubard BI, Williamson DF, Gail MH. Excess deaths associated with underweight, overweight, and obesity. *JAMA*. 2005;293(15):1861-1867.
43. Flegal KM, Kit BK, Orpana H, Graubard BI. Association of all-cause mortality with overweight and obesity using standard body mass index categories: a systematic review and meta-analysis. *JAMA*. 2013;309(1):71-82.
44. Di Angelantonio E, Bhupathiraju SN, Wormser D, et al. Body-mass index and all-cause mortality: individual-participant-data meta-analysis of 239 prospective studies in four continents. *Lancet*. 2016;388(10046):776-786.
45. Fontaine KR, Redden DT, Wang C, Westfall AO, Allison DB. Years of life lost due to obesity. *JAMA*. 2003;289(2):187-193.
46. Sjöström L, Narbro K, Sjöström CD, et al. Effects of bariatric surgery on mortality in Swedish obese subjects. *N Eng J Med*. 2007;357(8):741-752.

47. Adams TD, Gress RE, Smith SC, et al. Long-term mortality after gastric bypass surgery. *N Eng J Med.* 2007;357(8):753-761.
48. Eliasson B, Liakopoulos V, Franzén S, et al. Cardiovascular disease and mortality in patients with type 2 diabetes after bariatric surgery in Sweden: a nationwide, matched, observational cohort study. *Lancet Diabet Endocrinol.* 2015;3(11):847-854.
49. Arterburn DE, Olsen MK, Smith VA, et al. Association between bariatric surgery and long-term survival. *JAMA.* 2015;313(1):62-70.
50. Reges O, Greenland P, Dicker D, et al. Association of bariatric surgery using laparoscopic banding, Roux-en-Y gastric bypass, or laparoscopic sleeve gastrectomy vs usual care obesity management with all-cause mortality. *JAMA.* 2018;319(3):279-290.
51. Kauppila JH, Tao W, Santoni G, et al. Effects of obesity surgery on overall and disease-specific mortality in a 5-country population-based study. *Gastroenterology.* 2019;157(1):119-127.e111.
52. Gribsholt SB, Thomsen RW, Svensson E, Richelsen B. Overall and cause-specific mortality after Roux-en-Y gastric bypass surgery: a nationwide cohort study. *Surg Obes Relat Dis.* 2017;13(4):581-587.
53. Davidson LE, Adams TD, Kim J, et al. Association of patient age at gastric bypass surgery with long-term all-cause and cause-specific mortality. *JAMA Surg.* 2016;151(7):631-637.
54. Sowemimo OA, Yood SM, Courtney J, et al. Natural history of morbid obesity without surgical intervention. *Surg Obes Relat Dis.* 2007;3(1):73-77.
55. Mackenzie H, Markar SR, Askari A, et al. Obesity surgery and risk of cancer. *Br J Surg.* 2018;105(12):1650-1657.
56. Bailly L, Fabre R, Pradier C, Iannelli A. Colorectal Cancer risk following bariatric surgery in a nationwide study of French individuals with obesity. *JAMA Surg.* 2020.
57. Schauer DP, Feigelson HS, Koebnick C, et al. Bariatric surgery and the risk of cancer in a large multisite cohort. *Ann Surg.* 2019;269(1):95-101.
58. Sjöström L, Gummesson A, Sjöström CD, et al. Effects of bariatric surgery on cancer incidence in obese patients in Sweden (Swedish Obese Subjects Study): a prospective, controlled intervention trial. *Lancet Oncol.* 2009;10(7):653-662.
59. Zhang K, Luo Y, Dai H, Deng Z. Effects of bariatric surgery on cancer risk: evidence from meta-analysis. *Obes Surg.* 2019:1-8.

SECTION 9

Other Issues

59

MBSAQIP Accreditation

Yong Choi, MD, and James Dickerson, MD

A 46-year-old female presents to your office to discuss bariatric surgery. Her body mass index (BMI) is 42 kg/m^2. She has hypertension, which is controlled with two medications. She has tried various attempts at weight loss to include diets, medications, and exercise. As she prepares for surgery, she has read about bariatric centers of excellence (COEs) and the Metabolic and Bariatric Surgery Accreditation and Quality Improvement Program (MBSAQIP) accreditation. She is considering either a sleeve gastrectomy or gastric bypass but wants to know the differences between an accredited and a nonaccredited hospital.

1. Which of the following is a standard for a hospital to attain MBSAQIP accreditation?

A. Annual volume of 75 cases per year
B. Critical care support
C. Data collection on 5% of the bariatric cases performed
D. Surgeon designated as Fellow of the American Society of Metabolic and Bariatric Surgery (ASMBS)

2. Since the creation of accreditation for bariatric surgery COEs, which of the following statements is true?

A. The Centers for Medicare and Medicaid Services restrict coverage for bariatric patients to COE.
B. Studies have shown lower mortality after bariatric surgery in COEs.
C. There is clear evidence of longer length of stay after bariatric surgery in non-COE hospitals.
D. Access to care is restricted due to the creation of MBSAQIP accreditation.

3. Hospital accreditation for bariatric surgery has the expressed purpose of promoting patient safety and improving outcomes. Which of the following contributes to the achievement of these goals?

A. The development of best clinical practices and techniques for bariatric surgery
B. Elimination for a need of detailed patient counseling
C. Patient experience as a model for risk stratification
D. No need for long-term data collection

4. Which of the following is true regarding MBSAQIP accreditation?

A. COEs must perform a minimum of 125 stapled bariatric procedures per year.
B. The Metabolic and Bariatric Surgery (MBS) Committee must include all surgeons and proceduralists performing procedures for the treatment of metabolic or obesity-related diseases.
C. Bariatric call coverage must be done by certified bariatric surgeons.
D. COEs are only required to provide emergency coverage for the patients that they have operated on.

ANSWERS

1. **B.** As the number of bariatric surgeries performed in the United States have grown over the years, there has been increased attention placed on the development of core factors that help improve outcome. Recently, the ASMBS and the American College of Surgeons (ACS) had their own criteria for hospitals obtaining accreditation as COEs in bariatric surgery. However, the two societies joined to create one national accreditation standard called the MBSAQIP.[1]

   There are 7 core standards for accreditation under MBSAQIP. These standards are case volume, commitment to quality care, appropriate equipment and instruments, critical care support, continuum of care, data collection, and continuous quality improvement process.[2] Bariatric surgeons can now become a fellow of the ASMBS. While this displays added commitment to the care of obese patients, it is not a requirement for accreditation. Various studies have shown improved outcome for bariatric patients in accredited centers.[1,3-5]

   While surgical volume is an important aspect of accreditation, centers can attain accreditation with 25 stapled bariatric cases for low-acuity centers and 50 stapled bariatric cases for a comprehensive program. Data collection is also a vital aspect of a bariatric center. In fact, a key factor that accreditation provides is the ability to collect data and monitor the programs. This allows for self-improvement and adherence to evidence-based practice of bariatric surgery.[1] Accreditation also provides a surgeon with strong arguments to ensure that the hospital administration supports the program and provides the proper equipment and medical support necessary for the program to be successful.

2. **B.** In 2006, the Centers for Medicare and Medicaid Services (CMS) required all covered patients to undergo bariatric surgeries only at COEs. At that time, a center could become accredited through either the ACS or the ASMBS.[6] However, in 2013, after review of various studies, the CMS reversed its decision. The CMS eliminated the requirement for all bariatric surgeries to be performed at bariatric COEs. They concluded that the requirement for surgeries to be performed in COEs would not improve the overall health outcomes for their beneficiaries and may limit access to care.

   Various studies, though, have shown lower mortality for bariatric surgery done in hospitals accredited as COEs. Stroh et al. reported a statistically significant lower rate of 30-day mortality in certified hospitals,[3] and several other studies have supported this.[1,2,4,7] In addition, the Bariatric Outcomes Longitudinal Database (BOLD) showed a decrease in mortality after bariatric surgery.[8] This database is made possible by data collection from hospitals accredited as COEs. Various factors may contribute to the decrease in mortality but some observations may point to the core standards that all accredited institutions possess (case volume, commitment to quality care, appropriate equipment and instruments, critical care support, continuum of care, data collection, and continuous quality improvement process).[2]

   In the literature, the length of stay appears to be similar in accredited or high-volume centers versus nonaccredited or low-volume centers.[7,9,10] This is a difficult outcome to measure because there can be multiple factors that can contribute to length of stay.

   With the institution of bariatric COEs, there was concern about access to care, especially in rural areas. However, while more patients with private insurance undergo bariatric surgery, there has been an increase in the rate of publicly insured patients undergoing bariatric surgery from 2005 to 2016 from 10.2% to 19%. There has also been an increase in access to bariatric surgery seen in some underserved populations.[6] While studies need to be performed on what factors may prolong wait times or hinder access to surgery, there is no clear evidence that the institution of an MBSAQIP COE accreditation has limited access to bariatric surgery.

3. **A.** In the early 2000s, as a result of the increasing number of bariatric procedures performed and their inherent perioperative risk, there was considerable emphasis surrounding the issues of patient safety and clinical outcomes. The ACS achieved success in improving patient care by the accreditation of Trauma and Cancer Centers throughout the Unites States. A similar result was sought when the ASMBS created the COE in bariatric surgery programs.[1] The goal of the accreditation process is to ensure a standardized mechanism for consistent performance and outcome assessment.[5]

   The observed improvements in patient outcomes after accreditation can be attributed to the COE commitment to the long-term care of bariatric patients.[2,5,7]

Appropriate surgeon experience and leadership, bariatric-trained personnel, specialized equipment, critical care support, adherence to clinical pathways, and outcome reporting are critical to patient safety and improved outcomes.[5]

The accreditation process has allowed bariatric centers to participate in long-term data collection and monitoring. This process is an integral component of self-improvement and evidence-based practices. The databases have been used to identify modifiable risk factors such as smoking and super-obesity that lead to postoperative complications. They have also been used to analyze the safety and efficacy of relatively new procedures such as the sleeve gastrectomy.[1] Large databases allow for better evaluation of low-frequency events by enhancing analytical power, which allow investigators to exponentially increase the power that can be applied to statistical analysis of the data. This increase in power can help answer critical bariatric surgery outcome questions.[8] Accurate data can be used for risk stratification rather than using patient experience alone. Although underserved populations such as black and Hispanic Americans demonstrate higher rates of obesity, they are less likely to undergo bariatric surgery.[6] Medicare and Medicaid patients who are considered a higher risk for perioperative complications also experience lower rates of bariatric surgery.[5] These rates have not improved since the institutions of COEs.[5,9]

4. **B.** Under the MBSAQIP, there are several designations of accreditation. To achieve a designation of MBSAQIP Comprehensive Center, Comprehensive Center with Obesity Medicine Qualifications, or Comprehensive Center with Adolescent and Obesity Medicine Qualifications, a center must perform a minimum of 50 bariatric stapling procedures annually. A MBSAQIP Low Acuity Center is required to perform a minimum of 25 bariatric procedures per year. A MBSAQIP Adolescent Center must perform a minimum of 15 stapling procedures annually on adolescents only or utilize an MBSAQIP verified co-surgeon.

The MBS Committee is considered the primary forum for continuous quality improvement. At a minimum, the committee must consist of the following members: MBS Director, MBS Coordinator, MBS Clinical Reviewer, all surgeons and proceduralists at the facility performing procedures for the treatment of metabolic or obesity-related diseases, and a representative from the facility's administration who is involved in the care or oversight of metabolic and bariatric patients. If a center is accredited with Adolescent Qualifications, the center must establish a Pediatric Medical Advisor. A center that is accredited with Obesity Medicine Qualifications must establish an Obesity Medicine Director.

Accredited facilities must maintain various on-site and consultative services required for the care of metabolic and bariatric patients. This includes immediate availability of personnel capable of administering advanced cardiovascular life support. The MBS Committee and Director are responsible for ensuring the center's resources and experience are appropriate for their patient selection. MBSAQIP Comprehensive Centers must be able to provide on-site CCU and/or ICU support, endoscopy, and diagnostic and interventional radiology services. Centers accredited under all other designation levels are eligible to provide these services either on-site or through transfer agreements.

It is the responsibility of the MBSAQIP-accredited centers to provide call coverage for all metabolic and bariatric patients presenting to the facility, even if the center did not perform the patient's principal metabolic and bariatric procedure(s). Call coverage must be provided 24 hours a day and 365 days per year. All surgeons performing metabolic and bariatric surgery at the center must have qualified call coverage by a colleague who is responsible for the emergency care of metabolic and bariatric patients in the absence of the primary surgeon. This must include call coverage for the full range of complications associated with metabolic and bariatric surgery. If the center's call coverage involves one or more general surgeons who are not privileged to perform metabolic and bariatric surgery, the surgeon covering must be credentialed with general surgery privileges and have undergone adequate education and training as determined by the center's MBS Committee.[10]

REFERENCES

1. DeMaria EJ, Chaar ME, Rogers AM, et al. American Society for Metabolic and Bariatric Surgery position statement on accreditation of bariatric surgery centers endorsed by the Society of American Gastrointestinal and Endoscopic Surgeons. *Surg Obes Relat Dis.* 2016;12:946-954.
2. Azagury D, Morton JM. Bariatric surgery outcomes in US accredited vs non-accredited centers: a systemic review. *J Am Coll Surg.* 2016;223(3):469-477.

3. Stroh C, Kockerling F, Lange V, et al. Does certification as bariatric surgery center and volume influence the outcome in RYGB – data analysis of German bariatric surgery registry. *Obes Surg*. 2017;27:445-453.
4. Kwon S, Wang B, Wong E, et al. The impact of accreditation on safety and cost of bariatric surgery. *Surg Obes Relat Dis*. 2013;9:617-622.
5. Telem DA, Talamini M, Altieri M, et al. The effect of national hospital accreditation in bariatric surgery on perioperative outcomes and long-term mortality. *Surg Obes Relat Dis*. 2015;11:749-757.
6. Kuo LE, Simmons KD, Kelz RR. Bariatric centers of excellence: effect of centralization on access to care. *J Am Coll Surg*. 2015;221(5):914-922.
7. Gebhart A, Young M, Phelan M, et al. Impact of accreditation in bariatric surgery. *Surg Obes Rel Dis*. 2014;10:767-773
8. Demaria EJ, Pate V, Warthen M, et al. Baseline data from American Society for Metabolic and Bariatric Surgery-designated Bariatric Surgery Centers of Excellence using the Bariatric Outcomes Longitudinal Database. *Surg Obes Relat Dis*. 2010;6:347-355.
9. Markar SR, Penna M, Karthikesalingan A, et al. The impact of hospital and surgeon volume on clinical outcome following bariatric surgery. *Obes Surg*. 2012;22:1126-1134.
10. Livingston EH. Bariatric surgery outcomes at designated centers of excellence vs. nondesignated programs. *Arch Surg*. 2009;144:319-325.

60

Support Groups

Teresa LaMasters MD, and Paul Davidson, PhD

A support group meeting is held once a month for an established metabolic and bariatric surgery program. It has an in-person, town hall open forum style available to bariatric patients, support persons, or others interested in considering surgery. Some of the people attending may have had bariatric surgery with a different bariatric program. A surgeon is often present for the first part of the support group to answer questions (45 minutes). There is an interim time for networking, vegetable sampling, protein and vitamin sampling, and time to shop at the free clothing exchange (30 minutes). The final portion of the support group is a topic based with a guest speaker (45 minutes). The surgeon portion of the program can be streamed online and recorded for later viewing by private members—only access.

1. **During a town hall–style meeting there is a risk of getting the same questions repetitively. This may make people feel it is a waste of time. What is an effective strategy the surgeon or facilitator can use to maintain the value of education to the attendees?**
   A. Keep the answers to questions from the group as brief as possible.
   B. Give the most specific answer possible for the question.
   C. Allow the same person in the group to ask as many questions as they want without addressing others in the room.
   D. Expand the answer from a narrow focus to include a broader related topic for education, especially regarding the underlying disease of obesity.
   E. Refrain from taking any questions from the attendees following a topic presentation to keep the focus on the presenter only.

2. **An established bariatric program has noticed that attendance and engagement in the support group have been declining. Which one of the following is true regarding methods to increase engagement and attendance at the support group?**
   A. Bariatric Surgery Anniversary Celebrations are not effective.
   B. A 5K fun walk/run may increase donations but does not increase engagement.
   C. Live streaming a support group via a restricted website is an effective way to increase engagement.
   D. A consistent facilitator, short meetings, and publicizing attendance increases attendance.
   E. Providing weekly in person small groups is a cost-effective and efficient way to communicate and increase attendance.

3. **Inevitably, difficult interpersonal issues may arise, and this can be a challenge for the support groups. Handling problematic group behaviors entails:**
   A. Waiting a few sessions to see if the problem goes away
   B. Addressing monopolizers but letting silent members work their way into the discussion
   C. Letting the group be part of the solution
   D. Patient advisory panels that will limit staff involvement
   E. Eliminating anonymous surveys to elicit feedback

4. **Which of the following is true regarding online support groups?**
   A. They are not effective at delivering factual information
   B. They adequately provide tangible support like cooking classes
   C. They do not adequately provide emotional support and encouragement
   D. They can provide advice on coping strategies following surgery
   E. They do not allow for flexibility of timing or location

5. **Regarding support groups, which of the following is true?**
   A. Attendance of support groups following bariatric surgery is associated with increased weight loss.
   B. Attending one support group meeting in the year following surgery has the same benefit for weight loss as attending five or more support groups in the first postsurgery year.
   C. Having a parent who has undergone bariatric surgery makes adolescents more likely to attend support groups.
   D. Support groups do not improve management of other chronic diseases.
   E. Attending individual psychotherapy visits makes adolescent patients more likely to attend clinic follow up visits after bariatric surgery.

ANSWERS

1. **D.** Support groups are a required component of a comprehensive accredited center in the American College of Surgeons' Metabolic and Bariatric Surgery Accreditation and Quality Improvement Program (MBSAQIP).[1] It is further recommended that all postoperative bariatric patients attend support groups. MBSAQIP accredited centers must provide regularly scheduled, organized, and supervised support groups for metabolic and bariatric patients. Regularly scheduled support groups must be made available a minimum of every 2 months and can be in-person, web-based, or teleconferenced. All support group activities must be documented, including group location, meeting time, supervisor, curriculum, and number of people in attendance. Other activities, including online forums, exercise instruction, and clothing sales must be noted but do not require full documentation.[1]

Obesity is recognized a complex chronic progressive disease. At the core, obesity is a disease of the brain, which tightly regulates hunger, satiety, and metabolism through neurohormonal pathways. In people with obesity, the brain has set the "normal" level of fat storage and weight regulation too high. The brain then uses many sophisticated pathways to allow the body to defend this higher "normal" weight.[2,3] Physiology is a critical component of the disease of obesity; however, it is important to address other components contributing to the disease as well, such as behavioral elements. There are several avenues to address the various factors to lead to the most successful outcome after metabolic bariatric surgery. One of the ways to address several of these components is through support groups.

Support groups and additional methods of patient encouragement are important in the successful management of many chronic conditions. Because obesity is also a chronic progressive disease, providing additional support has been shown to be a critical contribution to the successful management of the disease. Support groups have demonstrated consistent benefits for both weight loss and other outcomes following the surgical treatment of obesity.[4,5]

The presence of a bariatric surgeon at the support group has been shown to significantly increase the engagement of patients. The surgeon can provide education on many topics, including the physiology of obesity, comorbid health conditions, changes related to bariatric surgery, addressing weight regain, and the use of medications in combination with surgery.

It is important for a surgeon who is presenting or facilitating to manage group dynamics when allowing for a town hall open forum–style structure. Allowing a single person to ask multiple questions in a row can be very disengaging for others in the group. A large group usually includes a wide diversity in background, types of surgical procedures, and timing from surgery. When providing an answer that is broad, it is more likely to be relevant to more members of the group rather than a brief, specific answer to a question. It allows the opportunity to turn a specific question into a broader educational point.

There are many different structures that can be utilized to deliver the content effectively. These may include presurgery groups, combined pre- and postsurgery groups, postsurgery groups, adolescent groups, online groups, peer led groups, and mentorship style groups.[4,5]

The scenario presented demonstrates a combined pre- and postsurgery group with a large group structure. It also incorporates opportunity for smaller group networking and connection with the multidisciplinary team from the bariatric surgery program. An additional benefit is the tangible support provided through vitamin/supplement tasting, and a clothing exchange. A barrier in the scenario provided is the once a month timing. The use of an online streaming and recorded version of a portion of the program improves access and can potentially extend the educational benefits. A mixed benefit of the open support group structure is the opportunity for members to bring guests who may or may not have had bariatric surgery in another program. These members from outside the group may benefit and contribute to the group as well as act as ambassadors for treatment of people with obesity and may be more motivated to make their own health-related changes. The potential drawback of inclusion of these individuals can arise if the education they have received previously is conflicting with what the program is teaching, or if they are spreading misinformation. The facilitator must be aware of the potential of misinformation originating from outside the core group and be prepared to handle that situation.

2. **C.** Special events can increase the sense of community with people undergoing a major life change with a shared experience. Creating social connections has been proven to increase attendance at support groups and to make patients feel part of a cohesive program. Such events include a 5K fun walk/run, a fashion show, and anniversary celebrations. They normalize the patient experience and help to reinforce the lifestyle and self-image changes that patients undergo. They also support long-term follow-up care with the original bariatric surgery program by maintaining a connection with the multidisciplinary team.[4,6–8]

   Providing a weekly in person support group led by a facilitator would be of clear value to the members but would be less cost-effective regarding staff resource utilization. The use of a social media platform with use restricted to approved members can live stream the support group and keep a recording available of presentations for members to watch later. An added benefit is the fact that social media is either free or comes at minimal cost. It is important to recognize that personal material may not be appropriate for rebroadcast, and that any recorded presentation involving patients who may be seen or heard may require a release of information form from the hosting facility. Other internet-based platforms can also be used for webinars that can share the screen materials from the presenter and be recorded for later viewing can also be a cost-effective solution.[9–12]

   There can be several issues and barriers to navigate when incorporating social media and online technology. The protection of member privacy is the most important factor to address. One strategy to protect member privacy is to have the camera focused only on the presenter without showing anyone else present. As mentioned earlier, use release of information forms as required by your institution if patients will be seen during the broadcast. Be sure that the presenter or surgeon repeats aloud any questions from the audience so that they can be heard by the viewing audience. It is important to understand the specifications and limitations of the technology that will be used, including potential capacity issues of the software. Planning ahead and testing prior to the event will also increase the likelihood of successful incorporation of new technology.[9–12]

   Offering flexible meeting times, novel topics, and a structured agenda has been empirically validated to show an increase in group attendance. Offering flexibility in scheduling allows for individuals to go to an earlier or a later group, which limits commitments such as work or school from preventing attendance. Offering novel topics is consistently a factor in patients' desires to belong to such a group. Topics covering physical health, diet, behavioral issues, physical activity, relationships, and addressing the challenges of adopting a bariatric lifestyle provide opportunities for a wide variety of programming. Lastly, a structured agenda allows individuals to develop a sense of security and familiarity with the process, which increases comfort in attending.[4,13] Using the same facilitator, short meetings, and publicizing attendance does not seem to increase participation.

3. **C.** The heart of running any successful support group involves providing an environment of safety for all members. It is only within the confines of a safe space that individuals will feel comfortable revealing their true feelings about situations. In nearly all group settings, problematic behaviors and destabilizing dynamics can arise. From those who remain silent during a meeting, those who dominate sessions, open conflict, or the expression of strong

emotions, these pose challenges which need to be addressed by the facilitator. The one thing that proves to be deleterious to group functioning is waiting for the problem to go away without addressing it within the group structure. In the case of conflicts, monopolizing, or silence, there is commonly an unstated need that must be addressed openly to move on in a healthy fashion. One of the great strategies in addressing problems is to let the group help bring the issues out in the open and expressing how members feel about the difficulty and what they would like to see happen. In addition, the facilitator becomes responsible to communicate to the group through words and actions that they are going to make sure that the group is a safe place by not allowing personal attacks, establishing confidentiality, and making sure that group members understand and will abide by the expectations to stay involved.[4]

It is important that support groups are flexible in their programming and adapt to member needs. Soliciting feedback is an important component to keeping the group fresh and relevant. It is possible to obtain feedback through surveys delivered either electronically or on paper. These surveys have an advantage of anonymity and may increase response rates. It can be helpful to share the information learned and plans for any changes with the larger group once a decision has been made. Closing the feedback loop with the larger group can increase engagement and participation in future surveys.

A patient advisory panel can also be a useful source of information and guidance on topics and structure to keep the support group relevant. It frequently requires more staff involvement to manage this type of group; however, it may yield very useful feedback.[9–11,14,15]

4. **D.** Online support groups have become very popular and can serve an important group by allowing for flexibility of timing, decreasing barriers related to travel or location, and add a variable of anonymity. Online support groups are missing other components that can provide important support to patients. Online support groups tend to be successful at delivering information, advice on coping strategies related to changes following surgery, and emotional support and encouragement. It is not as successful at providing networking with like-minded people, improved self-esteem, or tangible support. Tangible support may include protein and vitamin sampling, cooking classes, a clothing exchange, and continued contact with the multidisciplinary team and bariatric surgery program specifically.[10,12,15]

One way to provide this support can be through the presence of more than one multidisciplinary team member at the group who can also answer questions. The presence of a dietitian to answer diet or vitamin supplement questions can be very helpful. In addition, providing samples of different vitamins and protein supplements for patients to try can be very valuable.[4] Of note, many vitamin and protein supplement companies are willing to send free samples to a program for patients to try before purchase.

5. **A.** Attendance at support groups postsurgery has been repeatedly linked to greater weight loss in patients following Roux-en-Y gastric bypass (RYGB) and laparoscopic adjustable gastric banding (LAGB).[6,13,16–18]

A salient finding has been a "dose effect," with patients who attended five or more meetings the first year after surgery losing more weight.[19] Patients who reported regular attendance at postsurgical support groups had more than double the likelihood of a successful postsurgical weight loss outcome (92% vs. 40%). These findings were noted with moderate adherence to dietary recommendations.[4,16,19] The authors did feel that for those reporting "low moderate" adherence, regular attendance at a support group (either in-person or online) would be highly encouraged.[16] Support groups have been demonstrated to have some benefit for weight loss and prevention of weight regain as well as a positive outcome for other patient reported outcome measures (PROM).[13,16,20]

Several factors have been identified as barriers for adolescents. Adolescents may not have the ability to transport themselves or have control of their schedule. The distance from their home to the support group may be important due to relying on others' availability and transportation to the support group location. A higher initial BMI prior to surgery was a negative predictive factor for support group attendance, possibly related to self-esteem or self-confidence. And finally, having a parent who has undergone bariatric surgery was also a negative predictor. This factor may be related to a desire for increased independence and control of their personal life-changing journey, or a sense that they have a built-in support system at home.[21]

Increased multidisciplinary support and support groups have been demonstrated to improve management of chronic diseases including obesity, congestive heart failure, diabetes, and chronic pulmonary disease. The Reynolds systematic review of chronic disease management showed that the self-management system (SMS) was the most commonly tested intervention.[22] The SMS had the greatest proportion of studies demonstrating a significant result for one or more outcome measure categories for all diseases examined in the review.[22-27]

Regular attendance >4 times after bariatric surgery was correlated with higher bariatric clinic follow-up visit attendance at 6-months and 1-year postsurgery for adolescents.[21] Attending individual psychotherapy visits had a correlation similar to support group attendance with weight loss post bariatric surgery but was not specifically identified to correlate with adherence to clinic follow-up visit attendance for teens.[28] Increased clinic follow-up visits may effectively engage patients more actively in following their treatment plan, and allows for more rapid intervention in the event that something isn't going well.[29]

REFERENCES

1. The Metabolic and Bariatric Surgery Accreditation and Quality Improvement Program (MBSAQIP), Oct 2019. Version 3. Standards, Optimal Resources for Metabolic and Bariatric Surgery 2019. Standard 8 Education: Professional and Community Outreach, 8.1 Support Groups. https://www.facs.org/quality-programs/mbsaqip/standards. Accessed March 1, 2020.
2. Harris RB. Role of set-point theory in regulation of body weight. *FASEB J.* 1990;4(15):3310-3318. doi:10.1096/fasebj.4.15.2253845
3. Kaplan LM, Seeley RJ, Harris JL. Myths associated with obesity and bariatric surgery. Bariatric surgery: beyond restriction and malabsorption. Myth 1: "Weight can be reliably controlled by voluntarily adjusting energy balance through diet and exercise." *Bariatric Times.* 2012;9(4):12-13.
4. ASMBS Bariatric Surgery Support Group Facilitator Manual. July 2015. https://asmbs.org/resources/asmbs-bariatric-surgery-support-group-facilitator-manual. Accessed March 1, 2020.
5. Rudolph A, Hilbert A. Post-op behavioral management in bariatric surgery: a systematic review and meta-analysis of randomized controlled trials. *Obes Rev.* 2013;14:292-302.
6. Orth W, Madan A, Taddeucci R, et al. Support group meeting attendance is associated with better weight loss. *Obes Surg.* 2008;18:391-394.
7. Monkhouse S, Choudry M, Sergeant T, Woodcock S. Do Bariatric patient support groups influence short-term surgical outcomes? An investigation into the true value of bariatric patient support groups. *Bariat Surg Prac Patient Care.* 2013;8:1-5.
8. Hameed S, Salem V, Tan TM, et al. Beyond weight loss: establishing a postbariatric surgery patient support group—what do patients want? *J Obes.* 2018 Feb 14. doi:10.1155/2018/8419120
9. Cranwell J, Seymour-Smith S. Monitoring and normalizing a lack of appetite and weight loss. A discursive analysis of an online support group for bariatric surgery. *Appetite.* 2012;58:873-881.
10. Atwood M, Friedman A, Meisner B, Cassin S. The exchange of social support on online bariatric surgery discussion forums: a mixed-methods content analysis. *Health Comm.* 2018;33(5):628-635.
11. Koball A, Jester D, Domoff S, Kallies K, Grothe K, Kothari S. Examination of bariatric Facebook support groups: a content analysis. *Surg Obes Relat Dis.* 2017;13(8):1369-1375.
12. Frost RL, Rickwood DJ. A systematic review of the mental health outcomes associated with Facebook use. *Comp Human Behav.* 2017;76:576-600.
13. Livhits M, Mercado C, Yermilov I, et al. Is social support associated with greater weight loss after bariatric surgery?: a systematic review. *Obes Rev.* 2011;12:142-148.
14. Groller KD, Teel C, Stegenga KH, El Chaar M. Patient perspectives about bariatric surgery unveil experiences, education, satisfaction, and recommendations for improvement. *Surg Obes Relat Dis.* 2018;14(6):785-796. doi:10.1016/j.soard.2018.02.016
15. Wright KB. Communication in health-related online social support groups/communities: a review of research on predictors of participation, applications of social support theory, and health outcomes. *Rev Comm Res.* 2016;4:65-87.
16. Robinson A, Adler A, Stevens HB, Darcy AM, Morton JM, Safer D. What variables are associated with successful weight loss outcomes for bariatric surgery after one year? *Surg Obes Relat Dis.* 2014;10(4):697-704. doi:10.1016/j.soard.2014.01.030
17. Kaiser K, Franks S, Smith A. Positive relationship between support group attendance and one-year postoperative weight loss in gastric banding patients. *Surg Obes Relat Dis.* 2011;7:89-93.
18. Song Z, Reinhardt M, Buzdon M, Liao P. Association between support group attendance and weight loss after Roux-en-Y gastric bypass. *Surg Obes Relat Dis.* 2008;4:100-103.
19. Beck N, Johannsen M, Stoving R, et al. Do postoperative psychotherapeutic interventions and support groups influence weight loss following bariatric surgery? A systematic review and meta-analysis of randomized and nonrandomized trials. *Obes Surg.* 2012 Aug 30. doi:10.1007/s11695-012-0739-4
20. Lemstra M, Bird Y, Nwankwo C, Rogers M, Moraros J. Weight loss intervention adherence and factors promoting adherence: a meta-analysis. *Patient Prefer Adherence.* 2016;10:1547-1559.

21. Sawhney P, Modi A, Jenkins T, et al. Predictors and outcomes of adolescent bariatric support group attendance. *Surg Obes Relat Dis*. 2013;9:773-779.
22. Reynolds R, Dennis S, Hasan I, et al. A systematic review of chronic disease management interventions in primary care. *BMC Fam Pract*. 2018;19(11). doi:10.1186/s12875-017-0692-3
23. World Health Organization. Global status report on noncommunicable diseases. 2014. http://www.who.int/nmh/publications/ncd-status-report-2014/en/. Accessed March 28, 2020.
24. World Health Organization. Noncommunicable diseases country profiles 2018. Geneva: World Health Organization; 2018. License: CC BY-NC-SA 3.0 IGO. Accessed March 28, 2020.
25. Rothman AA, Wagner EH. Chronic illness management: what is the role of primary care? *Ann Intern Med*. 2003. doi:https://doi.org/10.7326/0003-4819-138-3-200302040-00034.
26. National Heart, Lung, and Blood Institute. Clinical Guidelines on the Identification, Evaluation, Treatment of Overweight and Obesity in Adults. (NIH publication 98-4083). The Evidence Report. 1998 Sep. http://www.nhlbi.nih.gov/guidelines/obesity/ob_gdlns.pdf.
27. Pollack A. AMA recognizes obesity as a disease. *New York Times*. June 18, 2013 http://nyti.ms/1Guko03. Accessed November 20, 2015.
28. Beck N, Johannsen M, Stoving R, et al. Do postoperative psychotherapeutic interventions and support groups influence weight loss following bariatric surgery? A systematic review and meta-analysis of randomized and nonrandomized trials. *Obes Surg*. 2012 Aug 30. doi:10.1007/s11695-012-0739-4.
29. Jones L, Cleator J, Yorke J. Maintaining weight loss after bariatric surgery when the spectator role is no longer enough. *Clin Obes*. 2016;6(4):249-258.

61

Exercise after Bariatric Surgery

Julietta Chang, MD

A 38-year-old female with type 2 insulin-dependent diabetes and a body mass index (BMI) of 42 kg/m^2 is undergoing workup for a laparoscopic Roux-en-Y gastric bypass (RYGB).

1. Three months prior to her surgery, she asks whether she should join her local gym now or after her gastric bypass. Which of the following is correct?

A. Exercise prior to surgery does not increase weight loss postoperatively.
B. Exercise tolerance increases with structured exercise programs preoperatively, and these changes are also durable after surgery.
C. The amount of physical activity (PA) that patients engage in before surgery does not determine their level of PA postoperatively.
D. In bariatric patients, experts recommend either aerobic or strength training exercise rather than a combination of both to avoid overuse injury.

2. One month postoperatively, her incisions are well healed and she asks for advice about lifestyle modifications after surgery to aid in physical fitness. Which statement is accurate?

A. Protein supplementation with aerobic exercise can help increase muscle strength after surgery.
B. Consistent PA does not prevent the loss of muscle mass during the rapid weight loss.
C. Postoperative dual energy x-ray absorptiometry (DEXA) scans tend to show decreased bone mineral density at the lumbar spine and hip after surgery even with exercise.
D. Resistance training is recommended only after weight loss plateaus.

3. Her insulin requirements shortly after surgery were immediately halved, and now 6 months postoperatively, she remains on metformin 1000 mg twice daily with a glycated hemoglobin (HbA1c) of 6.0. She is wondering if she will eventually be able to stop her metformin. Which of the following is correct?

A. Improved insulin sensitivity in the immediate postoperative period is independent of weight loss.
B. Exercise has minimal effect on glycemic control.
C. Improved hepatic insulin sensitivity leads to increased gluconeogenesis.
D. Skeletal muscle is responsible for 25% of glucose uptake after a meal.

4. It has been 18 months since her surgery and unfortunately her weight loss has plateaued at a BMI of 35 kg/m^2. When asked about exercise, she reports she is "always on her feet," but admits that she lacks a scheduled exercise routine due to a busy work schedule. Which of the following is accurate?

A. This far after surgery, she will not be able to reverse her plateaued weight loss.
B. There can be significant improvement in BMI with a structured exercise program.
C. A patient's reported PA levels are generally accurate.
D. Recommended exercise includes 90 minutes of intense aerobic exercise and 60 minutes of intense resistance training weekly.

ANSWERS

1. **B.** Studies have shown that patients are most motived to exercise before their bariatric surgery. One study by Baillot et al. enrolled patients prior to bariatric surgery in a structured exercise program incorporating both aerobic exercise and strength training.[1] During this preoperative period, patients improved in objective parameters of fitness such as the 6-minute walk test (distance covered in 6 minutes), as well as in weight loss. In addition, there were significant improvements in patient-reported measures such as fear of injury/anxiety toward exercise as well as emotions, social interactions, and sexual function.

   Prospective studies have also shown that patients tend to maintain their preoperative levels of PA after surgery, and so it is productive to start patients on an exercise regimen prior to their surgery. The same aforementioned group followed their study group 1 year postoperative and compared PA levels to usual care patients, and found that the patients in the prescribed exercise group continued to have higher levels of PA as measured by pedometers with lower BMIs compared to control.[2]

2. **A.** Weight loss after bariatric surgery is ideally from loss of fat mass. Excessive loss of fat free mass (FFM) including muscle, bone, and organs can lead to a decrease in resting energy expenditure and may lead to weight regain, sarcopenia, and osteoporosis.[3] Decrease in muscle mass and muscle strength has also been linked to decreased functional capacity.[4]

   To mitigate the loss of FFM, studies have been performed to determine the effects of exercise programs on postoperative body composition.[5] Both aerobic and resistance training increases loss of fat-mass, but resistance training leads to greater preservation of muscle mass as well. Studies also show that the addition of whey protein supplementation in addition to resistance exercise after weight loss surgery has been shown to increase muscle strength more than either protein supplementation or exercise alone.[4]

   Bariatric surgery has been reported to negatively impact bone health, likely due to ongoing vitamin D deficiency that leads to increased bone turnover. A randomized study observed the effects of vitamin D, calcium, and protein supplementation in addition to consistent exercise in post-RYGB and sleeve gastrectomy patients. A DEXA scan showed significant decrease in bone mineral density in the nonintervention group more than in the intervention group, and there was also an increase in bone turnover markers such as parathyroid hormone levels in this group.[6]

3. **A.** Early in the pathogenesis of type 2 diabetes there is increased insulin resistance in peripheral tissues including muscle and fat as well as hepatic resistance. Dramatic improvements in glycemic control are observed perioperatively after RYGB before significant weight loss. This is likely due to improved hepatic insulin sensitivity leading to increased insulin clearance as well as decreased hepatic gluconeogenesis.[7,8]

   Peripheral insulin sensitivity in tissues such as muscle and fat mirrors significant weight loss, and thus may take up to 1 year to improve. Skeletal muscle is responsible for up to 80% of glucose uptake following a meal. Because of this physiology, exercise programs after bariatric surgery have been shown to improve glycemic control after RYGB with resultant increase in muscle mass.[9]

4. **B.** Studies show that weight regain or inadequate weight loss leads to decreased physical function and diminished ability to perform activities of daily living. However, after bariatric surgery, structured exercise programs have demonstrated improvements in both exercise tolerance and weight loss even in previously inactive patients.[10]

   Unfortunately, patients' self-reported PA varies widely with objective measurements. For example, one study comparing accelerometer-measured versus self-reported PA levels found that although patients significantly report greater exercise after their RYGB, this unfortunately was not confirmed by the patients' individual accelerometers.[11] Therefore, the clinician should use objective measures of PA such as pedometers, rather than questionnaires, when assessing adequate exercise in their postbariatric patient. They recommended that exercise for postbariatric patients is 150 min/week of moderate level exercise with a combination of both aerobic and resistance-training exercises.

REFERENCES

1. Baillot A, Mampuya W, Comeau E, Méziat-Burdin A, Langlois M. Feasibility and impacts of supervised exercise training in subjects with obesity awaiting bariatric surgery: a pilot study. *Obes Surg.* 2013;23(7):882-891.
2. Baillot A, Vallée C, Mampuya W, Dionne I, et al. Effects of a pre-surgery supervised exercise training 1 year after

bariatric surgery: a randomized controlled study. *Obes Surg*. 2018;28(4):955-962.

3. Coen PM, Goodpaster BH. A role for exercise after bariatric surgery? *Diabetes Obes Metab*. 2016;18(1):16-23.
4. Oppert JM, Bellicha A, Roda C, et al. Resistance training and protein supplementation increase strength after bariatric surgery: a randomized controlled trial. *Obesity*. 2018;26(11):1709-1720.
5. Hassannejad A, Khalaj A, Mansournia MA, Rajabian Tabesh M, Alizadeh Z. The effect of aerobic or aerobic-strength exercise on body composition and functional capacity in patients with BMI ≥35 after bariatric surgery: a randomized control trial. *Obes Surg*. 2017;27(11):2792-2801.
6. Muschitz C, Kocijan R, Haschka J, et al. The impact of vitamin D, calcium, protein supplementation, and physical exercise on bone metabolism after bariatric surgery: the BABS study. *J Bone Mineral Res*. 2016;31(3):672-682.
7. Svane MS, Bojsen-Møller KN, Madsbad SS, Holst JJ. Updates in weight loss surgery and gastrointestinal peptides. *Curr Opin Endocrinol Diabet Obes*. 2015;22(1):21-28.
8. Holst JJ, Madsbad S, Bojsen-Møller KN, et al. Mechanisms in bariatric surgery: gut hormones, diabetes resolution, and weight loss. *Surg Obes Relat Dis*. 2018;14(5):708-714.
9. Shah M, Snell PG, Rao S, Adams-Huet B, et al. High-volume exercise program in obese bariatric surgery patients: a randomized, controlled trial. *Obesity*. 2011;19(9):1826-1834.
10. Herring LY, Stevinson C, Carter P, et al. The effects of supervised exercise training 12-24 months after bariatric surgery on physical function and body composition: a randomised controlled trial. *Int J Obes*. 2017;41(6):909-916.
11. Berglind D, Willmer M, Tynelius P, Ghaderi A, Näslund E, Rasmussen F. Accelerometer-measured versus self-reported physical activity levels and sedentary behavior in women before and 9 months after Roux-en-Y gastric bypass. *Obes Surg*. 2016;26(7):1463-1470.

62

Body Contouring Surgery

Darya D. Kazei, MD, Laure-Anne Van Loon, MD, Samuel M. Manstein, MD, Nargiz Seyidova, MD, MHQS, and Samuel J. Lin, MD, MBA

A 42-year-old female patient with a history of massive weight loss, and a current a body mass index (BMI) of 30 kg/m^2, arrives for her consultation. Her weight has been stable for the last 3 months. The patient suffers from excess skin around her waist, pannus, and has a significant amount of epigastric laxity that she finds aesthetically displeasing. She would like to be considered for an abdominoplasty.

1. What is considered to be the ideal BMI for a patient who wishes to undergo postbariatric body contouring surgery?

A. <25 kg/m^2
B. 25 to 30 kg/m^2
C. 30 to 35 kg/m^2
D. 35 to 40 kg/m^2
E. >40 kg/m^2

2. What is the most common complication after body contouring surgery in postbariatric patients?

A. Hematoma
B. Seroma
C. Dehiscence
D. Deep venous thrombosis
E. Cellulitis

3. What is the best type of abdominoplasty for this patient?

A. A short scar abdominoplasty
B. A fleur-de-lis abdominoplasty
C. High lateral tension abdominoplasty
D. Circumferential abdominoplasty
E. Abdominoplasty with umbilical transection

4. What constitutes Zone II of the Huger classification of the abdominal blood supply?

A. The area that is fed anteriorly by the vertically oriented deep epigastric arcade
B. The lateral aspect of the abdominal wall (flanks) that are fed by the six lateral intercostal and four lumbar arteries
C. The superficial epigastric, superficial external pudendal, and superficial circumflex iliac systems
D. Superior aspect of the abdomen fed by arterial branches directly off the thoracic aorta.
E. Inferior portion of the abdomen fed by the deep external pudendal artery.

ANSWERS

1. B. Among patients undergoing body contouring surgery following massive weight loss, higher BMI (>32 kg/m^2) is related to increased complications.[1–3] This higher complication rate can be attributed to the increased need for tissue resection among this patient population.[4] Patients achieving massive weight loss through a gastric bypass potentially suffer from nutritional deficiency, which could negatively influence wound healing, putting them even more at risk for postoperative complications.[4] Most postoperative complications are minor, mainly being wound dehiscence and formation of seromas.[5] Furthermore, patients with a BMI of >32 kg/m^2 at time of body contouring surgery reported less pleasing aesthetic results. According to the literature, patients with a BMI between 25 and 30 kg/m^2 are most satisfied with postoperative aesthetic results.[6,7] Plastic surgeons should carefully consider the timing of surgery; the patient should be weight-stable a minimum of 3 months, usually around 12 to 18 months following their weight-loss surgery.[8]

2. **C.** Although seroma and hematoma formation are common complications of postbariatric surgery, by far the most common complication is dehiscence of the wound.[5,7,9] The rates of complications in post-massive-weight-loss body-lift procedures are dehiscence (32.5%), seroma (16.5%), infection (3.50%), bleeding (3.00%), deep vein thrombosis (2.00%), and pulmonary embolism (1.00%).[7]

3. **B. A mini- or short scar abdominoplasty:** the patient most suited for a short scar abdominoplasty will have a mild to moderate problem confined to the lower abdomen. For example young women with a preexisting Pfannenstiel incision. See Figure 62-1.

   A fleur-de-lis abdominoplasty: this procedure the ability create a maximum improvement of body shape and to reduce the circumference of the waist. This is done by eliminating horizontal and vertical excess tissue of the lower and upper abdomen. This technique is suitable for patients suffering from a tissue surplus of the lower and particularly of the upper abdomen (epigastric laxity), often after massive weight loss. Massive weight loss is often described as a loss of 50% or more of excess weight above the patient's ideal weight.[10] This is what is described in the case example.[11-13]

   High lateral tension abdominoplasty: this procedure not only treats the abdomen, but also the hips and the lateral thigh. It is suitable for patients that expect more than an abdominal tightening and is often applicable for patients after massive weight loss.

   Circumferential abdominoplasty: this option not only treats the anterior loose skin but also the posterior side. This is suitable for patients who have undergone massive weight loss and need more than just anterior tightening.

   Abdominoplasty with umbilical transection: this technique is suited for patients with longer distances of between the umbilicus and symphysis. For example this is for suitable for patients who have an unnatural high umbilical position.

4. **C.** Zone I: The area that is fed anteriorly by the vertically oriented deep epigastric arcade.

   Zone II: The superficial epigastric, superficial external pudendal, and superficial circumflex iliac systems. See Figure 62-2.

   Zone III: The lateral aspect of the abdominal wall (flanks) that are fed by the six lateral intercostal and four lumbar arteries.[8,14]

   Bariatric surgeons can help prepare a patient for body contouring through routine screening of their nutritional status during the postoperative period. Protein, iron, vitamin B12, folate, and many other vitamins are known deficiencies following bariatric surgery.[15]

   Close monitoring, dietary supplementation, and consultation with a nutritionist should be performed by the bariatric team to ensure proper wound healing during body contouring procedures. Bariatric surgeons should minimize the size of scars because blood supply to these areas can be limited, which could impact skin integrity following the elevation of abdominal flaps. Contraindications to post–bariatric plastic surgery include active smoker, large fluctuations in weight, BMI >35, poor nutritional status, severe medical comorbidities, unrealistic expectations, and limited psychiatric work-up.[8]

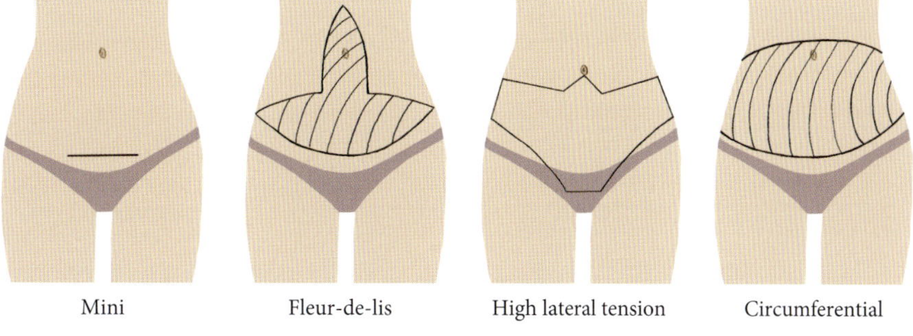

Figure 62-1 Types of abdominoplasty.

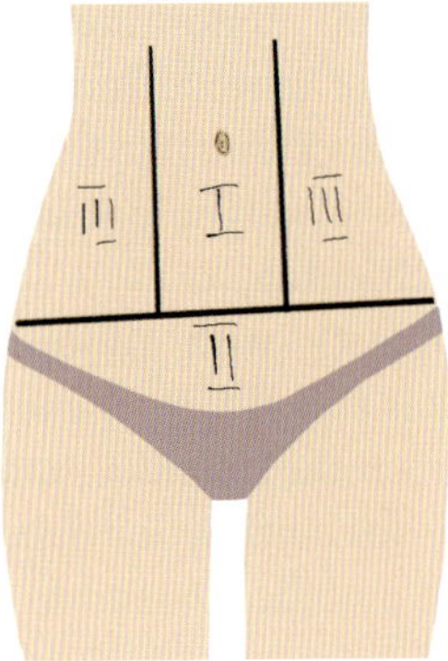

Figure 62-2 Abdominoplasty zones. Huger classification zones of abdominal blood supply; Labled Zones I, II, and III.

REFERENCES

1. Matory WE Jr, O'Sullivan J, Fudem G, Dunn R. Abdominal surgery in patients with severe morbid obesity. *Plast Reconstr Surg*. Dec 1994;94(7):976-87. doi:10.1097/00006534-199412000-00011
2. Vastine VL, Morgan RF, Williams GS, et al. Wound complications of abdominoplasty in obese patients. *Ann Plast Surg*. Jan 1999;42(1):34-9. doi:10.1097/00000637-199901000-00006
3. Coon D, Gusenoff JA, Kannan N, El Khoudary SR, Naghshineh N, Rubin JP. Body mass and surgical complications in the postbariatric reconstructive patient: analysis of 511 cases. *Ann Surg*. Mar 2009;249(3):397-401. doi:10.1097/SLA.0b013e318196d0c6
4. Sebastian JL. Bariatric surgery and work-up of the massive weight loss patient. *Clin Plast Surg*. Jan 2008;35(1):11-26. doi:10.1016/j.cps.2007.08.004
5. Garcia Botero A, Garcia Wenninger M, Fernandez Loaiza D. Complications After Body Contouring Surgery in Postbariatric Patients. *Ann Plast Surg*. Sep 2017;79(3):293-297. doi:10.1097/SAP.0000000000001109
6. Aly AS, Cram AE, Chao M, Pang J, McKeon M. Belt lipectomy for circumferential truncal excess: the University of Iowa experience. *Plast Reconstr Surg*. Jan 2003;111(1):398-413. doi:10.1097/01.PRS.0000037873.49035.2A
7. Nemerofsky RB, Oliak DA, Capella JF. Body lift: an account of 200 consecutive cases in the massive weight loss patient. *Plast Reconstr Surg*. Feb 2006;117(2):414-30. doi:10.1097/01.prs.0000197524.18233.bb
8. Neligan P. *Plastic Surgery, Volume 2, Aesthetic Surgery, Chapter 30: Post Bariatric Reconstruction*. 2013.
9. Poodt IG, van Dijk MM, Klein S, Hoogbergen MM. Complications of Lower Body Lift Surgery in Postbariatric Patients. *Plast Reconstr Surg Glob Open*. Sep 2016;4(9):e1030. doi:10.1097/GOX.0000000000001030
10. Shrivastava P, Aggarwal A, Khazanchi RK. Body contouring surgery in a massive weight loss patient: An overview. *Indian J Plast Surg*. Oct 2008;41(Suppl):S114-29.
11. Dellon AL. Fleur-de-lis abdominoplasty. *Aesthetic Plast Surg*. 1985;9(1):27-32. doi:10.1007/bf01570680
12. Friedman T, O'Brien Coon D, Michaels J, et al. Fleur-de-Lis abdominoplasty: a safe alternative to traditional abdominoplasty for the massive weight loss patient. *Plast Reconstr Surg*. May 2010;125(5):1525-35. doi:10.1097/PRS.0b013e3181d6e7e0
13. Ramsey-Stewart G. Radical "Fleur-de-Lis" Abdominal after Bariatric Surgery. *Obes Surg*. Nov 1993;3(4):410-414. doi:10.1381/096089293765559124
14. Neligan P. Plastic Surgery, Volume 2, Aesthetic Surgery, Chapter 25: Abdominoplasty Procedures. 2013;
15. Bloomberg RD, Fleishman A, Nalle JE, Herron DM, Kini S. Nutritional deficiencies following bariatric surgery: what have we learned? *Obes Surg*. Feb 2005;15(2):145-54. doi:10.1381/0960892053268264

63

Abdominal Wall Hernias

Brent D. Matthews, MD, and Matthew N. Marturano, MD

A 54-year-old female with a body mass index (BMI) of 41.2 kg/m^2 is in the office for preoperative consultation regarding surgical management of her obesity- and weight-related comorbidities. She has diabetes mellitus and smokes one pack of cigarettes a day (30 pack-years). Her HgbA1c is 8.6%. She is moderately compliant with her Metformin and diabetic diet. Four years ago, she underwent sigmoid colectomy and primary anastomosis for complicated diverticulitis. After developing a postoperative wound infection, she now has an asymptomatic 3 cm × 10 cm lower midline, reducible incisional hernia.

1. What steps must be done prior to surgery for this patient?

A. Aggressive preoperative management of modifiable risk factors including BMI, glycemic control, and tobacco use
B. Preoperative abdominal and pelvic computed tomography (CT) scan to evaluate the hernia for size and contents
C. Preoperative screening abdominal ultrasound for cholelithiasis
D. Colonoscopy
E. Mammogram

2. Which of the following is true regarding the choice of bariatric operation you will offer for this patient?

A. Whichever bariatric operation best fits the patient's overall goals.
B. Laparoscopic Roux-en-Y gastric bypass (RYGB) because it provides the most durable weight loss and control of type 2 diabetes.
C. Laparoscopic sleeve gastrectomy (SG) because it does not involve manipulation of the small intestine.
D. Laparoscopic gastric banding (LAGB) to avoid violating the gastrointestinal tract so that the ventral hernia can be repaired simultaneously with permanent, synthetic mesh.
E. Whatever bariatric operation is offered, a concomitant hernia repair requires biologic or biosynthetic mesh.

3. The patient mentions that she has previously had her ventral hernia repaired five times and it has again recurred. After reconsideration of this additional patient information, which of the following is the best option for this patient?

A. Open ventral incisional hernia repair and RYGB.
B. Laparoscopic ventral incisional hernia repair and laparoscopic RYGB.
C. Open ventral incisional hernia repair and sleeve gastrectomy.
D. Open ventral incisional hernia repair and panniculectomy followed by a staged laparoscopic bariatric procedure.
E. Laparoscopic sleeve gastrectomy followed by a staged ventral hernia repair.

4. Regarding laparoscopic bariatric surgery followed by delayed ventral incisional hernia repair, which of the following is correct?

A. For patients with large fascial defects, you should bridge the defect during the laparoscopic bariatric surgery or risk small bowel obstruction during the period of rapid weight loss.

B. Asymptomatic incarcerated omentum in a ventral hernia defect should be removed during the laparoscopic bariatric surgery.
C. Primary suture repair using a suture passer is adequate for hernias smaller than 5 cm.
D. Laparoscopic intraperitoneal onlay mesh (IPOM) placement with biologic mesh during the laparoscopic bariatric surgery has higher recurrence rate but reduces the risk of potential mesh infection.
E. Previous intraperitoneal onlay mesh (IPOM) for a ventral incisional hernia repair is a contraindication to laparoscopic bariatric surgery.

ANSWERS

1. **A.** The concept of prehabilitation describes optimizing patient's comorbidities prior to surgery in order to maximize clinical outcomes for surgery. Using standardized protocols to improve modifiable risk factors before surgery has been shown to decrease wound complication and mesh infection rates.[1-5] In addition, preoperative weight loss, smoking cessation, and glycemic control can reduce patient's wound complications postoperatively.[6]

Inadequate control of blood sugar is defined as a HgbA1C >7.3% within the last 3 months or average fingerstick blood sugars >180 mg/dL. Without adequate control, the body's ability to heal is altered and the patient is at higher risk of wound breakdown. The risk can be predicted with deterioration of blood sugar control.[7] Tobacco use also correlates with inferior surgical wound outcomes because perioperative tobacco use can triple the rate of wound necrosis.[8] Furthermore, bariatric surgery patients have an increased risk of wound complications due to the clean-contaminated wound classification related to gastrointestinal anastomosis and the preoperative BMI qualifying patients for weight loss surgery. In fact, for every one-point increase in BMI, there exhibits 1.066 times increase in wound complications.[2,9]

Diagnosis of a ventral incisional hernia is typically made during the preoperative history and physical examination. Diagnostic imaging studies include ultrasound, provocative ultrasound [dynamic abdominal sonography for hernia (DASH)], CT with and/or without Valsalva, and magnetic resonance imaging (MRI).[10,11] These imaging studies may be useful in assessing the characteristics of the hernia such as size and contents (Figure 63-1) and to augment the physical exam. Imaging is especially helpful in morbidly obese patients with a large pannus, when the defect is small or contents are incarcerated in the hernia preventing assessment or definitive diagnosis of an abdominal wall defect. This patient has a large, reducible ventral incisional hernia. Thus diagnosis of the ventral incisional hernia was made preoperatively. Intraoperative assessment of the hernia defect will guide overall management (repair technique vs. staged repair). For nonmidline hernias, imaging is helpful to delineate the abdominal and pelvic anatomy as alternative techniques such as bone anchor fixation may be required. Abdominal and pelvic CT scanning is not useful in assessing the presence or character of intrabdominal adhesions however, determining anatomical landmarks and associations preoperatively is imperative.

Finally, while it is always important to screen patients for health issues that they are at risk for such as colon and breast cancer, it is not imperative that this be done prior to undergoing bariatric surgery. While prophylactic cholecystectomy has been championed by some bariatric surgeons, its use is still controversial. In their meta-analysis, Warschkow et al. determined that of 6,048 obese patients who underwent RYGB without concomitant cholecystectomy, the rate of subsequent cholecystectomy was only 6.8%. They concluded that prophylactic cholecystectomy during RYGB should be avoided in patients and exclusively performed in patients with symptomatic biliary disease.[12]

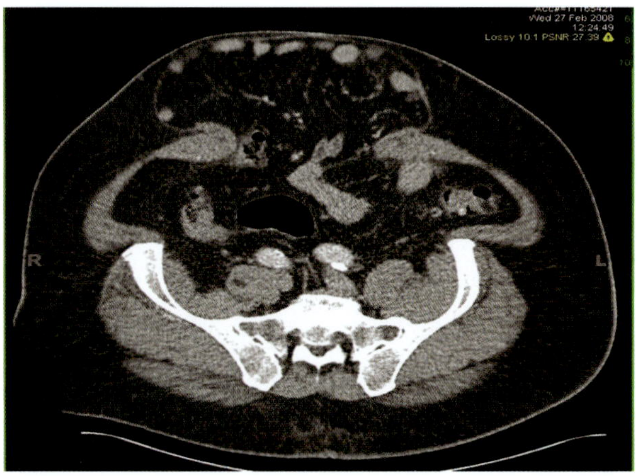

Figure 63-1 Axial cut of CT abdomen and pelvis. Infraumbilical midline hernia defect with intra-abdominal contents. Diagnosis of this hernia is made preoperatively but additional imaging can help determine contents of hernia sac.

2. **A.** Based on this patient's past surgical history of wound infection and development of a hernia, she most likely underwent a partial colectomy for complicated diverticulitis. The three most common bariatric procedures for patients undergoing hernia surgery are laparoscopic RYGB, laparoscopic SG, and LAGB.[13] Of these, RYGB is the only procedure that entails small bowel manipulation. In their retrospective analysis, Major et al. demonstrated that although there was increased operative time in laparoscopic RYGB patients who had undergone previous abdominal surgeries, there was no increased risk of adverse postoperative outcomes. In addition, the most significant difference in operative time was related to patients who had previous operations in both the upper and lower abdomen, for which this patient has not. They did not find a difference in operative times or outcomes in patients who underwent laparoscopic SG.

   Traditionally, RYGB does provide the most durable weight loss.[14] This could be of benefit in patients with ventral incisional hernia as one of the risk factors for recurrence is obesity. However, there is no data to suggest that the extent of weight loss significantly reduces recurrence. Laparoscopic SG is another appropriate bariatric surgery option for this patient.

   Inherently, violation of the gastrointestinal tract (clean-contaminated or contaminated wound classification) during ventral incisional hernia repair increases the risk for wound complications and the need for subsequent reoperation and/or mesh explantation. Many surgeons will utilize biologic or absorbable synthetic mesh if repairing a ventral hernia during a clean-contaminated or contaminated procedure. Rosen et al. describe the safe application of biologic and biosynthetic mesh in patients for ventral incisional hernia repair in patients who underwent concomitant gastrointestinal surgery. Nevertheless, they also witnessed a recurrence rate of 31.3% in these patients.[15–17] Conversely, a number of retrospective case series have shown implantation of synthetic mesh at the time of stapled bariatric surgery to be safe.[18–23] Acute wound morbidity and long-term outcomes such as mesh infection and/or need for mesh explantation versus hernia recurrence are important variables to consider. Any patient-centered, shared decision-making process has to balance clinical outcomes, quality of life for the patient, and healthcare cost. At this time, the American Society for Metabolic and Bariatric Surgery and the Americas Hernia Society do not have guidelines or a position statement for selection of mesh reinforcement in concomitant bariatric and hernia surgery.[2,10,24] Thus, any of the above procedures is considered safe and effective in this patient and choice should be based on the patient's goals.[6,11,25]

3. **E.** Many hernia patients with morbid obesity are not good candidates for combined laparoscopic bariatric surgery and ventral hernia repair. These include but are not limited to large abdominal wall defects, loss of abdominal domain, extensive, known intestinal adhesive disease, active wound complications, or incarcerated ventral hernias containing small or large intestine (Figure 63-2). This also includes patients with multiple recurrences after previous repairs. Mesh is likely to be present in these wounds as well. In such patients, aggressive medical weight loss prior to hernia repair is a desirable means to optimize hernia repair outcomes.

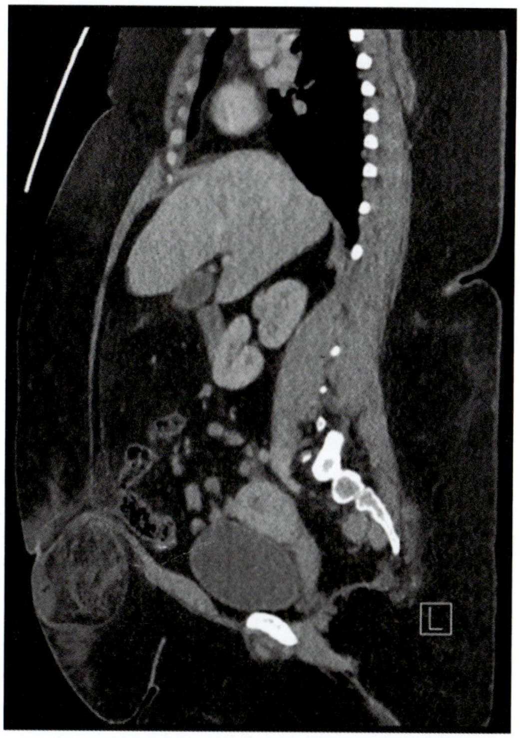

Figure 63-2 Infra-umbilical incisional hernia with incarcerated intra-abdominal contents. Many patients that are not suitable for combined hernia and bariatric weight loss surgery include but are not limited to large abdominal wall defects, loss of abdominal domain, extensive, known intestinal adhesive disease, active wound complications, or incarcerated ventral hernias containing the small or large intestine.

In the first Italian Consensus on Laparoscopic Ventral Incisional Hernia Repair, Cuccerullo et al. recommend increased caution with hernia defects greater than 10 cm but do not determine such hernias to be an absolute contraindication to bariatric surgery.[26] As with any procedure, patient characteristics and surgeon experience play a critical role in operative planning and success. In addition, although they describe higher conversion rates to open, increased complications, and more recurrences when attempted laparoscopic in patients with multiply recurrent ventral hernias, patients with multiply recurrent ventral hernias are not an absolute contraindication to laparoscopic repair. In this patient with multiple previous ventral incisional hernia repairs, who may require mesh explantation, an open ventral repair is most likely safer.

In patients with morbid obesity and a ventral hernia that is not amenable to laparoscopic repair, a staged approach is recommended. Weight loss, whether through surgery or multidisciplinary medical management, prior to ventral hernia repair is expected to improve hernia repair outcomes. Bariatric surgery appears to provide far more significant and rapid weight loss than other modalities and may be the option of choice for selected patients with morbid obesity and large abdominal wall hernias.[5,10,13]

Panniculectomy may be combined with open ventral incisional hernia repair to eliminate dystrophic skin, decrease tension upon the healing incision, and spare patients a second anesthetic after peak weight loss is achieved. However, panniculectomy combined with ventral incisional hernia repair increases the risk of postoperative wound infections.[10,27–29] In addition, performing open ventral incisional hernia repair followed by a staged gastrointestinal procedure could put the patient at risk of wound and mesh infection from the subsequent operation.

4. **D.** Dual stage bariatric surgery, defined as bariatric weight loss surgery followed by delayed ventral hernia repair, is a safe and effective approach to manage a patient's morbid obesity and hernia. Owei et al. describe that in morbidly obese patients, both surgical and medical complications are significantly more likely to occur.[30] In addition, Heniford et al. found patients who underwent laparoscopic ventral incisional hernia repair with a BMI >40 recurred significantly more frequently than those with lower BMI.[31] One of the obvious benefits to dual-staged repair is significant weight loss preoperatively that can optimize their comorbidities prior to ventral incisional hernia repair to offer optimal durability.[32]

Although small bowel obstructions have been described during the period of rapid, surgically induced weight loss, these typically occur within small-sized hernia defects (Figure 63-3).[33,34]

In patients with large defects, some authors recommend leaving the hernia undisturbed. However, for defects that are small, there exhibits higher risk of incarceration and thus should be temporized in some way. These small hernias can be easily temporized with suture passer closure with the expectation of recurrence (Figure 63-4). The patient will subsequently undergo definitive hernia repair. The Italian Consensus Conference lists this as any hernia 3 cm or less, and in a retrospective series, Newcomb has had success with 2 cm or less.[23,28]

Incarcerated omentum within a ventral hernia defect can be managed in multiple ways. If symptomatic, the omentum should be reduced and the hernia defect closed and reinforced in a standard fashion. However, routine removal of omentum without repairing the fascial defect invites incarceration of bowel and subsequent postoperative morbidity such as small bowel obstruction and/or anastomotic or staple line leak. An omental patch to temporize ventral hernias allows weight loss surgery

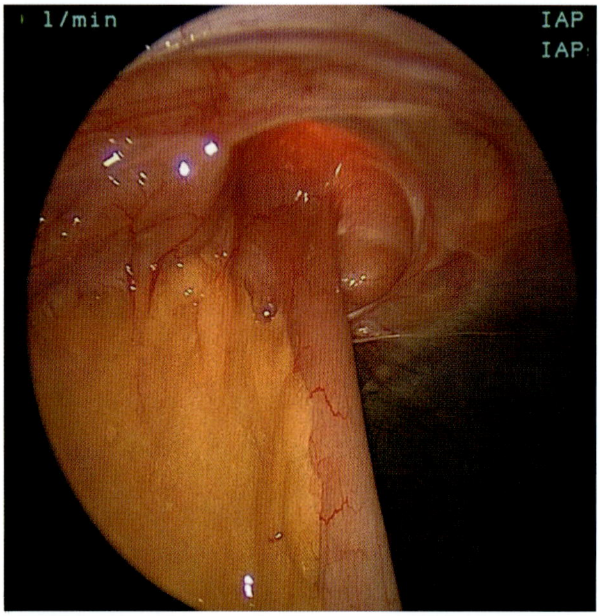

Figure 63-3 Intraoperative findings.

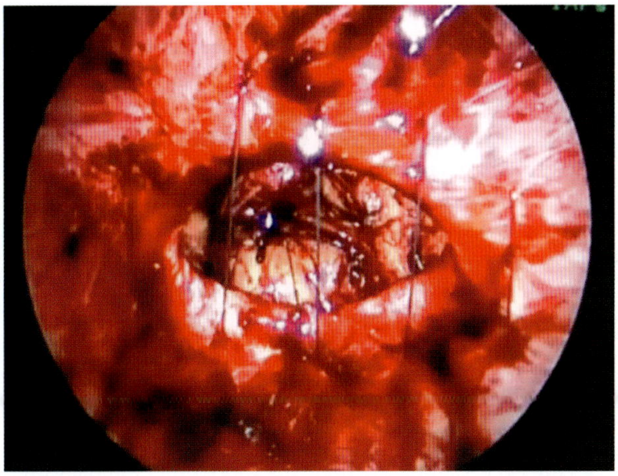

Figure 63-4 This small fascial defect can be closed intraoperatively using a suture passer as shown. This allows a staged procedure because the bariatric weight loss surgery can be performed followed by definitive hernia repair at a later date. Primary closure with a suture passer should be expected to recur.

to be completed and subsequent delayed, but definitive ventral hernia repair.

Mesh choice when repairing CDC class 2 (clean-contaminated) and greater is controversial[35] and the use of biologic mesh for infection risk-reduction is recommended as a Grade 2 (weak recommendation) by the Ventral Hernia Working Group (VHWG).[36] As previously stated, the American Society for Metabolic and Bariatric Surgery and the Americas Hernia Society do not have guidelines or a position statement for selection of mesh reinforcement in concomitant bariatric and hernia surgery. Regardless, biologic prostheses are commonly used in the setting of contaminated fields or in high-risk patients. This is due to biologic mesh's ability to support revascularization, which has been hypothesized to aid in its resistance to infection. Overall, the recommendation of the VHWG is to reinforce the primary fascial closure of a ventral hernia with a prosthetic repair material. Choice of synthetic or biologic mesh should be based on patient risk factors, surgeon experience, and cost.

Choice of bariatric surgery amongst these patients should not change based on staged approach. Patients who are amenable to laparoscopic bariatric surgery should undergo choice of procedure based on the individual patient centered discussion and can be temporized as previously discussed.

REFERENCES

1. Augenstein VA, Colavita PD, Wormer BA, et al. CeDAR: Carolinas equation for determining associated risks. *J Am Coll Surg*. 2015. doi:10.1016/j.jamcollsurg.2015.07.145
2. Heniford BT, Park A, Ramshaw BJ, Voeller G, Hunter JG, Fitzgibbons RJ. Laparoscopic repair of ventral hernias: nine years' experience with 850 consecutive hernias. *Ann Surg*. 2003. doi:10.1097/01.sla.0000086662.49499.ab
3. Poulose BK, Shelton J, Phillips S, et al. Epidemiology and cost of ventral hernia repair: making the case for hernia research. *Hernia*. 2012. doi:10.1007/s10029-011-0879-9
4. Stearns E, Plymale MA, Davenport DL, et al. Early outcomes of an enhanced recovery protocol for open repair of ventral hernia. *Surg Endosc*. 2018. doi: 10.1007/s00464-017-6004-0.
5. Mechanick JI, Youdim A, Jones DB, et al. Clinical practice guidelines for the perioperative nutritional, metabolic, and nonsurgical support of the bariatric surgery. *Surg Obes Related Dis*. 2013. doi:10.1016/j.soard.2012.12.010
6. Knapp N, Jedrzejewski B, Martindale R. Abdominal wall procedures: the benefits of prehabilitation. *Plastic Aesthet Res*. 2020. doi:10.20517/2347-9264.2019.69
7. Schauer PR, Kashyap SR, Wolski K, et al. Bariatric surgery versus intensive medical therapy in obese patients with diabetes. *N Engl J Med*. 2012. doi:10.1056/NEJMoa1200225
8. Sørensen LT. Wound healing and infection in surgery. *Ann Surg*. 2012. doi:10.1097/sla.0b013e31824f632d
9. Sauerland S, Korenkov M, Kleinen T, Arndt M, Paul A. Obesity is a risk factor for recurrence after incisional hernia repair. *Hernia* 2004. doi:10.1007/s10029-003-0161-x
10. Kroese LF, Sneiders D, Kleinrensink GJ, Muysoms F, Lange JF. Comparing different modalities for the diagnosis of incisional hernia: a systematic review. *Hernia*. 2018. doi:10.1007/s10029-017-1725-5
11. Earle D, Roth JS, Saber A, et al. SAGES guidelines for laparoscopic ventral hernia repair. *Surg Endosc*. 2016. doi:10.1007/s00464-016-5072-x
12. Warschkow R, Tarantino I, Ukegjini K, et al. Concomitant cholecystectomy during laparoscopic Roux-en-Y gastric bypass in obese patients is not justified: a meta-analysis. *Obes Surg*. 2013. doi:10.1007/s11695-012-0852-4.
13. Lo Menzo E, Hinojosa M, Carbonell A, Krpata D, Carter J, Rogers AM. American Society for Metabolic and Bariatric Surgery and American Hernia Society consensus guideline on bariatric surgery and hernia surgery. *Surg Obes Relat Dis*. 2018. doi:10.1016/j.soard.2018.07.005
14. Maciejewski ML, Arterburn DE, Van Scoyoc L, et al. Bariatric surgery and long-term durability of weight loss. *JAMA Surg*. 2016. doi:10.1001/jamasurg.2016.2317
15. Cozacov Y, Szomstein S, Safdie FM, Lo Menzo E, Rosenthal R. Is the use of prosthetic mesh recommended in severely obese patients undergoing concomitant abdominal wall hernia repair and sleeve gastrectomy? *J Am Coll Surg*. 2014. doi:10.1016/j.jamcollsurg.2013.12.008
16. Rosen MJ, Aydogdu K, Grafmiller K, Petro CC, Faiman GH, Prabhu A. A multidisciplinary approach to medical weight loss prior to complex abdominal wall

reconstruction: is it feasible? *J Gastrointest Surg*. 2015. doi:10.1007/s11605-015-2856-6

17. Rosen MJ, Bauer JJ, Harmaty M, et al. Multicenter, prospective, longitudinal study of the recurrence, surgical site infection, and quality of life after contaminated ventral hernia repair using biosynthetic absorbable mesh: The COBRA study. *Ann Surg*. 2017. doi:10.1097/SLA.0000000000001601
18. Datta T, Eid G, Nahmias N, Dallal RM. Management of ventral hernias during laparoscopic gastric bypass. *Surg Obes Relat Dis*. 2008. doi:10.1016/j.soard.2008.03.246
19. Schuster R, Curet MJ, Alami RS, Morton JM, Wren SM, Safadi BY. Concurrent gastric bypass and repair of anterior abdominal wall hernias. *Obes Surg*. 2006. doi:10.1381/096089206778392374
20. Chan DL, Talbot ML. Synchronous ventral hernia repair in bariatric patients. *Obes Surg*. 2014. doi:10.1007/s11695-014-1241-y
21. Raziel A, Sakran N, Szold A, Goitein D. Concomitant bariatric and ventral/incisional hernia surgery in morbidly obese patients. *Surg Endosc*. 2014. doi:10.1007/s00464-013-3310-z
22. Majumder A, Winder JS, Wen Y, Pauli EM, Belyansky I, Novitsky YW. Comparative analysis of biologic versus synthetic mesh outcomes in contaminated hernia repairs. *Surgery (United States)*. 2016. doi:10.1016/j.surg.2016.04.041
23. Rosen MJ. Polyester-based mesh for ventral hernia repair: is it safe? *Am J Surg*. 2009. doi:1016/j.amjsurg.2008.11.003
24. Cobb WS, Kercher KW, Heniford BT. The argument for lightweight polypropylene mesh in hernia repair. *Surg Innovat*. 2005. doi:10.1177/155335060501200109
25. Major P, Droś J, Kacprzyk A, et al. Does previous abdominal surgery affect the course and outcomes of laparoscopic bariatric surgery? *Surg Obes Relat Dis*. 2018. doi:10.1016/j.soard.2018.03.025
26. Cuccurullo D, Piccoli M, Agresta F, et al. Laparoscopic ventral incisional hernia repair: evidence-based guidelines of the first Italian Consensus Conference. *Hernia*. 2013. doi:10.1007/s10029-013-1055-1
27. Moreno-Egea A, Campillo-Soto Á, Morales-Cuenca G. Does abdominoplasty add morbidity to incisional hernia repair? A randomized controlled trial. *Surg Innovat*. 2016. doi:10.1177/1553350616646480
28. Fischer JP, Basta MN, Wink JD, Wes AM, Kovach SJ. Optimizing patient selection in ventral hernia repair with concurrent panniculectomy: An analysis of 1974 patients from the ACS-NSQIP datasets. *J Plastic Reconstruct Aesthet Surg*. 2014. doi:1016/j.bjps.2014.07.001
29. Fischer JP, Wink JD, Tuggle CT, Nelson JA, Kovach SJ. Wound risk assessment in ventral hernia repair: generation and internal validation of a risk stratification system using the ACS-NSQIP. *Hernia*. 2015. doi:10.1007/s10029-014-1318-5
30. Owei L, Swendiman RA, Torres-Landa S, Dempsey DT, Dumon KR. Impact of body mass index on minimally invasive ventral hernia repair: an ACS-NSQIP analysis. *Hernia*. 2019. doi:10.1007/s10029-019-01944-6
31. Tsereteli Z, Pryor BA, Heniford BT, Park A, Voeller G, Ramshaw BJ. Laparoscopic ventral hernia repair (LVHR) in morbidly obese patients. *Hernia*. 2008. doi:10.1007/s10029-007-0310-8
32. Newcomb WL, Polhill JL, Chen AY, et al. Staged hernia repair preceded by gastric bypass for the treatment of morbidly obese patients with complex ventral hernias. *Hernia*. 2008. doi:1007/s10029-008-0381-1
33. Eid GM, Mattar SG, Hamad G, et al. Repair of ventral hernias in morbidly obese patients undergoing laparoscopic gastric bypass should not be deferred. *Surg Endosc Other Intervent Techniq*. 2004. doi:10.1007/s00464-003-8915-1
34. Bonatti H, Hoeller E, Kirchmayr W, et al. Ventral hernia repair in bariatric surgery. *Obes Surg*. 2004. doi:10.1381/096089204323093444
35. Majumder A, Winder JS, Wen Y, Pauli EM, Belyansky I, Novitsky YW. Comparative analysis of biologic versus synthetic mesh outcomes in contaminated hernia repairs. *Surgery (United States)*. 2016. doi:10.1016/j.surg.2016.04.041
36. Breuing K, Butler CE, Ferzoco S, et al. Incisional ventral hernias: Review of the literature and recommendations regarding the grading and technique of repair. *Surgery*. 2010. doi: 10.1016/j.surg.2010.01.008

64

Bariatric Surgery and Transplant

Eduardo Pirolla, MD, PhD, and Danbee Kim, MD

A 45-year-old male with a body mass index (BMI) of 52 kg/m^2, obstructive sleep apnea, hypertension, prediabetes, and Child–Pugh class C cirrhosis from fatty liver disease is being considered for liver transplant.

1. **Which of the following is true regarding the patient's candidacy for transplant surgery?**
   A. Transplant surgery is contraindicated in patients with super morbid obesity.
   B. Obesity class I, II, and III obesity patients have similar outcomes after liver transplantation.
   C. Type 2 diabetes mellitus does not worsen survival after liver transplantation.
   D. Transplantation done for nonalcoholic steatohepatitis (NASH)-related cirrhosis has worse outcomes than done for hepatitis C-related cirrhosis.

2. **The patient is also being considered for bariatric surgery. This patient has biopsy-confirmed cirrhosis and a MELD score of 10. Which of the following is true regarding bariatric surgery in this patient?**
   A. Roux-en-Y gastric bypass (RYGB) is contraindicated.
   B. Sleeve gastrectomy is the only bariatric surgical option.
   C. Surgery should not be performed in patients with cirrhosis and this patient should undergo transplant surgery first.
   D. Ingastric balloon therapy is a good option in preparation for transplant.

3. **During the evaluation and work-up for both of these procedures, the patient's condition worsens over the period of a few months. His MELD score is now 25 and his HgbA1C is 10.7%. A two-dimensional cardiac echocardiogram shows normal wall motion and an ejection fraction of 50%. He can meet six metabolic equivalents (METS) and his electrocardiogram is normal. The hepatologist and bariatrician have done all that they can regarding medical management of his cirrhosis and metabolic diseases. Which of the following statements is best option?**
   A. He has low-to-medium cardiac risk so a liver transplant should be done first.
   B. His metabolic syndrome elevates his transplant graft survival risk, so a sleeve gastrectomy should be done first.
   C. Bariatric surgery should be done concomitantly with a liver transplant.
   D. Because of his MELD score, liver transplantation should be done first.

4. **If this patient had end-stage renal disease instead of NASH-related cirrhosis and was a candidate for renal transplantation, which of the following statements is true?**
   A. Class III obesity is not a contraindication to transplant in these patients.
   B. Simultaneous bariatric surgery and renal transplant should never be done.
   C. Bariatric surgery done prior to renal transplant reduces the risk of graft failure and overall mortality.
   D. End-stage renal disease increases the risk of bariatric surgery complications.

ANSWERS

1. **A.** Fatty liver disease progressing to NASH-related cirrhosis is the most common indication for liver transplantation today. This means that many transplant surgery candidates are obese and with metabolic disease. This is felt to make them higher risk for surgery due to a cardiovascular event. It is not clear, however, if NASH-related cirrhosis patients are indeed any higher risk than those who undergo transplant for non–NASH-related reasons.[1] Obesity itself is not an independent predictor for poor transplant outcome because those with class I, II, and III obesity have the same outcomes as normal BMI individuals.[2,3]

   Patients with NASH-related cirrhosis do have a higher risk of cardiovascular events and sepsis after transplant but obesity alone is not an independent risk factor for poor transplant outcomes.[4] Type 2 diabetes mellitus, however, is considered a predictor of poor outcomes. In addition, super morbid obesity is a predictor of worse outcomes, although the data for this is not nearly as robust.[5] The main reason to do bariatric surgery prior to liver transplant is to reduce their cardiac risk and control their diabetes.

   While there are certain factors in obese patients that may make them higher-risk candidates for liver transplant, there is data to suggest that NASH-related transplantation does not predict worse overall outcomes than transplant done for malignancy, alcoholism, hepatitis C, or acute hepatic necrosis.[6] Ultimately, the decision to transplant an obese patient depends on their overall physiology. While obesity and obesity related diseases like type 2 diabetes and hypertension are important, they are not contraindications to transplantation.

2. **D.** NASH-related cirrhotic obese patients are likely to be considered for both bariatric procedures and transplant procedures. Several different bariatric procedures have been documented as safe to perform prior to transplant surgery including the RYGB. The sleeve gastrectomy is the most commonly used procedure, mostly due to the concern of anastomotic disruption and complications that may be present in the RYGB or duodenal switch such as decreased medicine absorption and the inability to access the biliary tree endoscopically. For patients who need cardiac risk reduction and better control of their comorbid obesity conditions prior to transplant, most available bariatric procedures can be done including the RYGB and the duodenal switch, along with their variants. However, the sleeve gastrectomy is by far the most preferred option by bariatric surgeons.

   The presence of cirrhosis itself is not a contraindication to surgery and compensated cirrhosis in Child–Pugh class A and B patients have similar outcomes after bariatric surgery as do non-cirrhosis patients. The data is not as clear in Child-Pugh class C patients. On the other hand, uncompensated cirrhosis is a relative contraindication to bariatric surgery.

   Endoscopic therapy for weight loss including intragastric balloon placement has been described for NASH and prior to transplant.[7] In general, intragastric balloon therapy has not been efficacious for long-term weight loss with only around 30% to 40% of patients maintaining significant weight loss after the balloons are removed. However, they do show about 30% excess weight loss when they are in place.[8] As such, they can be very practical for short-term weight loss needs such as prior to transplantation. Interestingly, they can also improve liver function tests and the amount of liver fibrosis.[9]

3. **C.** The timing of when to perform metabolic surgery in relation to transplant surgery is controversial, not clear, and not backed by high-quality evidence. As such, providers must consider each patient individually and with a multidisciplinary approach. In general, liver transplant candidates with metabolic syndrome have the highest risk of postoperative complications including surgical site infections and wound dehiscence. While obesity is associated with metabolic syndrome, obesity alone is again not a predictor of worse outcomes from liver transplantation surgery. Thus the reason to perform bariatric/metabolic surgery prior to transplant would be to decrease the risk of postoperative complications and cardiac risk. Since this patient appears to have a low cardiac risk based on their echocardiogram, ability to reach six METS, and electrocardiogram, it is not imperative that he undergoes bariatric surgery first. Furthermore, his MELD score is very high >15 and thus his risk for postoperative complications precludes performing a bariatric procedure first. Finally, bariatric surgery is contraindicated in patients with uncompensated cirrhosis and portal hypertension.[10] The other disadvantage of performing bariatric surgery first is that it may also delay placing the patient on the transplant list due to protein malnutrition.[11]

On the other hand, this patient is super morbidly obese with a BMI >50 kg/m^2 and is newly diagnosed with type 2 diabetes. As stated earlier, super morbidly obese patients and those with type 2 diabetes are higher risk for postoperative complications, so performing a liver transplant first is likely to result in complications including graft loss. In addition, performing bariatric surgery on patients who are on chronic steroids and other immunosuppressant medications increases the risk of wound complications and anastomotic or staple line dehiscence. Finally, performing bariatric surgery after transplantation has the least amount of published data.[12]

In a select group of patients, a concomitant transplant and bariatric surgery should be done. These patients are at high-risk for complications from both disease processes: cirrhosis and obesity-related diseases. This patient can be best treated by performing a bariatric procedure at the same time as liver transplantation. The sleeve gastrectomy is again recommended for this. In addition to its less complicated technique, there is less issue with absorption of medications and access to the common bile duct endoscopically as there would be with the RYGB or other bypass-like operations. In this patient with a high-MELD, difficult to control diabetes, and a very high BMI, performing simultaneous procedures lends to better long-term outcomes for the obesity-related disease and no worse outcomes for the cirrhosis and transplant.

4. C. There are several differences between renal and hepatic transplantation as it pertains to obese patients. First and foremost, class III obesity is an absolute contraindication to renal transplant surgery owing to its higher complication rates in these patients.[13] As such, more and more centers are using bariatric surgery prior to performing renal transplantation because it increases the number of candidates.[14] Moreover, when compared with non-metabolic surgery controls with obesity, performing metabolic surgery before transplantation reduced the risks of graft failure and overall mortality by almost 70% and 45%, respectively.[15]

Like liver surgery, bariatric surgery has been used before, during, and after renal transplantation. The optimal timing is not known for all patients. There are reports of concomitant procedures noting an overall faster recovery.[16] In end-stage liver disease or those with high-MELD scores or uncompensated cirrhosis, bariatric surgery was contraindicated; but end-stage renal disease does not increase the relative risk of postoperative complications in bariatric procedures.[17]

REFERENCES

1. Tsochatziz E, et al. International liver transplantation consensus statement on end-stage liver disease due to NASH and liver transplantation. *Transplantation*. 2019;103(1):45-57.
2. Charlton MR, Burns JM, Pedersen RA, et al. Frequency and outcomes of liver transplantation for nonalcoholic steatohepatitis in the United States. *Gastroenterology*. 2011;141: 1249-1125.
3. Sadler EM, Mehta N, Bhat M, et al. Liver transplantation for NASH-related hepatocellular carcinoma versus non-NASH etiologies of hepatocellular carcinoma. *Transplantation*. 2018;102:640-647.
4. Dodge JL, Roberts J, Brandman D. Weighing the risks: morbid obesity and diabetes are associated with increased risk of death on the liver transplant waiting list. *Liver Int*. 2018;38:553-563.
5. Detry O, Seydel B, Kohnen L, et al. Liver transplant is feasible is super-obese patients: a case report. *Transplant Proc*. 2009;41(8):3430-3431.
6. Afzali A, Berry K, Ioannou GN. Excellent posttransplant survival for patients with nonalcoholic steatohepatitis in the United States. *Liver Transpl*. 2012;18:29-37.
7. Salomone F, Sharaiha RZ, Boskoski I. Endoscopic bariatric and metabolic therapies for non-alcoholic fatty liver disease; evidence and perspectives. *Liver Int*. 2020;40(6): 1262-1268.
8. Neto MG, Silva LB, Grecco E, et al. Brazilian intragastric balloon consensus statement (BIBC); practical guidelines based on experience of over 40,000 cases. *Surg Obes Relat Dis*. 2018;14:151-159.
9. Bazerbachi F, Vargas EJ, Mounajjed T, et al. Impact of single fluid-filled intragastric balloon on metabolic parameters and nonalcoholic steatohepatitis: a prospective paired endoscopic ultrasound guided core liver biopsy at the time of balloon placement and removal. *Gastroenterology*. 2018;154(6):suppl1:S-1360.
10. Diwan TS, Rice TC, Heimbach JK, Schauer DP. Liver transplantation and bariatric surgery: timing and outcomes. *Liver Transplantation*. 2018;24:1280-1287.
11. Lee Y, Tian C, Lovrics O, et al. Bariatric surgery before, during, and after liver transplantation: a systematic review and meta-analysis. *Surg Obes Relat Dis*. 2020;16(9): 1336-1347.
12. Verhoeff K, Dang JT, Modasi A, Switzer N, Birch DW, Karmali S. Bariatric Surgery Outcomes in Patients with Previous Organ Transplant: Scoping Review and Analysis of the MBSAQIP. *Obes Surg*. 2021;31(2):508-516.
13. Cohen JB, Lim MA, Tewksbury CM, et al. Bariatric surgery before and after kidney transplantation: long-term weight loss and allograft outcomes. *Surg Obes Relat Dis*. 2019;15:935-941.

14. Al-Bahri S, Fakhry TK, Gonzalvo JP, Murr MM. Bariatric surgery as a bridge to renal transplantation in patients with end-stage renal disease. *Obes Surg.* 2017;27(11):2951-2955.
15. Kim Y, Jung AD, Dhar VK, et al. Laparoscopic sleeve gastrectomy improves renal transplant candidacy and post-transplant outcomes in morbidly obese patients. *Am J Transplant.* 2018;18(2):410-416.
16. Montgomery JR, Telem DA, Waits SA. Bariatric surgery for prospective living kidney donors with obesity? *Am J Transplant.* 2019;19:2415-2420.
17. Sheetz KH, Woodside KJ, Shahinian VB, Dimick JB, Montgomery JR, Waits SA. Trends in bariatric surgery procedures among patients with ESKD in the United States. *Clin J Am Soc Nephrol.* 2019;14:1193-1199.

Index

Page numbers followed by "f" indicate figures; those followed by "t" indicate tables.

C